Clinical Aspects and Management of Aging

Clinical Aspects and Management of Aging

Editor: Mason Button

AMERICAN
MEDICAL PUBLISHERS
www.americanmedicalpublishers.com

AMERICAN
MEDICAL PUBLISHERS
www.americanmedicalpublishers.com

Cataloging-in-Publication Data

Clinical aspects and management of aging / edited by Mason Button
p. cm.
Includes bibliographical references and index.
ISBN 978-1-63927-581-6
1. Older people--Diseases--Treatment. 2. Older people--Medical care. 3. Older people--Rehabilitation.
4. Geriatrics. 5. Aging. I. Button, Mason.
RC953.5 .C55 2023
615.547--dc23

American Medical Publishers,
41 Flatbush Avenue,
1st Floor, New York,
NY 11217, USA

ISBN 978-1-63927-581-6 (Hardback)

Contents

Preface

Aging is the process of getting older and it is generally related with dynamic changes in the physiological, biological, psychological, social and environmental processes. It occurs when the single cells in an organism cease to populate or divide. It increases the risk of various diseases in humans, such as cardiovascular disease, cancer and stroke. Maintaining a good lifestyle is helpful in delaying and preventing aging. Higher consumption of fruits, vegetables, fish, nuts, and monounsaturated fatty acids such as olive oil can reduce the mortality risk. Consumption of foods items such as alcohol, sugar, fried food, processed meats and refined carbohydrates accelerates aging. Physical exercise, avoiding chronic stress, and taking appropriate sleep helps in increasing the life expectancy. This book aims to understand the clinical perspectives of aging. Experts and students actively engaged in research on aging will find it full of crucial and unexplored information on the management of aging. The extensive content of this book provides the readers with a thorough understanding of the topic.

Significant researches are present in this book. Intensive efforts have been employed by authors to make this book an outstanding discourse. This book contains the enlightening chapters which have been written on the basis of significant researches done by the experts.

Finally, I would also like to thank all the members involved in this book for being a team and meeting all the deadlines for the submission of their respective works. I would also like to thank my friends and family for being supportive in my efforts.

Editor

1

Comparison of the Change in Diastolic Dysfunction after Transcatheter Atrial Septal Defect Closure between Asymptomatic Younger and Older Age Groups

Lucy Youngmin Eun [1], Han Ki Park [2,*] and Jae Young Choi [1,*]

1 Division of Pediatric Cardiology, Department of Pediatrics, Yonsei University College of Medicine, Seoul 03722, Korea; lucyeun@yuhs.ac

2 Division of Cardiovascular Surgery, Department of Thoracic and Cardiovascular Surgery, Yonsei University College of Medicine, Seoul 03722, Korea

* Correspondence: HANK@yuhs.ac (H.K.P.); cjy0122@yuhs.ac (J.Y.C.)

Abstract: Transcatheter device closure of a secundum atrial septal defect (ASD) is followed by a noticeable change in the left atrium (LA) and left ventricle (LV) over a long-term follow-up. This study aimed to assess the remodeling of the atrial and ventricular myocardium with respect to diastolic function in adult ASD patients. Around 38 asymptomatic patients (age: 48.6 ± 17.1 years, range: 23–69 years) diagnosed with ASD during routine health check-up and who underwent ASD device closure with the Amplatzer septal occluder were included in this retrospective study, and their medical records (containing echocardiographic data) were reviewed. The defect size was 21.77 + 6.79 mm, while the balloon measurement of the defect was 24.29 ± 6.64 mm. The patients were divided into two groups, namely, Group I (with 18 patients aged <50 years [mean: 33.06 ± 9.43 years] and Group II (with 20 patients aged ≥50 years [mean: 62.55 ± 7.54 years]). Comparison of echocardiographic data collected before closure and at a follow-up 2 years later revealed significant differences between pre-closure and post-closure states in the left ventricular end-diastolic dimension (40.76 ± 3.28 vs. 43.39 ± 3.52), left ventricular mass (99.64 ± 28.81 vs. 116.57 ± 32.03), and right ventricular pressure (36.88 ± 12.20 vs. 31.81 ± 11.11). Tissue Doppler measurements were significantly decreased 2 years after closure, while the post-closure E/E′ was higher than the pre-closure E/E′ (11.58 ± 4.80 vs. 8.79 + 3.19, $p < 0.005$). In both groups, mitral A and tissue Doppler E′, A′, and S′ values decreased post-closure, while the E/E′ was higher in Group II than in Group I at both pre-closure and long-term follow-up measurements (pre-closure: 9.60 ± 5.15 vs. 7.41 ± 1.42, $p < 0.003$; post-closure: 13.03 + 4.05 vs. 10.49 ± 3.95, $p < 0.02$). The LA size and LV function exhibited recognizable remodeling after transcatheter ASD closure. Because the LV preload elevation (i.e., E/E′) after ASD closure can be pronounced in older patients, caution should be provided more in older patients than in younger patients. Hence, it may be beneficial to close the ASD at an earlier age in adults even after a late diagnosis; a relatively younger age may be more suited for adaptation to the remodeling process to protect the myocardial function. Careful consideration should be given to the previous underloaded left heart after long-term closure.

Keywords: atrial septal defect; adult; transcatheter device closure; echocardiography; LA; LV

---

1. Introduction

In recent years, an increasing number of cases with atrial septal defect (ASD) have been treated using transcatheter device occlusion. Beneficial for hemodynamic improvement, it is a safe procedure that is associated with lesser complications than conventional surgical procedures [1,2]. However, some elderly patients develop diastolic heart failure (HF) after occlusion [3,4].

Left-to-right inter-atrial shunting through the ASD causes right and left heart volume overload [5], and changes in the left atrium (LA) and left ventricle (LV) are observed during a long-term follow-up after transcatheter closure of ASD. Moreover, owing to age-related differences in LV diastolic dysfunction, the baseline hemodynamics and hemodynamic changes induced by transcatheter ASD closure are different between younger and older patients [6]. Therefore, it is necessary to clarify whether HF in elderly transcatheter occlusion patients is related to senile changes or to the impact of device closure.

The purpose of this study was to assess cardiac function including diastolic function after transcatheter atrial septal defect closure in asymptomatic younger and older patients with ASD.

2. Experimental Section

Patient Enrollment and Data Measurement

Thirty-eight patients (age: 48.6 ± 17.1 years, range: 23–69 years) incidentally diagnosed with ASD during routine health check-up, and who were indicated for ASD treatment and underwent ASD closure with the Amplatzer Septal Occluder, were included in this retrospective study. All the patients were asymptomatic.

The patients' medical records, including the echocardiographic data collected before closure and 2 years after closure during a follow-up, were reviewed. The patients were divided into two groups according to their ages: Group I consisted of 18 patients <50 years old (33.06 ± 9.43 years) and Group II consisted of 20 patients ≥50 years old (62.55 ± 7.54 years).

The echocardiographic data comprised the LV inflow velocity, early and late mitral inflow velocities with the ratio of early diastole to atrial contraction (E/A), tissue Doppler image (TDI) findings, and all conventional measurements such as the LV and right ventricular (RV) diameters, LV ejection fraction (LVEF), LV mass, and LA volume. The LVEF was calculated using the Teichholz formula, while the mitral inflow pattern was assessed using the peak velocity during E and A, the ratio of E to A, and the E deceleration time. Myocardial velocities were obtained by tissue Doppler measurements (TDI) of the septal E′, septal A′, septal S′, septal E/E′, lateral E′, lateral A′, lateral S,′ and lateral E/E′, then all the TDI values were presented with the average of septal and lateral measurements.

The pre- and post-closure data were compared. Furthermore, these data were also compared between the two groups.

3. Study Design and Statistical Analysis

All statistical analyses were performed using SPSS version 23.0 for Windows (SPSS Inc., Chicago, IL, USA). Data are expressed as means ± SD. Paired t tests were used to analyze changes in the continuous variables between baseline and follow-up assessments; accordingly, the pre-closure and post-closure baseline characteristics were compared using a paired t test. Differences between Groups I and II were assessed using an unpaired t test. The Wilcoxon signed-rank test was used to compare variables between the baseline and follow-up assessments. p-values <0.05 were considered statistically significant.

4. Ethics Statement

This study was approved by the Yonsei University College of Medicine Institutional Review Board and the Research Ethics Committee of Severance Hospital (study approval number: 2020-0699-001). All research was performed in accordance with the relevant guidelines and regulations. The requirement for written informed consent was waived by the Institutional Review Board owing to the retrospective study design.

5. Results

Thirty-eight patients were indicated for ASD closure. The defect size was 21.77 + 6.79 mm and the balloon measurement was 24.29 ± 6.64 mm, with RV volume overload and without pulmonary hypertension.

The post-closure measurements of left ventricular end-diastolic dimension (LVEDD) and the LV mass were greater than their pre-closure measurements. The post-closure RV pressure was lower than the pre-closure RV pressure (Table 1). LA volume and the LA volume index increased after closure, although, this increase was not statistically significant. However, the older age patients showed different trend of LA volume and LA volume index over time rather than younger age patients (Table 2). The myocardial velocities significantly decreased after closure. Furthermore, the post-closure measurements of E′, A′, and S′ were lower than their pre-closure measurements. The estimated post-closure LV filling pressure (E/E′) was higher than the pressure in the pre-closure state (Table 1).

In Group I, the post-closure measurements of the LVEDD, LV mass, and mass index were higher than their pre-closure measurements. The post-closure RV pressure was lower than the pre-closure RV pressure. The post-closure measurements of TDI E′ and S′ were lower than their pre-closure measurements; however, A′ was higher at post-closure than at pre-closure. The estimated post-closure E/E′ was higher than the pre-closure E/E′ (Table 2) (Figure 1).

In Group II, the pre-closure measurements of LVEDD, LV mass, and mass index were higher than their pre-closure measurements. The post-closure RV pressure was lower than the pre-closure RV pressure. The TDI E′ and S′ at post-closure were lower than those at pre-closure; however, the post-closure A′ was higher than the pre-closure A′. The estimated post-closure E/E′ was higher than the pre-closure E/E′ (Table 2) (Figure 1).

Table 1. Comparison of echocardiographic data collected before and after atrial septal defect closure (N = 38).

N = 38	Pre-Closure	Post-Closure (2-Year Follow-Up)	p-Value
LVEDD (mm)	40.76 ± 3.28	43.39 ± 3.52	0.001
LVESD (mm)	26.86 ± 2.98	27.79 ± 3.11	0.11
LVEF (%)	66.41 ± 5.56	68.69 ± 5.08	0.48
LV mass (g)	99.64 ± 28.81	116.57 ± 32.03	0.01
LV mass Ix (g/m^2)	61.23 ± 16.22	71.09 ± 16.07	0.01
LA volume (mL)	42.83 ± 15.67	45.48 ± 14.57	0.24
LA vol Ix (mL/m^2)	26.1 ± 9.03	27.98 ± 8.99	0.20
RVSP (mmHg)	36.88 ± 12.20	31.81 ± 11.11	0.04
Mitral E (cm/s)	81.55 ± 19.54	84.79 ± 23.62	0.28
Mitral A (cm/s)	55.59 ± 12.90	60.68 ± 21.95	0.14
DT (ms)	191.68 ± 47.40	197.85 ± 50.62	0.31
TDI E′ (cm/s)	9.91 ± 2.87	8.12 ± 2.91	0.008
TDI A′ (cm/s)	8.83 ± 2.34	7.81 ± 1.72	0.03
TDI S′ (cm/s)	9.96 ± 2.55	8.06 ± 1.69	0.004
E/E′	8.79 ± 3.19	11.58 ± 4.80	0.005

LV: left ventricle, LA: left atrium, LVEDD: left ventricular end-diastolic dimension, LVESD: left ventricular end-systolic dimension, LVEF: left ventricular ejection fraction, RV: right ventricle, RVSP: right ventricular systolic pressure, DT; Deceleration time, E; peak early inflow velocity, A; peak late inflow velocity, TDI: tissue Doppler imaging, E′; peak early diastolic velocity, A′; peak late diastolic velocity, S′: peak systolic velocity.

Table 2. Comparison of echocardiographic data collected before and after atrial septal defect closure in Group I (N = 18) and Group II (N = 20).

	Group I (<50 Years Old) (n = 18)	Group II (≥50 Years Old) (n = 20)	p-Value
Age (years)	33.06 ± 9.43	62.55 ± 7.54	NA
LVEDD pre	40.44 ± 3.50	41.15 ± 3.08	0.28
post	44.43 ± 3.44	42.63 ± 3.47	0.07
LVESD pre	26.69 ± 2.87	27.08 ± 3.23	0.36
post	28.5 ± 3.41	27.26 ± 2.84	0.13
LVEF pre	66.19 ± 5.94	66.69 ± 5.28	0.40
post	68.86 ± 6.01	68.58 ± 4.44	0.43
LV mass pre	89.69 ± 21.43	111.89 ± 32.68	0.02
post	113.24 ± 35.5	119.02 ± 29.97	0.31
LV mass Ix pre	54.93 ± 11.48	68.98 ± 18.2	0.008
post	68.73 ± 21.18	72.83 ± 12.75	0.24
LA volume pre	36.07 ± 10.24	51.15 ± 17.49	0.003
post	38.16 ± 15.87	50.87 ± 11.09	0.005
LA volume Ix pre	21.89 ± 6.31	31.28 ± 9.37	0.001
post	23.17 ± 9.88	31.52 ± 6.48	0.003
RVSP pre	33.14 ± 6.97	41.47 ± 15.66	0.03
post	25.18 ± 6.31	36.6 ± 11.48	0.001
Mitral E pre	84.06 ± 17.2	82.71 ± 22.5	0.17
post	78.46 ± 22.37	86.32 ± 24.88	0.33
Mitral A pre	50.56 ± 11.17	49.78 ± 23.84	0.005
post	62.9 ± 12.08	69.64 ± 15.88	0.004
DT pre	189.67 ± 48.19	208.71 ± 65.9	0.40
post	194.00 ± 48.33	189.84 ± 35.5	0.15
TDI E′ pre	11.53 ± 2.38	9.92 ± 3.45	0.0001
post	7.93 ± 2.09	6.79 ± 1.44	0.0005
TDI A′ pre	8.09 ± 2.36	7.14 ± 1.29	0.02
post	9.91 ± 1.92	8.35 ± 1.87	0.02
TDI S′ pre	11.09 ± 2.55	8.86 ± 1.95	0.002
post	8.57 ± 1.80	7.47 ± 1.22	0.008
E/E′ pre	7.41 ± 1.42	9.60 ± 5.15	0.003
post	10.49 ± 3.95	13.03 ± 4.05	0.02

LV: left ventricle, LA: left atrium, LVEDD: left ventricular end-diastolic dimension, LVESD: left ventricular end-systolic dimension, LVEF: left ventricular ejection fraction, RV: right ventricle, RVSP: right ventricular systolic pressure, DT; Deceleration time, E; peak early inflow velocity, A; peak late inflow velocity, TDI: tissue Doppler imaging, E′; peak early diastolic velocity, A′; peak late diastolic velocity, S′: peak systolic velocity.

With conventional diastolic velocities, significant differences were observed in the inflow velocity of late atrial kick with mitral A between Groups I and II at both pre- and post-closure. Regarding tissue Doppler myocardial velocities, E′ decreased at post-closure in Groups I (pre-closure: 11.53 ± 2.38 vs. post-closure: 7.93 ± 2.09, $p = 0.008$) (Figure 1) and II (pre-closure: 9.92 ± 3.45 vs. post-closure: 6.79 ± 1.44, $p = 0.008$) (Figure 1). Both A′ and S′ decreased in Groups I and II post-closure. The E/E′ was more elevated in Group II than in Group I at both pre-closure and post-closure (pre-closure: 9.60 ± 5.15 vs. 7.41 ± 1.42, $p < 0.003$; post-closure: 13.03 + 4.05 vs. 10.49 ± 3.95, $p < 0.02$) (Table 2), also E/E′ was significantly elevated at post-closure in Group I (pre-closure: 7.41 ± 1.42 vs. post-closure: 10.49 ± 3.95, $p = 0.005$) and II (pre-closure: 9.60 ± 5.15 vs. post-closure: 13.03 + 4.05, $p = 0.005$) (Figure 1).

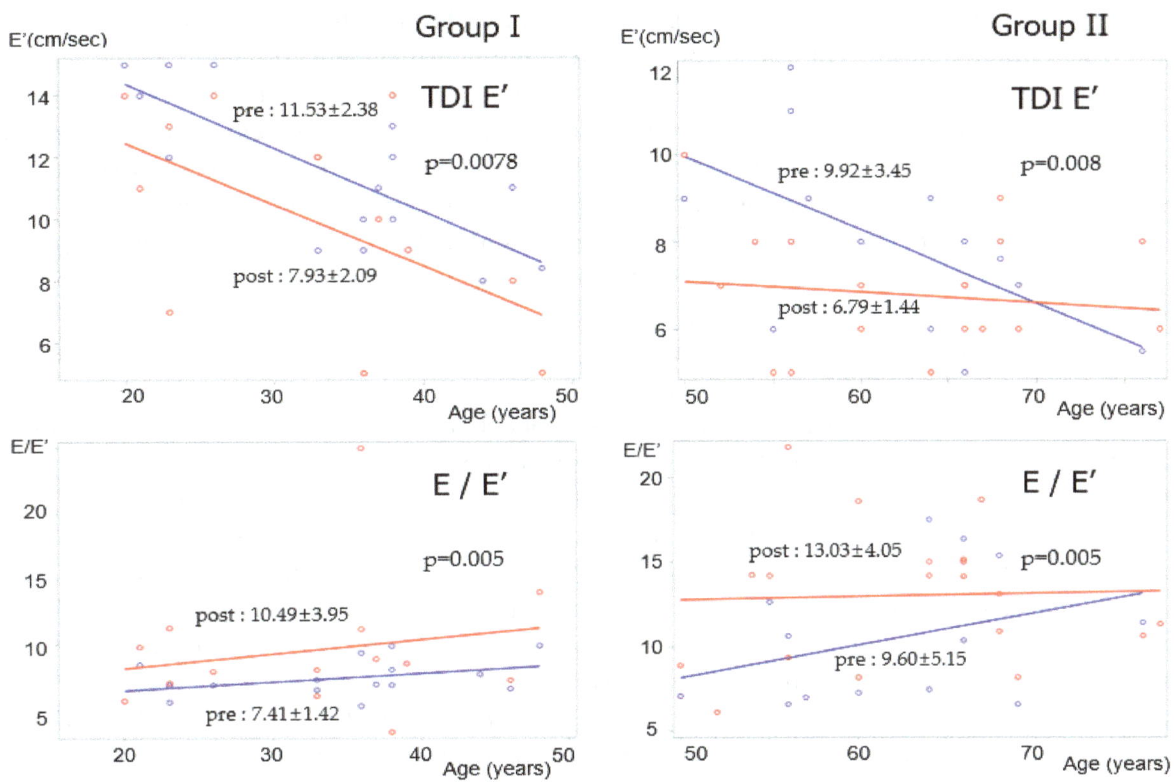

Figure 1. TDI E′ and E/E′ data as a function of age before and after atrial septal defect closure in Group I (N = 18) and Group II (N = 20). TDI: tissue Doppler imaging.

6. Discussion

Left-to-right inter-atrial shunting through the ASD causes right and left heart volume overload [5]. Even in asymptomatic patients, volume discrepancy and concomitant alteration between the left and right heart chambers progress with long-term shunting.

In patients presenting with senile LV dysfunction, left-to-right shunt in ASD could offer another inter-atrial route for LA flow instead of LV filling, and mask the abnormal increase of LA pressure and LV filling pressure [7]. Therefore, in these patients, ASD closure can increase the LV diastolic and LV filling pressures in the enlarged, volume-loaded left heart.

To exclude ASD patients with existing diastolic dysfunction, we included asymptomatic patients who believed that they did not have any heart diseases or cardiac dysfunction, and were incidentally diagnosed with ASD at routine health check-up without presenting with arrhythmias, right HF, or pulmonary hypertension. Surprisingly, the size of their ASDs were relatively large, and they presented with RV volume overload; the defect size was 21.77 + 6.79 mm and the balloon measurement was 24.29 ± 6.64 mm, certainly requiring treatment with device occlusion.

ASD closure causes a rapid left ventricular (LV) volume overload and a consequent surge in myocardial oxygen consumption, because of the abrupt stoppage of the left-to-right shunt. These important hemodynamic changes are generally tolerated in patients with normal LV function [8], but may be detrimental in patients with LV dysfunction [9] and in elderly patients with decreased LV compliance [3].

As we compared the echocardiographic measurements taken before procedure and 2 years after ASD closure, the LVEDD and LV mass were observed to have increased, while the RV pressure had lowered after closure. With ASD closure, the LV changed from being a long-standing underloaded chamber to a relatively enlarged chamber that was as normal as could be expected, while the RV changed from being a volume-overloaded ventricle with an elevated pressure to a reasonably-sized chamber with a reduced volume. Meanwhile, LA volume and the LA volume index showed the increased measurement after closure, even it was without statistical significance, however, the older age patients showed the variation of re-decreasing LA volume and LA volume index (Figure 1), which might be due to age-related alteration of LA pressure with diastolic functional change.

Furthermore, the post-closure increase of E/E′ implied a diastolic function decline with relaxation abnormality in all the patients in younger age and older age group (Table 2). Diastolic dysfunction may progress after ASD closure; as opposed to in younger patients of Group I, ASD closure in older patients of Group II resulted in further deterioration of baseline LV relaxation and increased the age-related LV stiffness, thereby further increasing the LV filling pressure. Luckily, no patients developed severe congestive HF in this study. This could be an adaptive phenomenon of post-closure myocardial adjustment with increased volume loading.

Previous studies that examined changes in relaxation using echocardiographic parameters measured before and after ASD device repair yielded inconsistent results. Hanseus KC et al. reported no significant changes in relaxation 1 or 2 days after ASD closure in both, the pediatric [10] and wider populations [11]; conversely, other studies have reported a decrease in the tissue Doppler spectral values in both these populations [12,13]. Meanwhile, Makino K et al. reported that LV diastolic function in post-closure ASD patients during the chronic phase was the same as that in healthy subjects aged below 50 years [14], however, LA dimension was larger, and the tissue Doppler E′ and E/E′ were significantly increased in the post ASD closure in elderly group of more than 50 years old. We also evaluated the patients grouping with below and equal or above the age of 50, followed for 2 years, the results revealed significant findings between two groups.

As Tomai F et al. reported for the case of ASD related with LV dysfunction, a real-time preprocedural evaluation of the hemodynamic effects with left-to-right shunt elimination may be useful for decision-making [15]. Even though our patients from health check-up were all asymptomatic, if we considered whether an intra-procedural balloon stress-test may be useful in unmasking latent diastolic impairment during the procedure, it might be helpful for expecting the hemodynamic changes with procedure [16].

The most prominent and consistent hemodynamic change after transcatheter ASD closure, and subsequent elimination of the inter-atrial shunt flow with device occlusion, is an increase in the LV preload with a simultaneous decrease in the RV volume. If LV diastolic dysfunction already existed before ASD closure, the LV cannot handle this acute elevation in preload after closure, resulting in a marked escalation of the LV end-diastolic pressure and pulmonary congestion [17]. Furthermore, ventricular diastolic myocardial stiffness is another important factor that can impact ventricular diastolic performance. Despite challenges in quantifying the diastolic chamber stiffness using echocardiography, Chen CH et al. published a study in which invasive ventricular pressure-volume measurement revealed a significant increase in age-related diastolic myocardial stiffness [18].

Therefore, older patients experience prominent diastolic dysfunction after ASD closure more frequently than younger patients, as demonstrated by our study results. Moreover, even asymptomatic patients exhibited a similar diastolic function change after ASD closure, without presenting with any cardiac function deterioration patterns before diagnosis. We believe that ASD closure in elderly patients with suspected or existing LV or RV dysfunction should be performed only after a meticulous consideration of the hemodynamic benefits and risks of closure [7,19].

The limitation of this study, due to the retrospective review of the patients from the regular health check-up, did not include blood test, especially brain natriuretic peptide (BNP) data, quality of life data with cardiac function including diastolic assessment long-term prior to ASD closure. Although it is not possible to investigate the functional change and myocardial analysis, all the included patients were asymptomatic without any cardiac disease, such as arrhythmias, right HF, or pulmonary hypertension. Further study will be necessary with the prospective design for the various aspects, not only for the diastolic function, but also with the quality of life with functional class, and other various comorbidities including diabetes, liver or kidney issues, comparing with healthy controls.

7. Conclusions

The LA size and LV function exhibited recognizable remodeling after transcatheter ASD closure. Because the LV preload elevation (i.e., E/E′) after ASD closure can be pronounced in older patients, caution should be provided more in older patients than in younger patients. It may be beneficial to close the ASD at an earlier age in adults even after a late diagnosis; a relatively younger age may be more suited for adaptation to the remodeling process to protect the myocardial function. In addition, vigilant early care would be helpful for the previous underloaded left heart by considering for latent diastolic impairment with the procedure.

Author Contributions: Conceptualization, L.Y.E., J.Y.C., H.K.P.; data curation, L.Y.E.; formal analysis, L.Y.E.; methodology, L.Y.E.; investigation, L.Y.E.; supervision, L.Y.E., J.Y.C.; validation, L.Y.E.; visualization, L.Y.E.; writing-original draft, L.Y.E.; writing-review and editing, L.Y.E., J.Y.C., H.K.P. All authors have read and agreed to the published version of the manuscript.

References

1. Du, Z.-D.; Hijazi, Z.M.; Kleinman, C.S.; Silverman, N.H.; Larntz, K. Comparison between transcatheter and surgical closure of secundum atrial septal defect in children and adults. *J. Am. Coll. Cardiol.* **2002**, *39*, 1836–1844. [CrossRef]
2. Eerola, A.; Pihkala, J.I.; Boldt, T.; Mattila, I.P.; Poutanen, T.; Jokinen, E. Hemodynamic improvement is faster after percutaneous ASD closure than after surgery. *Catheter. Cardiovasc. Interv.* **2007**, *69*, 432–441. [CrossRef] [PubMed]
3. Ewert, P.; Berger, F.; Nagdyman, N.; Kretschmar, O.; Dittrich, S.; Abdul-Khaliq, H.; Lange, P. Masked left ventricular restriction in elderly patients with atrial septal defects: A contraindication for closure? *Catheter. Cardiovasc. Interv.* **2001**, *52*, 177–180. [CrossRef]
4. Holzer, R.; Cao, Q.-L.; Hijazi, Z.M. Closure of a moderately large atrial septal defect with a self-fabricated fenestrated Amplatzer septal occluder in an 85-year-old patient with reduced diastolic elasticity of the left ventricle. *Catheter. Cardiovasc. Interv.* **2005**, *64*, 513–518. [CrossRef] [PubMed]
5. Masutani, S.; Senzaki, H. Left Ventricular Function in Adult Patients with Atrial Septal Defect: Implication for Development of Heart Failure After Transcatheter Closure. *J. Card. Fail.* **2011**, *17*, 957–963. [CrossRef] [PubMed]
6. Masutani, S.; Taketazu, M.; Ishido, H.; Iwamoto, Y.; Yoshiba, S.; Matsunaga, T.; Kobayashi, T.; Senzaki, H. Effects of age on hemodynamic changes after transcatheter closure of atrial septal defect: Importance of ventricular diastolic function. *Heart Vessel.* **2011**, *27*, 71–78. [CrossRef] [PubMed]
7. Shah, S.R.; Waxman, S.; Gaasch, W.H. The Impact of an Atrial Septal Defect on Hemodynamics in Patients with Heart Failure. *US Cardiol. Rev.* **2017**, *11*, 72. [CrossRef]
8. Shaheen, J.; Alper, L.; Rosenmann, D.; Klutstein, M.W.; Falkowsky, G.; Bitran, D.; Tzivoni, D. Effect of surgical repair of secundum-type atrial septal defect on right atrial, right ventricular, and left ventricular volumes in adults. *Am. J. Cardiol.* **2000**, *86*, 1395–1397. [CrossRef]
9. Tomai, F.; Gaspardone, A.; Papa, M.; Polisca, P. Acute left ventricular failure after transcatheter closure of a secundum atrial septal defect in a patient with coronary artery disease: A critical reappraisal. *Catheter. Cardiovasc. Interv.* **2002**, *55*, 97–99. [CrossRef] [PubMed]
10. Hanséus, K.; Björkhem, G.; Brodin, L.; Pesonen, E. Analysis of Atrioventricular Plane Movements by Doppler Tissue Imaging and M-Mode in Children with Atrial Septal Defects Before and After Surgical and Device Closure. *Pediatr. Cardiol.* **2002**, *23*, 152–159. [CrossRef] [PubMed]
11. Pascotto, M.; Santoro, G.; Caso, P.; Cerrato, F.; Caso, I.; Caputo, S.; Bigazzi, M.C.; D'Andrea, A.; Russo, M.G.; Calabrò, R. Global and Regional Left Ventricular Function in Patients Undergoing Transcatheter Closure of Secundum Atrial Septal Defect. *Am. J. Cardiol.* **2005**, *96*, 439–442. [CrossRef] [PubMed]
12. Pauliks, L.B.; Chan, K.-C.; Chang, D.; Kirby, S.K.; Logan, L.; DeGroff, C.G.; Boucek, M.M.; Valdes-Cruz, L.M. Regional myocardial velocities and isovolumic contraction acceleration before and after device closure of atrial septal defects: A color tissue Doppler study. *Am. Heart J.* **2005**, *150*, 294–301. [CrossRef] [PubMed]
13. Lange, A.; Coleman, D.M.; Palka, P.; Burstow, D.J.; Wilkinson, J.L.; Godman, M.J. Effect of catheter device closure of atrial septal defect on diastolic mitral annular motion. *Am. J. Cardiol.* **2003**, *91*, 104–108. [CrossRef]

14. Makino, K.; Hashimoto, G.; Makoto, S.; Hayama, H.; Otsuka, T.; Ikeda, N.; Iijima, R.; Hara, H.; Moroi, M.; Nakamura, M. Assessment of the left ventricular diastolic function after percutaneous atrial septal defect closure in chronic phase. *J. Am. Coll. Cardiol.* **2020**, *75*, 652. [CrossRef]
15. Tomai, F.; Andò, G.; De Paulis, R.; Chiariello, L. Real-time evaluation of the hemodynamic effects of atrial septal defect closure in adults with left ventricular dysfunction. *Catheter. Cardiovasc. Interv.* **2004**, *64*, 124–126. [CrossRef] [PubMed]
16. Miranda, W.R.; Hagler, D.J.; Reeder, G.S.; Warnes, C.A.; Connolly, H.M.; Egbe, A.C.; Taggart, N.W. Temporary balloon occlusion of atrial septal defects in suspected or documented left ventricular diastolic dysfunction: Hemodynamic and clinical findings. *Catheter. Cardiovasc. Interv.* **2019**, *93*, 1069–1075. [CrossRef] [PubMed]
17. Masutani, S.; Taketazu, M.; Mihara, C.; Mimura, Y.; Ishido, H.; Matsunaga, T.; Kobayashi, T.; Senzaki, H. Usefulness of Early Diastolic Mitral Annular Velocity to Predict Plasma Levels of Brain Natriuretic Peptide and Transient Heart Failure Development After Device Closure of Atrial Septal Defect. *Am. J. Cardiol.* **2009**, *104*, 1732–1736. [CrossRef] [PubMed]
18. Chen, C.-H.; Nakayama, M.; Nevo, E.; Fetics, B.J.; Maughan, W.; Kass, D.A. Coupled systolic-ventricular and vascular stiffening with age. *J. Am. Coll. Cardiol.* **1998**, *32*, 1221–1227. [CrossRef]
19. Takaya, Y.; Akagi, T.; Kijima, Y.; Nakagawa, K.; Watanabe, N.; Oe, H.; Taniguchi, M.; Ito, H. Echocardiographic Estimates of Left Ventricular Diastolic Dysfunction Do Not Predict the Clinical Course in Elderly Patients Undergoing Transcatheter Atrial Septal Defect Closure: Impact of Early Diastolic Mitral Annular Velocity. *J. Interv. Cardiol.* **2017**, *30*, 79–84. [CrossRef] [PubMed]

2

Typologies of Loneliness, Isolation and Living Alone are Associated with Psychological Well-Being among Older Adults in Taipei

Hui-Chuan Hsu

School of Public Health, Research Center of Health Equity, College of Public Health, Taipei Medical University, Taipei 11031, Taiwan; gingerhsu@tmu.edu.tw

Abstract: Background: Loneliness, isolation, and living alone are emerging as critical issues in older people's health and well-being, but the effects are not consistent. The purpose of this study was to examine the clustering of loneliness, isolation, and living alone, the risk factors and the associations with psychological well-being. Methods: The data were collected from the 2019 Taipei City Senior Citizen Condition Survey by face-to-face interviews and included a community-based sample (n = 3553). Loneliness, isolation, and living arrangement were analyzed by cluster analysis to define Loneliness-Isolation-Living-Alone clusters. Multinomial logistic regression was used to examine the factors related to Loneliness-Isolation-Living-Alone clusters, and linear regression was used to examine association of clusters with psychological well-being. Results: Five clusters of older adults were identified and named as follows: *Not Lonely-Connected-Others* (53.4%), *Not Lonely-Isolated-Others* (26.6%), *Not Lonely-Alone* (5.0%), *Lonely-Connected* (8.1%), and *Lonely-Isolated-Others* (6.9%). Demographics, financial satisfaction, physical function, family relationship, and social participation were related to the Loneliness-Isolation-Living-Alone clusters. Compared with the *Not Lonely-Connected-Others* cluster, the *Lonely-Connected* cluster and *Lonely-Isolated-Others* cluster had higher depressive symptoms and lower life satisfaction, and the *Not Lonely-Isolated-Others* cluster reported lower life satisfaction; the *Not Lonely-Alone* cluster was not different. Discussion: Loneliness and isolation are negatively associated with psychological well-being, and living arrangement is not the determinant to loneliness or isolation. Older adults are suggested to strengthen their informal social support, and the government may encourage social care and create an age friendly environment to reduce loneliness and isolation.

Keywords: loneliness; isolation; living arrangement; depressive symptoms; life satisfaction; psychological well-being; older adults

---

1. Introduction

Loneliness, isolation, and living alone (LIL) are emerging as critical issues in older people's health and well-being. Existing literature has examined the relationship of LIL with physical health, mental health and well-being [1–3]. Loneliness is a subjective feeling. It is often defined as a negative feeling due to a lack of intimate social relationships, especially the gap between what one wants and what one truly has regarding social relationships [4]. Isolation is defined as the psychological or physical distance between one individual and other people, or the gap in the social network. Isolation can be represented as lacking social connectedness [5], lacking meaningful, engaging, and quality social relationships in social contacts [6], or having subjective feelings of lacking belongingness or intimacy [6,7]. Living alone is one form of living arrangement that requires the social function or resources from the social network.

However, the effects of LIL are often intertwined, but the effects on health are not consistent. The purpose of this study was to identify the clusters of loneliness, isolation, and living alone and the associations of LIL patterns with psychological well-being.

The effects of LIL on health or well-being can be explained by stress [8]. Due to life events, stress influences an individual's hypothalamic-pituitary-adrenal axis in the endocrine and nervous systems, reduces immunity, and changes behavioral and cognitive status and is adjusted by an individual's resilience, coping ability and social support. Loneliness or isolation may be viewed as a long-term source of stress. When such stress effects last a long time, they may cause significant effects on health.

Past studies have explored the relationship of loneliness, isolation and living alone on the health and well-being of older people. LIL may cause depression, cardiovascular disease, reduced quality of life, low self-rated health, anxiety, reduced cognitive or physical function, frailty, insomnia, mortality, suicide, and work disability in older adults [1,3,9–21]. Such negative effects may be worse for individuals with lower education, lower income, and disability [16].

However, the effects of LIL on physical and psychological health are not consistent. Regarding cognitive function, Grande et al. found the effects of living alone related to mild cognitive impairment [22], but other studies from Evans et al. and Kuiper et al. indicated that the effect of living alone is not significant [13,23]. Yang et al. (2020) defines social isolation by living alone, family contact and social engagement, and social isolation showed direct effect on reduced cognitive functioning and through mediating by loneliness [24]. A longitudinal study shows that loneliness may affect cognitive function and increase the risk of dementia, but the isolation effects on cognitive function are not stable, and living alone is not significantly related to dementia [25]. Regarding emotional health, loneliness is found to be related to depressive symptoms but irrelevant to isolation [26]. A longitudinal study indicates that living alone is related to emotional loneliness, but living alone is not related to social isolation [27]. Another study found that living alone is related to depressive symptoms, but such an association is no longer significant when loneliness is controlled [28]. It seems that the effects of loneliness, isolation, and living alone on health and well-being may be different; they simply often happen together. It is necessary to examine their joint effects. Smith and Victor [29] used latent class analysis to examine the combinations of LIL and associations with physical and psychological health. They identified six groups of older people: no loneliness or isolation, moderate loneliness, living alone, moderate isolation, moderate loneliness and living alone, and high loneliness and moderate isolation. These groups were associated differently with physical function, self-rated health, chronic diseases, and depressive symptoms.

The factors related to LIL can be viewed by individual level (demographics, health and psychological characteristics), interpersonal level (family relationship and marital status), and society level (culture, social environment and age friendliness). The factors include age, sex, race, education, socioeconomic status, marital status or widowhood, working status, having children or not, social relationship with friends and neighbors, social anxiety, Internet use, self-rated health, disability, resilience, previous depression, and built environment [10,21,29–43]. In addition, social participation [44], activity engagement [45], bonding social capital [46], and religious belief or spirituality [47,48] may also be protective factors. Through participating in social activities, not only the social connection and social support are increased, but also the sense of achievement and feeling of belonging can be improved. In addition, the social environment may be related to loneliness or the effect of loneliness on well-being, such as public space walkability and accessibility [49].

Family relationships are especially important for a family-centered culture such as the traditional culture in Taiwan. According to tradition, Taiwanese people expect to live with family members, to be financially supported by their adult children in old age as a performance of filial piety. In the tradition, older people also did not expect to work or participate in social groups in the old age. However, due to modernization and change of social values, the rate of living with children or grandchildren has reduced in recent decades. Older people who live alone or only live with their spouse are more likely to be male, and also provide and received less support from those who live with family [50]. Loneliness and social isolation are not just lack of companionship, but also represent a state of mind: the gap between desire and reality in the context of culture [51]. In the family-centered Taiwanese culture, the feeling of loneliness may be affected by the gap of expectation and reality of family support. At the same time, the active aging concept is raised and social participation is promoted and gradually accepted among older people in Taiwan society. Age-friendly environments are advocated by World Health Organization [52] and applied in local governments in Taiwan. Age friendliness is found to be related to older people's well-being [53] and physical domain of health-related quality of life [54]. Therefore, not only may LIL combined with an individual's characteristics affect well-being, age friendliness should be considered as a factor to mental well-being.

Despite the existing findings about the relationship of LIL with health and well-being, only a few studies have tried to identify the intertwined relationship of LIL [29], and the inconsistent effects of LIL on health and well-being need further investigation. Therefore, the purpose of this study was to identify the possible combinations of loneliness, isolation, and living alone among community-based older adults and to examine the effects of LIL combinations on psychological well-being in the case of Taipei city.

2. Materials and Methods

2.1. *Data and Sample*

The data used for the present study were secondary data collected by face-to-face interviews for the "2019 Taipei City Senior Citizen Condition Survey". The sample was drawn from citizens whose household was registered in Taipei city. The community-based sample was drawn by stratified sampling (by age and sex stratification in the 12 districts of Taipei city) and systematic sampling (by address and age), and the institutional sample was drawn by stratified random sampling by different types of institutions (nursing homes and long-term care facilities). In total, the completed sample was composed of 3853 persons (3553 persons in the community and 300 persons in institutions). In this current study, only data from the community-based sample were included in the analysis (n = 3553). The data was deidentified when released. The study obtained the approval of the Taipei Medical University Joint Institutional Review Board (No. N202010050).

2.2. *Measures*

2.2.1. The Main Independent Variables: LIL

Loneliness was measured by one item from the CES-D scale (do you feel lonely?) [55], and the score was defined as yes (sometimes or often, one to seven days a week)/no (never), as the application of previous research [12,24]. Living alone was defined by the living arrangement, coded as living alone, and living with others in the household. Isolation was defined by the frequency of informal social contact, by asking the respondents, "How often do you have social interaction with friends, relatives, or colleagues, including meeting in person, by telephone, or internet in the past three months? (Interaction because of work does not count)". The social contact frequency was measured as never, less than once a month, once a month, two to three times a month, once a week, two to six times a week, or every day. If an individual had social contact less than once per week, he or she was described as isolated.

2.2.2. The Dependent Variables

Psychological well-being included two variables: depressive symptoms and life satisfaction. Life satisfaction was scored from 1 to 5 to represent very unsatisfactory to very satisfactory. The other dependent variable was depressive symptoms, which were measured by the CES-D 11-item scale [55] except for the loneliness item. In this survey, each item was scored 1 to 3, so the total 10 items scored from 10 to 30.

2.2.3. Other Covariates

Demographics included age (age 60–64, 65–74, and 75+), sex, education (illiterate, informal education or elementary school, primary high school, senior high school, college/university or above), financial satisfaction (scored 1–5, indicating very unsatisfied to very satisfied), and working status (yes/no).

Health condition variables included self-rated health (score 1–5, indicating worst to excellent), chronic disease numbers (endocrine disease, neuropsychiatry disease, cardiovascular disease, respiratory system disease, digestive system disease, skin disease, skeletal or joint disease, urinary and reproductive system disease, injuries, and other chronic disease), cognitive function, activities of daily living (ADLs), and instrumental activities of daily living (IADLs). Cognitive function was measured by Short Portable Mental State Questionnaire (SPMSQ) [56], scored 0 to 10. ADLs included six items: dressing, transferring, walking indoors, using a toilet, taking a bath, and eating. Each item was measured for performance difficulty and scored 0 to 3. The total score ranged from 0 to 18; a high score indicated more difficulties. IADLs included nine items: shopping for groceries, preparing food, using a telephone, going out by transportation, managing money, doing light housework, doing heavy housework, taking medicine, and doing laundry. Each item was measured by the difficulty, scored 0 to 3; the total score of the difficulties was from 0 to 27.

Social support and social participation included marital status (having a spouse or not), children (yes/no), participation in volunteering (yes/no), political participation (yes/no), religious activity (yes/no), other social group participation (yes/no), and satisfaction with family relationships (recoded as unsatisfied, no opinion or no family, and satisfied).

Age friendliness was measured by three items: how much do you think the public respects older people, does your neighborhood/community hold the events considering older people's needs, and do you think the products/services provided by society consider older people's needs? Total scores ranged from 5 to 15; a higher score indicated more age friendliness.

2.3. Analysis

The data analysis was conducted by IBM SPSS 22.0 (IBM, SPSS Inc., Chicago, IL, USA). Descriptive analysis and bivariate tests were conducted to examine the relationships among the variables. Loneliness, isolation, and living alone were analyzed by cluster analysis. The two-step cluster analysis in SPSS procedure was conducted to suggest the best cluster numbers, and then k-means cluster analysis was used to define the Loneliness-Isolation-Living Alone (LIL) clusters. Multinomial logistic regression was used to examine the factors related to LIL clusters. Linear regression was used to examine the relationship of the LIL cluster and other factors with depressive symptoms and life satisfaction.

3. Results

The sample characteristics are shown in Table 1. The participants who felt lonely represented 15.1% of the sample; 37.9% were isolated (having social contact less than once per week); and 6.4% were living alone. The bivariate analysis of loneliness, isolation, and living arrangement with the characteristics of the participants are shown in the Supplementary Table S1.

Table 1. Description of the sample.

Variables	*n* (*N* = 3553)	Mean (SD) or %
Age		
Age 60–64	1069	30.1%
Age 65–69	938	26.4%
Age 70–74	557	15.7%
Age 75–79	423	11.9%
Age 80–84	260	7.6%
Age 85+	296	8.3%
Sex		
Female	1941	54.6%
Male	1612	45.4%
Education		
Illiterate	166	4.7%
Informal education or elementary school	1055	29.7%
Primary high school	517	14.6%
Senior high school	938	26.4%
College/University or above	877	24.7%
Marital status		
No spouse	1123	31.6%
Having spouse	2430	68.4%
Children		
No children	207	83.3%
Having children	3346	16.7%
Financial satisfaction	3184	3.48 (0.78)
Working status		
No	2961	83.3%
Yes	592	16.7%
Self-rated health (1–5)	3184	3.55 (0.84)
Cognitive function (1–10)	3184	9.57 (0.98)
Chronic disease number (0–7)	3553	0.97 (0.96)
Activities of daily living (0–18)	3553	0.68 (2.87)
Instrumental activities of daily living (0–27)	3553	1.87 (5.44)
Depressive symptom1 (10–30)	3184	13.25 (2.68)
Life satisfaction (1–5)	3184	3.88 (0.74)
Age friendliness (3–15)	3164	10.45 (2.43)
Volunteering		
No	3397	95.6%
Yes	156	4.4%
Political participation		
No	3534	99.5%
Yes	19	0.5%
Religious activity		
No	3096	87.1%
Yes	457	12.9%
Other social groups		
No	3022	85.1%
Yes	531	14.9%
Family satisfaction		
Unsatisfied	121	3.8%
No family or no opinion	178	5.6%
Satisfied	2885	90.6%
Living arrangement		
Alone	229	6.4%
With others	3324	93.6%

Table 1. *Cont.*

Variables	n (N = 3553)	Mean (SD) or %
Loneliness		
Not lonely	2704	84.9%
Lonely	480	15.1%
Isolation		
Isolated (social contact < 1 per week)	1345	37.9%
Connected (social contact ≥ 1 per week)	2208	62.1%

Note: $N = 3553$. Missing cases are excluded listwise.

By the two-step cluster analysis, seven LIL clusters were suggested as presented in Table 2: Not Lonely, Connected, and with Others (53.4%); Not Lonely, Isolated, and with Others (26.6%); Not Lonely, Connected, and Alone (3.5%); Lonely, Connected, and with Others (7.1%); Lonely, Isolated, and with Others (6.9%); Lonely, Connected, and Alone (1.0%); and Not Lonely, Isolated, and Alone (1.4%). However, the sample size of the cluster 3, 6, and 7 was small, that was not suitable for further analysis. Thus, some of the small clusters were combined together, and in total five clusters were defined as presented in Table 3: *Not Lonely, Connected, and with Others (NLCO)*, 53.4%; *Not Lonely, Isolated, and with Others (NLIO)*, 26.6%; *Not Lonely and Alone (NLA)*, 5.0%; *Lonely and Connected (LC)*, 8.1%; and *Lonely, Isolated, and living with Others (LIO)*, 6.9%. The bivariate analysis of LIL clusters with the characteristics of the participants are shown in the Supplementary Table S2.

Table 2. Loneliness, isolation, and living alone (LIL) combination distribution of the community-based sample—seven clusters (%).

Variables	Cluster 1: (53.4%) [1]	Cluster 2: (26.6%) [2]	Cluster 3: (3.5%) [3]	Cluster 4: (7.1%) [4]	Cluster 5: (6.9%) [5]	Cluster 6: (1.0%) [6]	Cluster 7 (1.4%) [7]
Loneliness							
Not Lonely	100.0	100.0	100.0	0.0	0.0	0.0	100.0
Lonely	0.0	0.0	0.0	100.0	100.0	100.0	0.0
Isolation							
Isolated	0.0	100.0	0.0	0.0	100.0	0.0	100.0
Connected	100.0	0.0	100.0	100.0	0.0	100.0	0.0
Living arrangement							
Alone	0.0	0.0	100.0	0.0	15.4	100.00	100.0
With Others	100.0	100.0	0.0	100.0	84.6	0.0	0.0

Note: $N = 3184$. The clusters were grouped by two-stage cluster analysis. [1] Not Lonely, Connected, and with Others, [2] Not Lonely, Isolated, and with Others, [3] Not Lonely, Connected, and Alone, [4] Lonely, Connected, and with Others, [5] Lonely, Isolated, and with Others, [6] Lonely, Connected, and Alone, [7] Not Lonely, Isolated, and Alone.

Table 3. LIL combination distribution of the community-based sample—five clusters (%).

LIL Clusters	N (%)
Not Lonely-Connected-Others (NLCO)	1700 (53.4%)
Not Lonely-Isolated-Others (NLIO)	846 (26.6%)
Not Lonely-Alone (NLA)	158 (5.0%)
Lonely-Connected (LC)	259 (8.1%)
Lonely-Isolated-Others (LIO)	221 (6.9%)

Note: $N = 3184$. The clusters were grouped based on Table 2.

Table 4 shows the characteristics of the LIL clusters by the multinomial logistic regression analysis. Compared with the reference group the *Not Lonely-Connected-Others (NLCO)* cluster, the older adults who were in the *(Not Lonely-Isolated-Others (NLIO)* cluster were more likely to be lower educated

(OR = 0.905, $p < 0.05$), had worse self-rated health (OR = 0.826, $p < 0.01$), had worse cognitive function (OR = 0.866, $p < 0.01$), had lower financial satisfaction (OR = 0.707, $p < 0.001$), feeling less age friendliness (OR = 0.958, $p < 0.05$), be male (OR = 0.825, $p < 0.01$), had children (OR = 1.691, $p < 0.05$), not working (OR = 0.704, $p < 0.01$), and did not participate in other social groups (OR = 0.703, $p < 0.01$). The older adults in the *Not Lonely-Alone (NLA)* cluster were more likely to be higher educated (OR = 1.330, $p < 0.01$), had more chronic diseases (OR = 1.433, $p < 0.05$), did not have a spouse (OR = 0.002, $p < 0.001$), and reported lower family satisfaction or had no family (OR = 0.180, $p < 0.001$). The participants in the *Lonely-Connected (LC)* cluster were more likely to be higher educated (OR = 1.167, $p < 0.05$), had worse self-rated health (OR = 0.701, $p < 0.001$), had more IADL difficulties (OR = 1.095, $p < 0.01$), had more chronic diseases (OR = 1.327, $p < 0.01$), had a worse financial satisfaction (OR = 0.621, $p < 0.001$), be female (OR = 1.622, $p < 0.01$), did not have a spouse (OR = 0.414, $p < 0.001$), participated in other social groups (OR = 2.699, $p < 0.001$), and reported lower family relationship or did not have family (OR = 0.342, $p < 0.001$). The participants in the *Lonely-Isolated-Others (LIO)* cluster were more likely to have worse self-rated health (OR = 0.533, $p < 0.001$), had more IADL difficulties (OR = 1.094, $p < 0.05$), had a worse financial satisfaction (OR = 0.464, $p < 0.001$), were older than 75 years old (OR = 2.006, $p < 0.05$), did not have a spouse (OR = 0.492, $p < 0.001$), and reported lower family relationship or had no family (OR = 0.165, $p < 0.001$).

Table 4. Factors related to LIL combinations by multinomial logistic regression (odds ratios).

Factors	NLIO (Not Lonely, Isolated, with Others)	NLA (Not Lonely and Alone)	LC (Lonely and Connected)	LIO (Lonely, Isolated, with Others)
Education	0.905 *	1.330 **	1.167 *	0.931
Self-rated health	0.826 **	1.053	0.701 ***	0.533 ***
ADL difficulty	0.954	0.780	0.967	1.006
IADL difficulty	1.034	0.952	1.095 **	1.094 **
Chronic disease number	1.110	1.433 **	1.327 **	0.931
Cognitive function	0.866 **	0.930	0.919	0.883
Financial satisfaction	0.707 ***	1.016	0.621 ***	0.464 ***
Age friendliness	0.958 *	0.995	1.012	1.004
Age 65–74	1.062	1.064	0.853	1.123
Age 75+	1.274	1.395	0.851	2.006 **
Sex (female)	0.825 *	0.705	1.622 **	1.112
Marital status (having spouse)	0.929	0.002 ***	0.414 ***	0.492 ***
Children (yes)	1.691 *	0.815	0.957	0.807
Work (yes)	0.704 **	1.067	0.864	0.764
Volunteering (yes)	1.035	2.081	1.089	1.311
Religious activity (yes)	0.794	0.948	0.748	0.859
Other social group participation (yes)	0.703 **	0.822	2.699 ***	1.076
Family satisfaction (satisfied)	0.776	0.180 ***	0.342 ***	0.165 ***
Model fit	−2LL: intercept only = 7587.422; final model = 6363.982, Chi-square = 1223.440, df = 72, $p < 0.001$.			

Note: Analysis by multinomial logistic regression. Intercept is omitted from the table. −2LL: −2 log likelihood. The reference group: LIL (NLCO: *Not Lonely, Connected, and with Others*), sex (male), age (age 60–64), marital status (no spouse), children (no), volunteering (no), religious activity (no), other social group participation (no), family satisfaction (unsatisfied or no family). Ordinal or continuous variable: age, education, self-rated health, ADL difficulty, IADL difficulty, chronic disease number, cognitive function, financial satisfaction, age friendliness. * $p < 0.05$, ** $p < 0.01$, *** $p < 0.001$.

Table 5 shows the relationships of the LIL clusters and other factors with depressive symptoms and life satisfaction. Compared with those in the *NLCO* cluster, the older adults in the LC cluster ($\beta = 2.378$, $p < 0.001$) and in the LIO cluster ($\beta = 2.674$ $p < 0.001$) had higher depressive symptoms. In addition, who were younger, had children, not satisfied with family relationship or not family, lower financial satisfaction, worse self-rated health, more chronic diseases, more IADL difficulties, not participated in social groups and feeling lower age friendliness, had more depressive symptoms. The explained variance (R square) was 0.412.

Table 5. LIL and psychological health and well-being by linear regression.

Variables	Depressive Symptom		Life Satisfaction (a)		Life Satisfaction (b)	
	B	SE	B	SE	B	SE
Constant	17.945	0.507 ***	1.695	0.149 ***	2.711	0.173 ***
NLIO (not lonely, isolated, with others)	0.120	0.090	−0.058	0.026 *	−0.051	0.026
NLA (not lonely and alone)	0.055	0.189	0.007	0.056	0.010	0.055
LC (lonely and connected)	2.378	0.144 ***	−0.156	0.042 ***	−0.021	0.043
LIO (lonely, isolated, with others)	2.674	0.161 ***	−0.202	0.047***	−0.051	0.049
Age 65–74	−0.152	0.090	0.036	0.027	0.027	0.026
Age 75+	−0.472	0.118 ***	0.134	0.035 ***	0.107	0.034 **
Sex (male)	−0.068	0.080	−0.052	0.024 *	−0.056	0.023 *
Education	0.019	0.033	0.034	0.010 ***	0.035	0.010 ***
Marital status (having spouse)	−0.060	0.098	0.021	0.029	0.018	0.028
Children (yes)	0.523	0.169 **	−0.020	0.050	0.010	0.049
Family satisfaction (satisfied)	−0.665	0.136 ***	0.808	0.040 ***	0.770	0.039
Work (yes)	−0.116	0.104	<−0.001	0.031	−0.007	0.030 ***
Financial satisfaction	−0.296	0.053 ***	0.302	0.016 ***	0.285	0.015 ***
Self-rated health	−0.906	0.051 ***	0.065	0.015 ***	0.013	0.015
Chronic disease number	0.187	0.046 ***	−0.004	0.014	0.007	0.013
ADL difficulty	0.052	0.044	−0.012	0.013	−0.010	0.013
IADL difficulty	0.123	0.020 ***	−0.003	0.006	0.004	0.006
Cognitive function	−0.036	0.041	−0.006	0.012	−0.008	0.012
Volunteering (yes)	−0.150	0.176	0.014	0.052	0.005	0.051
Religious activity (yes)	−0.143	0.112	−0.015	0.033	−0.023	0.032
Other social group (yes)	−0.524	0.104 ***	0.048	0.031	0.018	0.030
Age friendliness	−0.035	0.016 *	0.013	0.005 **	0.012	0.005 *
Depressive symptoms	—	—	—	—	−0.057	0.005 ***
R square	0.412		0.345		0.369	

Note: Analysis by linear regression. The reference group: LIL (NLCO: the *Not Lonely-Connected-Others* cluster), age (age 60–64), sex (female), marital status (no spouse), children (no), family satisfaction (satisfied), working (no), volunteering (no), religious activity (no), other social group (no). Other variables are ordinal or continuous. * $p < 0.05$, ** $p < 0.01$, *** $p < 0.001$.

Regarding the model of life satisfaction, two models were analyzed. In Model (a), the older adults who were in the NLIO cluster (β = −0.058, $p < 0.05$), the LC cluster (β = −0.156, $p < 0.01$) and in the LIO cluster (β = −0.202, $p < 0.001$) had lower life satisfaction than the NLCO group. However, when depressive symptom was controlled in Model (b), the NLIO, LC and LIO clusters were not significant anymore. In addition, the older adults who were older than 75 years old, female, higher educated, satisfied with family relationship, having higher financial satisfaction, feeling more age friendliness, and having fewer depressive symptoms, reported higher life satisfaction. The explained variance (R'square) was 0.369.

4. Discussion

This study examined the intertwining relationship of loneliness, isolation, and living alone (LIL) to identify clusters among older adults and related factors, as well as the associations of the LIL clusters with depressive symptoms and life satisfaction in the case of Taipei city. Five LIL clusters were identified: *Not Lonely-Isolated-Others* (53.4%), *Not Lonely-Isolated-Others* (26.6%), *Not Lonely-Alone* (5.0%), *Lonely-Connected* (8.1%), and *Lonely-Isolated-Others* (6.9%). The factors related to LIL clusters included age, sex, education, physical function (IADLs), chronic disease numbers, marital status, having children, working status, family relationship satisfaction, financial satisfaction, and social participation. Compared with those in the *Not Lonely-Connected-Others* cluster, the older adults in the *Lonely-Connected* cluster and the *Lonely-Isolated-Others* cluster had more depressive symptoms and lower life satisfaction; the *Not Lonely-Isolated-Others* cluster did not have more depressive symptoms but reported lower life satisfaction; and the *Not Lonely-Alone* cluster was not significantly different.

4.1. Typology of LIL Cluster

The five LIL (*NLCO, NLIO, NLA, LC, LIO*) clusters show the mutual relationships of loneliness, isolation, and living alone. The typology is similar to what was found in the study of Smith and Victor [29], which identified six groups by latent class analysis, which indicated the different levels of loneliness and isolation. When controlling for other variables, living alone is not necessarily associated with feeling more isolated or lonely. This means that even if older adults live alone, they can still be socially active and connected. In other words, even though older people live with others, physical strain, poor family relationships, ignorance, or lack of social participation may make them isolated. The social welfare policy in Taiwan focuses on those living alone, but lonely or isolated older people are not noticed under the current system. The individual's living arrangement in itself may not be the most useful indicator for developing social care for older people.

4.2. Factors Related to LIL Clusters

The association of physical function with LIL clusters was found, but no connection was found with cognitive function. The factors related to the five LIL clusters included demographics, IADL difficulties, family relationships, marital status, and social participation. The older adults in the LC cluster and the LIO cluster had more IADL difficulties. The LIO cluster was older than other clusters. It is possible that frailty prevents older adults in the LIO cluster from interacting socially and participating in social life and thus makes them more isolated. Previous research indicates that ADL difficulties are related to loneliness [10,49]. This means that basic physical function limitations may not be the barriers to social connectedness or social participation in this sample, but IADLs need advanced physical function, which may be related to the activities of social interaction or social participation. Cognitive function was not significantly related to the LIL clusters except for the NLIO cluster. The lower cognitive function may be a challenge for the older adults to interact with other people, and thus they were more isolated. There may be two reasons that other clusters were not significantly related to LIL clusters. One reason is that the survey only investigated those who could respond and communicate. Another reason is that the measurement of cognitive function by the SPMSQ was not sensitive; most of the participants showed a high SPMSQ score, and there was no variation. Thus, cognitive function was not used as the dependent variable but was used as a controlling variable in the models. The older participants in the NLA cluster were not significantly different from the NLCO group in physical function or cognitive function. That means the NLA cluster adults are able to live independently and live alone.

Social network and family support are important factors in LIL clusters. Those who did not have spouses, had no family or were not satisfied with family relationships were more likely to be in the NLA, LC, and LIO clusters, i.e., living alone or feeling lonely. The results were consistent with previous studies [9,10,29–31]. The reason to live alone for the NLA cluster is probably because they did not have family or did not expect to live with family. Family relationship satisfaction was significant not only for those who did not have family, but also significant for those who had family or were living with family, especially the two lonely groups (LC and LIO). It is possible that the older adults have unfulfilled expectations on their family, and thus the feeling of loneliness was stronger.

The NLIO cluster needs further attention. The NLIO cluster was not significantly related to marital status; however, it was related to having children and working. The participants in the NLIO cluster also were more likely to be male, less likely to participate in social groups, and reported lower age friendliness. The NLIO cluster is similar to the isolated group in the study of Smith and Victor [29]. It is possible that the members of the NLIO cluster may live with family or have contact in their occupation, but they did not have much informal social interaction with family and friends, especially for older men. The lifestyle for NLIO cluster may be less socialized.

Participating in volunteering, religious activity were not different across cluster. Participating in other social groups were higher in the LC cluster (OR = 2.685) and lower in the NLIO cluster (OR = 0.703). Participating in social groups is one kind of social contact, which prevents older people from getting isolated by connecting with other people. Gale et al. [15] found that those who are socially isolated (no social contact and no social group participation) were more likely to be lonely. However, the effects of social group participation on its own on loneliness are not confirmed. One of the possible reasons for the association of loneliness and social group participation is that social group participation is a shallow interaction without engagement for the participants. Another explanation is that older adults participate in these social groups because they feel lonely and would like to reduce their loneliness by participation in a social group. Because this is a cross-sectional study, the causal relationship cannot be confirmed.

The *NLIO*, *LC*, and *LIO* older adults had lower financial satisfaction. The three clusters were either isolated or lonely. Chung et al. [57] define financial social exclusion as one type of social exclusion: financial strain may cause barriers in maintaining social relationships, and life satisfaction can be lower.

4.3. LIL Clusters and Psychological Well-Being

The two lonely cluster of older adults, LC and LIO, had more depressive symptoms and lower life satisfaction, which is consistent with previous studies [11,29,30,33,36]. When the depressive symptom variable was added, the effects of LIL clusters were not significant. That implies depressive symptoms are the mediators of loneliness to life satisfaction. The NLIO group did not report higher depressive symptoms, but they still showed significantly lower life satisfaction even when the depressive symptom was controlled for. The older adults in the NLIO cluster were isolated, had less family interaction and were more likely to be males. One explanation is that the NLIO cluster older adults did not recognize their loneliness [29]. The other explanation is that the social relationship was not positive for these older adults or there were unmet needs in their social relationship [39], or some of the older adults had social anxiety in social interactions [40]. Thus, social isolation did not influence their mental health (depressive symptoms). However, both isolated clusters (NLIO, LIO) had lower life satisfaction. Social connectedness is one of the indicators used to measure active aging [58], and social connectedness provides social capital, which is beneficial for resources and reciprocity [46]. Although not all social relationships are positive, having a moderate social network and appropriate social support may still be positive for well-being. The reasons for being isolated should be explored in qualitative research in the future.

Depressive symptoms and life satisfaction for the NLA older adults were not different from the NLCO cluster. Living alone is not necessarily equal to a lack of social connectedness and social participation [27], and loneliness but not living alone is associated with depressive symptoms [28]. It is also possible that the older adults in the NLA cluster may have intact physical function and cognitive function to live alone, and thus their psychological well-being was not affected by living arrangement. The NLA cluster also had higher education, indicating a better socioeconomic status and better chance to well-being. Although the older adults in the NLA cluster live alone or did not have family, if the living-alone adults have independent health and live in a meaningful, connected, and active lifestyle, their mental health and well-being can still be fine.

Lower financial satisfaction was related to more depressive symptoms and lower life satisfaction. A study from Europe indicates that individuals have more worries of retirement income if their country is projecting more population aging and more income inequality [59]. It seems that financial security is related to psychological well-being, especially when the older adults do not have confidence in social support, such as the *Lonely* or the *Isolated* older adults in this study. Old age policy should provide a good basis for pension and security for older people and trust in the government so that older people (especially isolated or lonely people) do not need to additionally worry about their financial security. In addition, age friendliness was related to lower depressive symptoms and higher life satisfaction, similar to previous research [53,54]. If the community or society is age-friendly, the older people would feel more comfortable and more willing in social interaction and social participation, which would thus reduce isolation and loneliness.

4.4. Limitations

There are some limitations in this study. First, the data were cross-sectional data. The causal relationships of LIL with other variables cannot be confirmed. Second, the sample was drawn from older adults living in Taipei city. Taipei city is an urban modern city. The infrastructure for an age-friendly environment is better, and the access to the health and community services is much abundant than in rural areas, which reduces the barrier of social connection and participation. However, the percentage of older adults living with children or grandchildren is lower than that of rural areas, and more social interactions with family, neighbors and friends may be more frequently in rural areas. In addition, the traditional culture in Taiwan is family-centered. Older people usually hope to live with family but not live alone. The results may not be generalizable to other areas, populations or cultures. Third, the data were from secondary data. There may be other confounders or related factors that are not available. For example, loneliness was measured by only a single item, just as past research using secondary data [12,24]. The single-item measure cannot describe loneliness in multiple dimensions. Cognitive function measurement may not be sensitive to detecting different levels of cognitive performance. There may be other confounders or related factors that are not available. Fourth, only the individual characteristics were included in the analysis. The social environment factors across the districts were not analyzed. There were district area differences in LIL clusters. The environmental factors may need further investigation.

5. Conclusions

The combinations of loneliness, isolation and living alone exhibit different typologies of the social lifestyle of older adults. Older adults who live alone are not necessarily isolated; isolated older adults do not necessarily feel lonely; older adults living with family can still be isolated or feel lonely. The LIL typologies provide information about the social lifestyle of older adults.

Social contact and social support, especially a good relationship with the family, may be the key to preventing loneliness and isolation. Older adults living with family may still feel lonely, with needs unfulfilled by their family. Older adults who feel lonely should be made aware of ways to prevent the negative impact of depression. An appropriate quantity of social contact and the quality of social relationships are both important. Older adults are suggested to strengthen their informal social support (including support from friends and neighbors in the community) in case the family support is not enough, and the government may encourage social care provided in the community as extra social support.

The barrier due to difficulty in physical function may prohibit social interaction or participation, and cause loneliness or isolation. An age-friendly environment would help remove such barriers regarding mobility. The financial security issue may also cause loneliness or isolation. Financial security should be addressed by the government, and a security net for older people should be built. In addition, not all social participation can reduce loneliness or isolation. That implies that meaningful engagement or participation is more important than shallow social interactions.

Finally, the causal relationship of loneliness, isolation and living alone with psychological well-being should be further investigated by better measurement and longitudinal studies, and the nature of isolation and the corresponding solution should be developed by qualitative research in the future.

Acknowledgments: The data was provided by the City Government of Taipei City, Taiwan, R.O.C. The interpretation and conclusions contained herein do not represent those of Taipei City.

References

1. Courin, E.; Knapp, M. Social isolation, loneliness and health in old age: A scoping review. *Health Soc. Care Comm.* **2017**, *25*, 799–812. [CrossRef] [PubMed]

2. Leigh-Hunt, N.; Bagguley, D.; Bash, K.; Turner, V.; Turnbull, S.; Valtorta, N.; Caan, W. An overview of systematic reviews on the public health consequences of social isolation and loneliness. *Public Health* **2017**, *152*, 157–171. [CrossRef] [PubMed]
3. Holt-Lunstad, J.; Smith, T.B.; Baker, M.; Harrs, T.; Stephenon, D. Loneliness and social isolation as risk factors for mortality: A meta-analytic review. *Perspect. Psychol. Sci.* **2015**, *10*, 227–237. [CrossRef] [PubMed]
4. Weiss, R. *Loneliness: The Experience of Emotional and Social Isolation*; MIT Press: Cambridge, MA, USA, 1973.
5. Nicholson, N.R.; Feinn, R.; Casey, E.A.; Dixon, J. Psychometric evaluation of the social isolation scale in older adults. *Gerontologist* **2020**, *60*, e491–e501. [CrossRef]
6. Nicolson, M.R. A review of social isolation: An important but underassessed condition in older adults. *J. Prim. Prev.* **2012**, *33*, 137–152. [CrossRef]
7. Ong, A.D.; Uchino, B.N.; Wethington, E. Loneliness and health in older adults: A mini-review and synthesis. *Gerontology* **2016**, *62*, 443–449. [CrossRef]
8. Campagne, D.M. Stress and perceived social isolation (loneliness). *Arch. Gerontol. Geriatr.* **2019**, *82*, 192–199. [CrossRef]
9. Coyle, C.E.; Dugan, E. Social isolation, loneliness and health among older adults. *J. Aging Health* **2012**, *24*, 1346–1363. [CrossRef]
10. Dahlberg, L.; Agahi, N.; Lennartsson, C. Lonelier than ever? Loneliness of older people over two decades. *Arch. Gerontol. Geriatr.* **2018**, *75*, 96–103. [CrossRef]
11. Domènech-Abella, J.; Mundó, J.; Haro, J.M.; Rubio-Valera, M. Anxiety, depression, loneliness and social network in the elderly: Longitudinal associations from the Irish Longitudinal Study on Ageing (TILDA). *J. Affect. Disord.* **2019**, *246*, 82–88. [CrossRef]
12. Donovan, N.J.; Wu, Q.; Rentz, D.M.; Sperling, R.A.; Marshall, G.A.; Glymour, M.M. Loneliness, depression and cognitive function in older U.S., adults. *Int. J. Geriatr. Psychiatr.* **2016**, *32*, 564–573. [CrossRef] [PubMed]
13. Evans, I.E.M.; Llewellyn, D.J.; Matthews, F.E.; Woods, R.T.; Bryane, C.; Clare, L.; On Behalf of the CFAS-Wales Research Team. Living alone and cognitive function in later life. *Arch. Gerontol. Geriatr.* **2019**, *81*, 222–233. [CrossRef] [PubMed]
14. Feng, Z.; Jones, K.; Phillips, D.R. Social exclusion, self-rated health and depression among older people in China: Evidence from a national survey of older persons. *Arch. Gerontol. Geriatr.* **2019**, *82*, 238–244. [CrossRef] [PubMed]
15. Gale, C.R.; Westbury, L.; Cooper, C. Social isolation and loneliness as risk factors for the progression of frailty: The English Longitudinal Study of Ageing. *Age Ageing* **2018**, *47*, 392–397. [CrossRef]
16. Klein, J.; von dem Kneesebeck, O.; Lüdecke, D. Social inequalities and loneliness as predictors of ageing well: A trend analysis using mixed models. *Int. J. Environ. Health* **2020**, *17*, 5314. [CrossRef]
17. Morris, Z.A. Loneliness as a Predictor of Work Disability Onset among Nondisabled, Working Older Adults in 14 Countries. *J. Aging Health* **2019**, *32*, 554–563. [CrossRef]
18. Nummela, O.; Seppänen, M.; Uutela, A. The effect of loneliness and change in loneliness on self-rated health (SRH): A longitudinal study among aging people. *Arch. Gerontol. Geriatr.* **2011**, *53*, 163–167. [CrossRef]
19. Stickley, A.; Koyanagi, A.; Leisalu, M.; Ferlader, S.; Sabawoon, W.; McKee, M. Loneliness and health in Eastern Europe: Findings from Moscow, Russia. *Public Health* **2015**, *129*, 403–410. [CrossRef]
20. Luchetti, M.; Terracciano, A.; Aschwanden, D.; Lee, J.H.; Stephan, Y.; Sutin, A.R. Loneliness is associated with risk of cognitive impairment in the Survey of Health, Ageing and Retirement in Europe. *Int. J. Geriatr. Psychiatr.* **2020**, *35*, 794–801. [CrossRef]
21. Emerson, E.; Fortune, N.; Llewellyn, G.; Stancliffe, R. Loneliness, social support, social isolation, and wellbeing among working age adults with and without disability: Cross sectional study. *Disabil. Health J.* **2020**. [CrossRef]
22. Grande, G.; Vetrano, D.L.; Cova, I.; Pomati, S.; Mattavelli, D.; Maggiore, L.; Cucumo, V.; Ghiretti, R.; Vanacore, N.; Mariani, C.; et al. Living alone and dementia incidence: A clinical-based study in people with mild cognitive impairment. *J. Geriatr. Psychiatr. Neurol.* **2018**, *31*, 107–113. [CrossRef] [PubMed]
23. Kuiper, J.S.; Smidt, N.; Zuidema, S.U.; Comijs, H.C.; Voshaar, R.C.O.; Zuidersma, M. A longitudinal study of the impact of social network size and loneliness on cognitive performance in depressed older adults. *Aging Ment. Health* **2020**, *24*, 889–897. [CrossRef] [PubMed]

24. Yang, R.; Wang, H.; Edelman, L.S.; Tracy, E.L.; Demiris, G.; Sward, K.A.; Donaldson, G.W. Loneliness as a mediator of the impact of social isolation on cognitive functioning of Chinese older adults. *Age Ageing* **2020**, *49*, 599–604. [CrossRef] [PubMed]
25. Holwerda, T.J.; Deeg, D.J.H.; Beekman, A.T.F.; van Tilburg, T.G.; Stek, M.L.; Jonker, C.; Schoevers, R.A. Feeling of loneliness, but not social isolation, predict dementia onset: Results from the Amsterdam Study of the Elderly (AMSTEL). *J. Neurol. Neurosurg. Psychiatr.* **2014**, *85*, 135–142. [CrossRef] [PubMed]
26. Grover, S.; Avasthi, A.; Sahoo, S.; Lakdawala, B.; Dan, A.; Nebhinani, N.; Dutt, A.; Tiwari, S.C.; Gania, A.M.; Subramanyam, A.A.; et al. Relationship of loneliness and social connectedness with depression in elderly: A multicentric study under the aegis of Indian Association for Geriatric Mental Health. *J. Geriatr. Ment. Health* **2018**, *5*, 99–106. [CrossRef]
27. O'Súilleabháin, P.S.; Gallagher, S.; Steptoe, A. Loneliness, living alone, and all-cause mortality: The role of emotional and social loneliness in the elderly during 19 years of follow-up. *Psychosom. Med.* **2019**, *81*, 521–526. [CrossRef]
28. Park, N.S.; Jang, Y.; Lee, B.S.; Chiriboga, D.A. The relation between living alone and depressive symptoms in older Korean Americans: Do feelings of loneliness mediate? *Aging Ment. Health* **2015**, *21*, 304–312. [CrossRef]
29. Smith, K.J.; Victor, C. Typologies of loneliness, living alone and social isolation, and their associations with physical and mental health. *Ageing Soc.* **2019**, *39*, 1709–1730. [CrossRef]
30. Beller, J.; Wagner, A. Disentangling loneliness: Differential effects of subjective loneliness, network quality, network size, and living alone on physical, mental, and cognitive health. *J. Aging Health* **2017**, *30*, 521–539. [CrossRef]
31. Bucher, A.; Neubauer, A.B.; Voss, A.; Oetzbach, C. Together is better: Higher committed relationships increase life satisfaction and reduce loneliness. *J. Happiness Stud.* **2019**, *20*, 2445–2469. [CrossRef]
32. Chou, K.L.; Cacioppo, J.T.; Kumari, J.; Song, Y.Q. Influence of social environment on loneliness in older adults: Moderation by polymorphism in the CRHR1. *Am. J. Geriatr. Psychiatr.* **2014**, *22*, 510–518. [CrossRef]
33. Aylaz, R.; Aktük, Ü.; Erci, B.; Öztürk, H.; Aslan, H. Relationship between depression and loneliness in elderly and examination of influential factors. *Arch. Gerontol. Geriatr.* **2012**, *55*, 548–554. [CrossRef]
34. Sacker, A.; Ross, A.; MacLeod, C.A.; Netuveli, G.; Windle, G. Health and social exclusion in older age: Evidence from understanding society, the UK household longitudinal study. *J. Epidemiol. Community Health* **2016**, *71*, 681–690. [CrossRef]
35. Shin, O.; Park, S.; Amano, T.; Kwon, E.; Kim, B.R. Nature of retirement and loneliness: The moderating roles of social support. *J. Appl. Gerontol.* **2019**. [CrossRef] [PubMed]
36. Santini, Z.I.; Fiori, K.L.; Feeney, J.; Tyrovolas, S.; Haro, J.M.; Koyanagi, A. Social relationship, loneliness and mental health among older men and women in Ireland: A prospective community-based study. *J. Affect. Disord.* **2016**, *204*, 59–69. [CrossRef] [PubMed]
37. Jarvis, M.A.; Padmanabhanunni, A.; Chipps, J. An evaluation of a low-intensity cognitive behavioral therapy mHealth-supported intervention to reduce loneliness in older people. *Int. J. Environ. Res. Public Health* **2019**, *16*, 1305. [CrossRef] [PubMed]
38. Yu, K.; Wu, S.; Chi, I. Internet use and loneliness of older adults over time: The mediating effect of social contact. *J. Gerontol. B Psychol. Sci. Soc. Sci.* **2020**, gbaa004. [CrossRef] [PubMed]
39. Tagahi, E.; Saito, Y.; Chan, A. Gender differences in the association between social relationships and loneliness among older adults in Singapore. *J. Popul. Res.* **2020**, *37*, 243–263. [CrossRef]
40. Hoffman, Y.S.G.; Grossman, E.S.; Bergman, Y.S.; Bodner, E. The link between social anxiety and intimate loneliness is stronger for older adults than for younger adults. *Aging Ment. Health* **2020**. [CrossRef]
41. Power, J.M.; Hannigan, C.; Hyland, P.; Brennan, S.; Kee, F.; Lawlor, B.A. Depressive symptoms predict increased social and emotional loneliness in older adults. *Aging Ment. Health* **2020**, *24*, 110–118. [CrossRef]
42. Yang, F.; Gyu, D. Predictors of loneliness incidence in Chinese older adults from a life course perspective: A national longitudinal study. *Aging Ment. Health* **2020**, *24*, 879–888. [CrossRef] [PubMed]
43. Domènech-Abella, J.; Mundó, J.; Leonardi, M.; Chatteriji, S.; Tobiasz-Adamczyk, B.; Koskinen, S.; Ayuso-Mateos, J.L.; Haro, J.M.; Olaya, B. Loneliness and depression among older European adults: The ole of perceived neighbourhood built environment. *Health Place* **2020**, *62*, 102280. [CrossRef] [PubMed]

44. Tilvis, R.S.; Routsalo, P.; Karppinen, H.; Strandberg, T.E.; Kautiainen, H.; Pitkala, K.H. Social isolation, social activity and loneliness as survival indicators in old age: A nationwide survey with a 7-year follow-up. *Eur. Geriatr. Med.* **2012**, *3*, 18–22. [CrossRef]
45. Zhao, M.; Gao, J.; Li, M.; Wang, K. Relationship between loneliness and frailty among older adults in nursing homes: The mediating role of activity engagement. *JAMDA* **2018**, *20*, 759–764. [CrossRef] [PubMed]
46. Jiang, D.; Hou, Y.; Hao, J.; Zhou, J.; Jiang, J.; Wang, Q. Association between personal social capital and loneliness among widowed older people. *Int. J. Environ. Health* **2020**, *17*, 5799. [CrossRef] [PubMed]
47. Cohen, A.B.; Johnson, K.A. The relation between religion and well-being. *Appl. Res. Qual. Life* **2017**, *12*, 533–547. [CrossRef]
48. Malone, J.; Dadswell, A. The role of religion, spirituality and/or belief in positive ageing for older adults. *Geriatrics* **2018**, *3*, 28. [CrossRef]
49. Bergefurt, L.; Kemperman, A.; van den Berg, P.; Borgers, A.; van der Waerden, P.; Oosterhuis, G.; Hommel, M. Loneliness and life satisfaction explained by public-space use and mobility patterns. *Int. J. Environ. Res. Public Health* **2019**, *16*, 4282. [CrossRef]
50. Liao, M.Y.; Yeh, C.J.; Lee, S.H.; Lioa, C.C.; Lee, M.C. Association of providing/receiving support on the mortality of older adults with different living arrangements in Taiwan: A longitudinal study on ageing. *Ageing Soc.* **2018**, *38*, 2082–2096. [CrossRef]
51. Morgan, T.; Wiles, J.; Moeke-Maxwell, T.; Black, S.; Park, H.J.; Dewes, O.; Williams, L.A.; Gott, M. 'People haven't got that close connection': Meanings of loneliness and social isolation to culturally diverse older people. *Aging Ment. Health* **2020**, *24*, 1627–1635. [CrossRef]
52. World Health Organization. *Global Age-Friendly Cities: A Guide*; World Health Organization: Geneva, Switzerland, 2007.
53. Au, A.; Lai, D.W.L.; Yip, H.M.; Chan, S.; Lai, S.; Chaudhury, H.; Scharlach, A.; Leeson, G. Sense of community mediating between age-friendly characteristics and life satisfaction of community-dwelling older adults. *Front. Psychol.* **2020**, *11*, 86. [CrossRef] [PubMed]
54. Hsu, H.C. Associations of City-Level Active Aging and Age Friendliness with Well-Being among Older Adults Aged 55 and over in Taiwan. *Int. J. Environ. Res. Public Health* **2020**, *17*, 4304. [CrossRef] [PubMed]
55. Radloff, L.S. The CES-D scale: A self-report depression scale for research in the general population. *Appl. Psychol. Meas.* **1977**, *1*, 385–401. [CrossRef]
56. Pfeiffer, E. Short Portable Mental Status Questionnaire for the assessment of organic brain deficit in elderly patients. *J. Am. Geriatr. Soc.* **1975**, *23*, 433–441. [CrossRef]
57. Chung, S.; Jeon, H.; Song, A.; Kim, J.H. Developmental trajectories and predictors of social exclusion among older Koreans: Exploring the multidimentional nature of social exclusion. *Soc. Ind. Res.* **2019**, *144*, 97–112. [CrossRef]
58. European Commission (EC); United Nations Economic Commission for Europe (UNECE). Active Aging Group. In *Active Ageing Index (AAI): Concept, Methodology and Final Results*; UNECE Grant No: ECE/GC/2012/003; UNECE: Vienna, Austria, 2013.
59. Hershey, D.A.; Henkens, K.; van Dalen, H.P. What drives retirement income worries in Europe? A multilevel analysis. *Eur. J. Aging* **2010**, *7*, 301–311. [CrossRef]

3

Dietary Patterns and their Association with Anxiety Symptoms among Older Adults: The ATTICA Study

Maria F. Masana [1,2,3], Stefanos Tyrovolas [1,2,4,*], Natasa Kollia [4], Christina Chrysohoou [5], John Skoumas [5], Josep Maria Haro [1,2], Dimitrios Tousoulis [5], Charalambos Papageorgiou [6], Christos Pitsavos [5] and Demosthenes B. Panagiotakos [4]

1 Parc Sanitari Sant Joan de Déu, Universitat de Barcelona, Fundació Sant Joan de Déu, 08007 Barcelona, Spain; mfmasana@gmail.com (M.F.M.); jmharo@pssjd.org (J.M.H.)
2 Instituto de Salud Carlos III, Centro de Investigación Biomédica en Red de Salud Mental, CIBERSAM, Monforte de Lemos 3-5, Pabellón 11, 28029 Madrid, Spain
3 Facultat de Medicina, Universitat de Barcelona, Casanova, 143, 08036 Barcelona, Spain
4 Department of Science of Dietetics and Nutrition, School of Health Science and Education, Harokopio University, 17671 Athens, Greece; natkollia@yahoo.gr (N.K.); dbpanag@hua.gr (D.B.P.)
5 First Cardiology Clinic, School of Medicine, University of Athens, 15772 Athens, Greece; chrysohoou@usa.net (C.C.); skoumasj@gmail.com (J.S.); tousouli@med.uoa.gr (D.T.); cpitsavo@med.uoa.gr (C.P.)
6 First Psychiatry Clinic, School of Medicine, University of Athens, 15772 Athens, Greece; cpapage@eginitio.uoa.gr
* Correspondence: s.tyrovolas@pssjd.org

Abstract: By 2050, the global population aged 60 years and over is expected to reach nearly 2.1 billion and affective disorders might be also expected to increase. Although nutrition has been related with affective disorders, there is a lack of studies assessing the relation between dietary habits and anxiety among European and Mediterranean older populations. In the present study, we aimed to evaluate the association between dietary habits, energy intake, and anxiety symptoms using data from 1128 Greek older adults (>50 years) without pre-existing cardiovascular disease (CVD) or any other chronic disease who participated in the ATTICA study. Various socio demographic lifestyle, bio-clinical (e.g., blood pressure), and psychological (e.g., depression) characteristics were used, and dietary habits as well as energy intake were calculated using standard procedures. Older people with anxiety were more likely to be sedentary, to be smokers, and to show symptoms of depression. The saturated fat and added sugars (SFAS) dietary pattern was associated with higher anxiety levels (non-standardized b (95% CI): 5.82 (0.03 to 11.61)). No association between energy intake tertiles and anxiety levels pictured in the later regression model. Moreover, female gender, family status, and depression were positively related to anxiety. Therefore, promoting healthy dietary habits could reduce anxiety symptoms of the older adults.

Keywords: snack; sugars; carbohydrate; energy intake; anxiety; older adults; Attica study; Greece

1. Introduction

The global population aged 60 years or over is expected to reach nearly 2.1 billion by 2050 due to reductions in fertility and a rise in life expectancy [1] resulting in an increased risk for non-communicable diseases such as cancer, dementia, and affective disorders (anxiety and depression). Particularly, affective disorders might be expected to be increased because older people living alone is continuously rising as a consequence of changes in societies, such as falling family size, family structure and less multigenerational living arrangements [2].

The estimated global prevalence for anxiety disorders was 7.3% (95% CI 4.8–10.9%) and considering socioeconomic factors and culture, the prevalence ranged from 5.3% (3.5–8.1%) to 10.4% (7.0–15.5%) in African and Euro/Anglo cultures, respectively [3]. However, anxiety disorders are frequently under-recognized and misdiagnosed. Consequently, individuals with an undiagnosed or misdiagnosed anxiety disorder may not receive the appropriate treatment, suffering a deterioration of quality of life and social ability [4]. Several risk factors have been related to anxiety, but the emergence of a health and social crisis due to the financial crisis and strict fiscal austerity in Europe (e.g., Greece, Portugal, and Spain) could have contributed to worsen mental health [5]. For instance, in Greece, worse health status was reported in older adults due to unhealthy changes in their lifestyle behaviours [6] and anxiety disorders were also reported to be the fourth cause of years lost due to disability (YLDs) [7].

Depression has shown to be the most common comorbid disorder with anxiety disorders [8], but a bidirectional prospective relationship with one another was also reported [9]. Although the relationship between anxiety and cognition remains unclear, some studies have shown that anxiety was associated with cognitive decline, specifically on spatial and verbal working memory [10], influencing positively in the progression of Mild Cognitive Impairment (MCI) to dementia [11,12]. Some other chronic diseases, such as gastrointestinal disorders (e.g., irritable bowel syndrome) [13], diabetes [14] and thyroid disorders [15] have been also related to anxiety disorders or/and elevated anxiety symptoms. Moreover, patients with cardiovascular disease (CVD) are more likely to show prevalent anxiety disorders compared to the general population, but anxiety disorders have been also reported to increase the CVD risk [16]. For instance, anxiety levels were directly associated with the 10 y CVD incidence (OR (95%CI): 1.03 (1.0–1.1)) in older Greek adults without previous CVD history [17]. Some common pathophysiological mechanisms seem to share anxiety and the interrelated comorbidities, such as increase of corticotropin-releasing factor (CRF) levels, dysregulation of the hypothalamic-pituitary-adrenal (HPA) axis [18], activation of the sympathetic nervous system, and increase of levels of proinflammatory cytokines [19,20].

In recent years, an increasing number of studies are providing evidence for diet as a modifiable risk factor for mental health problems, such as depression and anxiety, however there is a lack of data regarding the older adults, a vulnerable population subgroup that appears to have high prevalence of mental disorders. For instance, a dietary pattern characterized by consumption of vegetables, fruit, beef, lamb, fish, and whole-grain foods has been related to a lower risk of a diagnosis of anxiety, while a western dietary pattern characterized by consumption of foods such as meats and sugar has been associated with more psychiatric symptoms [21]. Later studies also found that an inadequate and poor diet quality (i.e., snack patterns, animal foods) [22] and high intake of alcohol [23] can contribute to an inadequate intake of nutrients leading to mental health problems.

To date, there is a lack of studies assessing the association between dietary habits, energy intake, and anxiety symptoms among older adults and specifically, among European and Mediterranean older populations. Therefore, the aim of the current study was to evaluate the relation between dietary patterns, energy intake, and anxiety in a sample of older people (50+ years old) living in the Attica region.

2. Methods

2.1. Study Population

In brief, ATTICA is a prospective, population-based, cohort study performed in Attica (Athens metropolitan region, Greece), which recruited 3042 non-institutionalized adults (Caucasians; women/men: 1528/1514; age: ≥18 years) without previous CVD. The enrolment of the participants was carried out during 2001–2002, and after that, two follow-up waves followed 5 (in 2006) and 10 years (in 2012) later. Random, multistage sampling based on the age and gender distribution of the reference population, as defined by the Hellenic National Statistical Service Census Survey of 2001, was applied. Sampling procedures anticipated enrolling only one participant per household, while institutionalized individuals were excluded from study participation. All participants underwent detailed baseline assessments which included medical history, physical examination, and blood sampling for biochemical measurements. Baseline CVD was excluded in all participants by the study physicians [24]. For the purposes of the present work, only baseline data for the study's sample of over 50 years old (i.e., $n = 1128$) men and women were used (there was no psychological assessment at follow-up examinations).

2.2. Sociodemographic and Life-Style Variables

The study questionnaire included demographic information such as age, gender, family status (married, divorced, widowed), financial status, and education level. The level of education (as a proxy of social status) was determined by years of schooling and classified into 3 groups: (1) <9 years; (2) up to high school or technical college (10–14 years); (3) university. Mean annual income during the past 3 years was also recorded.

Current smokers were defined as those who smoked at least one cigarette/day, never smokers as those who had never tried a cigarette in their life, and former smokers as those who had stopped smoking for at least one year. Occasional smokers (7 cigarettes/week) were recorded and combined with current smokers because of their small sample size. In order to evaluate more accurately the smoking habits, we calculated the pack-years (cigarette packs/day × years of smoking), adjusted for a nicotine content of 0.8 mg/cigarette.

The physical activity level of each participant was also assessed at baseline using the International Physical Activity Questionnaire (IPAQ; participants reporting no physical activities or exercise on the IPAQ were classified as physically inactive) [25].

2.3. Clinical and Biochemical Assessments

Standardized measurements of anthropometric parameters were performed by trained study researchers, including body weight and height, BMI (kg/m^2), and WC (cm). Resting arterial blood pressure (BP, average of 3 recordings in sitting position) was also measured, and participants exhibiting average BP ≥ 140/90 mmHg or taking antihypertensive medication(s) were categorized as hypertensive.

At baseline, fasting blood samples were obtained from all participants after overnight fasting. Triglyceride (TG), total cholesterol (TC) and high-density lipoprotein-cholesterol (HDL-C) levels were measured by a chromatographic enzymatic method using a Technicon automatic analyzer RA-1000 (Dade Behring, Marburg, Germany; corresponding intra- and inter-assay coefficients of variation (CV) were <4%, <9%, and <4%, respectively). Low-density lipoprotein-cholesterol (LDL-C) was calculated by the Friedewald formula [26]. Hypercholesterolemia was defined as TC > 200 mg/dL or treatment with lipid-lowering drug(s). Moreover, fasting blood glucose (FBG) levels were measured by a Beckman glucose analyzer (Beckman Instruments, Fullerton, CA, USA) and subjects with FBG >125 mg/dL or on antidiabetic treatment were classified as having diabetes.

2.4. Dietary Assessment

All participants underwent a detailed baseline dietary evaluation through the EPIC-Greek questionnaire [27], which is a validated semi-quantitative food-frequency questionnaire that was kindly provided by the Unit of Nutrition of Athens Medical School. The energy intake in kcal/day was also calculated based on the participants' responses in this questionnaire. Energy intake tertiles were also created, those in the 1st energy tertile were the participants consuming <1840 kcals/day.

All participants were asked to report the average intake (per week or day) of several food items that they consumed (during the last 12 months). Then, the frequency of consumption was quantified approximately in terms of the number of times a month this food was consumed. Thus, daily consumption multiplied by 30 and weekly consumption multiplied by 4 and a value of 0 was assigned to food items rarely or never consumed. Alcohol consumption was measured in wineglasses

(100 ml) and quantified by ethanol intake (grams per drink). One wineglass was considered equal to 12% ethanol concentration.

A dietary pyramid was developed to describe the Mediterranean dietary pattern [28]. This dietary pattern consist of: (a) daily consumption of non-refined cereals and products (whole grain bread, pasta, brown rice, etc.), vegetables (2–3 servings/day), fruits (6 servings/day), olive oil (as the main added lipid) and dairy products (1–2 servings/day); (b) weekly consumption of fish (4–5 servings/week), poultry (3–4 servings/week), olives, pulses, and nuts (3 servings/week), potatoes, eggs and sweets (3–4 servings/week) and monthly consumption of red meat and meat products (4–5 servings/month). The Mediterranean diet (MedDiet) is also characterized by moderate consumption of wine (1–2 wineglasses/day) and high monounsaturated to saturated fat ratio (>2).

A special diet score that assessed adherence to MedDiet was calculated. In particular, we assigned a score of 0 for rare or no consumption of food items that are close to this dietary pattern, 1 for 1 to 4 times/month, 2 for 5 to 8 times/month, 3 for 9 to 12 times/month, 4 for 13 to 18 times/month and 5 for almost daily consumption. On the other hand, for the consumption of foods that are away from this traditional diet, like meat and meat products, we assigned the opposite scores (i.e. 0 for almost daily consumption to 5 for rare or no consumption). For alcohol, we assigned a score of 5 for consumption of less than 3 wineglasses per day, a score of 0 for consumption of more than 7 wineglasses/day and scores of 1 to 4 for consumption of 3, 4–5, 6 and 7 wine glasses per day.

The calculation of the dietary inflammatory load of the participants' diet was according to the methodology and the rationale of the Dietary Inflammation Index (DII) that has been previously proposed by Shivappa and colleagues [29]. Thus, a Dietary Anti-Inflammation Index (D-AII) was developed based on participants' dietary habits. Detailed information on the D-AII has been reported in a previous ATTICA publication, by Georgousopoulou et al [30].

Aside from the classic indexes of MedDiet and D-AII, additional dietary patterns were defined for the daily dietary intake of the participants. Three main components were extracted using the principal components (PC) methods (Table 1). These were: (A) The lacto-fish-vegetarian (LFV) dietary pattern including the food components of vegetables, cereals, fruits, legumes, fish, and dairy products; (B) The meat-eaters dietary pattern including food components of all kinds of meat, read meat, and poultry; (C) The saturated fat and added sugars (SFAS) dietary pattern including the food components of sweets, soft drinks, nuts, and potatoes.

2.5. *Psychological Assessments*

Anxiety levels were assessed using the validated Greek translation of the 20 item, self-report State-Trait Anxiety Inventory (STAI) [31], the total score of which ranges from 20 to 80. Higher scores in this scale are indicative of more severe anxiety, and according to Spielberger's criteria, a score of 40 or higher reflects clinically relevant symptoms of anxiety.

Depressive symptomatology was assessed using a translated and validated version of the Zung Self-Rating Depression Scale (ZDRS) [32]. The ZDRS consists of 20 items that cover affective, psychological, and somatic symptoms, and ranges from 20 to 80. A subject with a ZDRS score below 50 is considered normal but with a score of 50 to 59, 60 to 69, or 70 or above is considered to suffer from mild, moderate, or severe depression, respectively.

Cognitive distortion symptomatology was assessed using a validated version of the cognitive distortions scale (CDS) [33]. This tool captures cognitive symptoms or distortions among individuals who have experienced inter-personal victimization: self-criticism, self-blame, helplessness, hopelessness, and preoccupation with danger.

2.6. *Bioethics*

The ATTICA study was approved by our institutional ethics committee and conformed to the ethical guidelines of the 1975 declaration of Helsinki. All participants were informed about the study protocol, and they provided written signed consent.

2.7. Statistical Analysis

To define the dietary patterns, factor analysis using the PC was applied [34]. Principal components were retained if their eigenvalues were greater than 1.0, a threshold that is commonly used as a cut-off to identify meaningful patterns. The resulting components were interpreted based on the variables with loadings above 0.3. Moreover, the Kaiser-Meyer-Olkin criterion was used as a measure of variables (components) inter-correlation and used as an indicator of internal consistency.

Normally distributed continuous variables are presented as mean values ± SD, and categorical variables as frequencies. Normality was tested using the Shapiro-Wilk criterion; the non-normally distributed variables are presented as median and 1st, 3rd tertile. Associations between categorical variables were tested by the chi-square test, whereas between continuous variables by the Pearson r or Spearman's rho coefficients for normally distributed and skewed variables, respectively. Continuous variables were tested for normality via P-P plots. For normally distributed variables, comparisons were performed by the student's t-test, after controlling for equality of variances by the Levene's test. For continuous variables without normal distribution, comparisons were performed by the non-parametric Mann-Whitney U-test. Previous literature was used as a guide for the selection of variables used for adjustment between dietary patterns and anxiety [35–37]. Multiple linear regression analyses were performed in order to evaluate the association between anxiety as the dependent outcome and a participant´s adherence to dietary patterns, adjusted for multiple confounders. All p-values are based on two-sided tests. Statistical analyses were performed with the Statistical Package for Social Sciences version 22 (SPSS Inc., Chicago, IL, USA).

3. Results

In Table 1 the component loadings and the eigenvalues from the factor analysis are presented. The size of eigenvalues strongly suggests the formation of three distinct dietary patterns, explaining 51.78% of the total variance of the information. The first dietary pattern could be characterized as the "lacto-fish-vegetarian", the second as the "meat-eaters" and the third as the "saturated fat and added sugars".

Table 1. Factor loadings of the food components included in the extracted dietary patterns.

Food Components	LFV Dietary Pattern	Meat-Eaters Dietary Pattern	SFAS Dietary Pattern
Vegetables	0.756	–	–
Fruit	0.653	–	–
Cereals	0.622	–	–
Legumes	0.609	–	–
Fish	0.579	–	–
Dairy Products	0.435	–	–
Total Meat	–	0.941	–
Red Meat	–	0.828	–
Poultry	–	0.708	–
Sweets	–	–	0.675
Soft Drinks	–	–	0.649
Nuts	–	–	0.648
Potatoes	–	–	0.523
Cumulative Variance explained (%)	25.675	41.609	51.788

Abbreviations: LFV, lacto-fish-vegetarian; and, SFAS, saturated fat and added sugars. In each factor only the components with values > 0.30 are included in the table.

The sociodemographic, lifestyle, and clinical characteristics of participants are presented by anxiety status in Table 2. Compared to the participants without anxiety, those with anxiety were more likely to be sedentary ($p = 0.001$), smokers ($p = 0.027$), and suffered depressive symptoms ($p < 0.001$). The rest of measured variables (i.e., age, gender, education, income, family status, diet, energy intake, BMI, hypertension, diabetes, hypercholesterolemia, and cognitive distortion) were not significantly associated with the level of anxiety.

Table 2. Baseline characteristics of the study sample 50+ years old, by anxiety status.

Characteristic	Total	No Anxiety	Anxiety	*p*
Sample size (*n*)	758	149	609	
Age (Mean ± SD)	59.67 ± 8.28	54.11 ± 4.31	54.68 ± 3.39	0.372
Sex				0.286
Female	41.6	37.3	45.9	
Male	58.4	62.7	54.1	
Education status (years of school) (Mean ± SD)	10.53 ± 3.96	12.43 ± 3.65	11.36 ± 4.15	0.100
Financial status (%)				0.151
Bad	12.8	8.0	17.6	
Poor	17.4	18.7	16.2	
Good	47.7	45.3	50.0	
Very good	22.1	28.0	16.2	
Family status (%)				0.580
Never married	10.7	10.7	10.08	
Married	78.5	80.0	77.0	
Divorced	7.4	8.0	6.8	
Widowed	3.4	1.3	5.4	
Current smoking (%)	46.3	37.3	55.4	0.027
Physically active (%)				0.001
Sedentary	52.3	38.7	66.2	
Physically active	47.7	61.3	33.8	
MedDiet (0–55)	23.02 ± 6.17	24.27 ± 5.25	24.03 ± 6.36	0.808
SFAS dietary pattern (Mean ± SD)	−0.32 ± 0.86	−0.189 ± 0.756	−0.33 ± 0.81	0.337
Meat-eaters dietary pattern (Mean ± SD)	−0.24 ± 0.76	−0.35 ± 0.55	−0.22 ± 0.77	0.294
LFV dietary pattern (Mean ± SD)	0.25 ± 0.98	0.29 ± 0.89	0.146 ± 1.09	0.434
Energy intake (kcal/day)	2409.38 ± 1019.19	2120.10 ± 693.15	2048.51 ± 855.46	0.617
D-AII (10–77)	32.61 ± 6.34	32.81 ± 6.04	32.44 ± 6.62	0.72
BMI (kg/m^2)	27.60 ± 4.25	26.87 ± 4.11	26.48 ± 3.29	0.532
Waist circumference (cm)	94.64 ± 18.87	95.58 ± 21.12	93.70 ± 16.70	0.57
Hypertension (%)	45.9	43.1	48.6	0.498
Diabetes (%)	10.1	8.0	12.2	0.399
Hypercholesterolemia (%)	51.0	46.7	55.4	0.286
Zung score (Mean ± SD)	35.17 ± 7.57	31.65 ± 6.30	38.54 ± 6.88	<0.001
Cognitive distortion score (Mean ± SD)	17.84 ± 24.35	11.36 ± 15.11	24.48 ± 30.35	0.073

Abbreviations: MedDiet, mediterranean diet; BMI, body mass index; LFV, lacto-fish-vegetarian; SFAS, saturated fat and added Sugars; diet anti-inflammatory index (D-AII).

As a first step, results of multi-adjusted analysis assessing the energy intake by tertiles on anxiety levels are presented in Table 3, without adjusting for dietary patterns. Initially the association between energy intake (kcals/day) as a continuous variable and anxiety levels was tested. Based on this analysis, it was observed that the higher levels of energy intake were positively related with higher anxiety levels (non-standardized b (95% CI): 0.01 (0.003 to 0.2)), after various adjustments (i.e., sex, smoking habits, physical activity, etc.) (data shown only in text). When the analysis was applied by energy intake tertiles, it was shown that the 1st energy intake tertile had an independent inverse association with anxiety levels as compared with the highest one (3rd tertile) (non-standardized b (95% CI): −11.65 (−22.83 to −0.48), $p = 0.04$). The 2nd energy intake tertile as compared with the 3rd tertile, was no related with anxiety levels (non-standardized b (95% CI): −7.61 (−18.55 to 3.34), $p = 0.16$). In addition, female gender (non-standardized b (95% CI): 11.96 (0.53 to 23.38), $p = 0.04$), family status (non-standardized b (95% CI): 18.17 (4.56 to 31.77), $p = 0.012$), and depression (non-standardized b (95% CI): 1.07 (0.27 to 1.87), $p = 0.01$) were positively related to higher anxiety levels. Cognitive distortion (non-standardized b (95% CI): 0.20 (0.09 to 0.32), $p = 0.001$) was also observed to be associated with the presence of anxiety symptoms, while physical activity was inversely related with anxiety levels (non-standardized b (95% CI): −8.58 (−15.90 to −1.25), $p = 0.02$). Finally, the results remained similar when basic metabolic rate was inserted as a confounding variable in the model.

Table 3. Correlates of anxiety among adults aged ≥ 50 years estimated by multivariable linear regression, in the ATTICA study, $n = 758$.

Variable	Non-Standardized b	95% CI
Female vs. male sex	11.96 *	0.53, 23.38
Education status (per 1 year)	0.87	−0.10, 1.85
Family status (married vs. other status)	18.17 *	4.56, 31.77
Financial status (high vs. low-medium)	−9.66 *	−19.32, −0.002
Physical activity (active vs. sedentary)	−8.58 *	−15.90, −1.25
Current smoking (yes vs. no)	−1.50	−9.40, 6.41
Energy intake (kcals)		
1st vs. 3rd tertile	−11.65 *	−22.83, −0.48
2nd vs. 3rd tertile	−7.61	−18.55, 3.34
BMI (per 1 kg/m^2)	0.91	−0.24, 2.06
Hypertension (yes vs. no)	1.68	−5.31, 8.68
Diabetes (yes vs. no)	1.88	−22.32, 26.09
Hypercholesterolemia (yes vs. no)	1.95	−5.16, 9.06
Depression (Zung scale)	1.07 *	0.27, 1.87
Cognitive distortion scale	0.20 **	0.09, 0.32

Data are presented as non-standardized coefficients (b) and their 95% confidence intervals (CIs). * $p < 0.05$, ** $p < 0.01$. Abbreviations: BMI, body mass index. Model is adjusted for all the covariates in the table.

As a next step, Table 4 illustrates the results from multiple linear regression analysis that evaluated the association between dietary patterns, energy intake and anxiety (models I and II). After adjusting for sociodemographic, lifestyle and clinical characteristics, as in Table 3, plus for confounding due to obesity, central obesity (waist circumference), and energy intake, the dietary pattern characterized by the consumption of saturated fats and added sugars (SFAS dietary pattern) was consistently associated with higher anxiety levels (non-standardized b (95% CI): 5.82 (0.03 to 11.61), $p = 0.04$) (Model II). Moreover, anxiety was positively associated with female gender (non-standardized b (95% CI): 21.06 (3.19 to 38.94), $p = 0.02$), and family status (non-standardized b (95% CI): 19.83 (2.47 to 37.19), $p = 0.02$). In addition, depressive symptomatology was related with higher level of anxiety (non-standardized b (95% CI): 1.88 (0.48 to 3.28), $p = 0.01$). Finally, LFV dietary pattern as well as meat-eaters and SFAS dietary patterns were replaced with the D-AII, a dietary index that is picturing pro- and anti-inflammatory dietary habits. In this additional analysis, there was not association between the D-AII and the anxiety levels ($p = 0.94$) (data shown only in text).

Table 4. Correlates of anxiety among adults aged ≥ 50 years estimated by additive multivariable linear regression (Model I and Model II), in the ATTICA study, $n = 758$.

Variable	Model I		Model II	
	Non-Standardized b	95% CI	Non-Standardized b	95% CI
Female vs. male sex	21.77	7.25, 36.28	21.06	3.19, 38.94
Education status (per 1 year)	1.92	0.29, 3.56	1.78	−0.07, 3.65
Family status (married vs. other status)	20.72	4.81, 36.63	19.83	2.47, 37.19
Financial status (high vs. low-medium)	−9.33	−19.61, 0.95	−9.84	−21.22, 1.53
Physical activity (active vs. sedentary)	−4.32	−13.35, 4.69	−4.00	−14.42, 6.41
Current smoking (yes vs. no)	−3.54	−12.30, 5.21	−2.42	−12.50, 7.66
LFV dietary pattern	−1.96	−9.05, 5.12	−1.20	−9.29, 6.88
Meat-eaters dietary pattern	3.41	−3.80, 10.62	3.33	−4.92, 11.59
SFAS dietary pattern	5.62	1.21, 10.02	5.82	0.03, 11,61
Obesity (yes vs. no)	19.22	0.51, 37.94	18.00	−4.52, 40.54
Waist circumference (cm)	−0.17	−0.45, 0.12	−0.16	−0.51, 0.18
Hypertension (yes vs. no)	5.70	−2.47, 13.87	5.17	−3.73, 14.08
Diabetes (yes vs. no)	−1.36	−26.13, 23.39	1.71	−26.53, 29.96

Table 4. *Cont.*

Variable	Model I		Model II	
	Non-Standardized b	95% CI	Non-Standardized b	95% CI
Hypercholesterolemia (yes vs. no)	1.96	−5.60, 9.54	2.67	−6.04, 11.40
Depression (Zung scale)	1.97	0.76, 3.17	1.88	0.48, 3.28
Cognitive distortion scale	0.14	−0.04, 0.37	0.16	−0.07, 0.39
Energy intake (kcals)	–	–		
1st vs. 3rd tertile	–	–	−0.48	−18.98, 18.02
2nd vs. 3rd tertile	–	–	−2.97	−16.80, 10.86

Data are presented as non-standardized coefficients (b) and their 95% confidence intervals (CIs). Abbreviations: LFV, lacto-fish-vegetarian; SFAS, saturated fat and added sugars. Model I and Model II are adjusted for all the respective covariates in the table.

4. Discussion

While anxiety is multi-factorial and mostly related with psychological, social and biological aspects [38], little is known about the contribution of holistic dietary patterns as preventive means of anxiety in older populations. Through factor analysis, three distinct dietary patterns were pictured (the LFV, the meat-eaters and the SFAS dietary patterns) among the older adults (50+ years old) of the ATTICA study. The present study reported that at an initial step, energy intake was related with anxiety levels among older adults. However, when the abovementioned dietary patterns were inserted in the analysis, it was reported that the SFAS dietary pattern was associated with higher levels of anxiety among older adults, while energy intake was no longer significant. Notably, this relation was independent of well-established risk factors such as depression, physical activity, and cognitive distortion. To the best of our knowledge, this is among the first studies to evaluate the association between dietary patterns, energy intake, and anxiety levels using a non-CVD, European, older population. These results point to the importance of specific dietary patterns in relation with anxiety and the public health actions needed to be taken with western older populations in which the burden of cognitive and mental disorders is increasing at alarming rates.

Older participants with anxiety from the Attica region in Greece were more likely to be smokers, sedentary and presented depressive symptoms, and this results are in agreement with the results of studies found in the literature. In particular, systematic reviews have reported that smoking [39] and depression [9] might be risk factors for the development of anxiety, but a bidirectional relationship has also been observed. Moreover, previous studies have suggested that a sedentary behavior (i.e., sitting time and screen time) is related to an increased risk for anxiety [40], and higher levels of anxiety were associated with increased diabetes risk among women but not among men [41].

Multi-adjusting analysis revealed an association between socio-economic and lifestyle factors and mental health problems with anxiety levels in older adults. In previous studies, associations between socio-economic and lifestyle factors have also reported. For instance, women with anxiety have reported lower socioeconomic status and income compared to men [42], and other risk factors such as stressful life events, chronic diseases, physical inactivity, depression, insomnia, and lower cognitive function have also been related to anxiety [43]. Regular physical activity has been related to reduced anxiety due to its impact on some pathological mechanisms, such as modulation of HPA and an increase of brain-derived neurotrophic factor (BDNF) levels and β-endorphins [44]. Smoking have been reported to activate the HPA axis increasing adrenocorticotropic hormone (ACTH) and cortisol [45], which have been related with anxiety [46]. However, in our fully adjusted regression analysis, physical activity, financial status and smoking habits did not remain significant. Anxiety has been also related to worse performance in some cognitive domains, such as spatial and verbal working memory [10], and bidirectional associations between anxiety symptomology and processing speed and attention have also reported in older adults [47]. Literature suggests that anxiety is highly comorbid with depression due to the overlap of symptomatology of both disorders increasing its severity and chronicity, and consequently, a worsening in the quality of life [48], but an inverse relationship between anxiety and reduced cognitive function have been also observed and explained by comorbid depression in non-demented elderly general population [49]. Therefore, older adults with healthy habits such as regular physical activity, healthy sleeping routine, and no smoking could contribute to maintain a good mental health reducing affective disorders, and consequently, reducing the deterioration of cognitive function.

Dietary habits are usually estimated using PC analysis and are reflecting the real behavior of the population [50]. To date various dietary patterns have been identified among older populations. Healthy dietary patterns (i.e., higher consumption of vegetables, fruits, poultry and fish), have been related with better quality of life, self-reported health, lower burden of morbidity as well as higher survival among the older adults [51,52]. However, until today, research on the effect of dietary patterns on the anxiety levels among older adults is sparse. In our analysis we extracted three major dietary patters (the LFV, the meat-eaters and the SFAS dietary patterns). Of them, only the SFAS dietary pattern characterized by the consumption of added sugars and saturated fats was related with higher anxiety levels, while no association was reported between the LFV and the meat-eaters dietary patterns. Furthermore, no relation was reported between anti-inflammatory dietary patterns (D-AII) and anxiety. These associations are partly in line with the literature, where mixed results are reported. For example, a previous ATTICA work focused only in women reported that increased consumption of sweets and meat products were associated with higher anxiety levels [35]. Other recent studies report that diets high in sugars, processed foods (i.e., meat products), and/or fats are related with higher anxiety levels through alterations of glucose, protein and energy homeostasis, and increases in inflammatory cytokines (i.e., IL-6, IL-1β, TNFα) and corticosterone [53,54]. Inverse associations have also been reported between anti-inflammatory dietary patterns [36], high intake of fruit and vegetables [37], and anxiety. Our analysis between energy intake tertiles and anxiety referred no association in the final regression model, although, some animal studies report an anxiolytic caloric restriction (CR) effect [55] contributing beneficially to brain microstructure integrity [56]. Further studies, especially with longitudinal data, are needed on dietary habits and anxiety levels among older adults to confirm our findings.

Anxiety disorders in high-income countries for the population over 70 years old in 2017 account for 1.41% of total YLDs (https://vizhub.healthdata.org/gbd-compare/). These associations combined with the fact that Western societies are ageing along with the increased epidemic of depression and cognitive problems raise major concerns about the need for early non-pharmacological measures (and promotion of lifestyle changes) in order to prevent anxiety among the older populations.

Strengths and limitations

The present study has several strengths since it is one of the few studies to evaluate the relation between dietary habits, energy intake, and anxiety in Mediterranean older adults. However, some limitations deserve mentioning. It should be acknowledged that the baseline/entry study examination was conducted once and hence, may be susceptible to a certain degree of measurement error. This observational study may have potential recall bias due to its cross-sectional design, and consequently, the nature of the study limits the possibility for etiological conclusions between dietary habits and anxiety. The assessment of dietary habits using as a tool the FFQ is known for certain bias. Furthermore, there might be several misinterpretations since the components extracted from a PC are sometimes subjective.

5. Conclusions

Our results report that a dietary pattern characterized by saturated fats and added sugars (SFAS) seems to be related to higher anxiety in older adults living in Greece while energy intake was not related with anxiety in the fully adjusted model. Further studies and longitudinal data analysis are needed to better address this interesting question on the role of dietary habits in the symptomatology of anxiety among older populations.

Author Contributions: Conceptualization, M.F.M. and S.T. Data curation, N.K. Formal analysis, M.F.M., S.T., N.K., and D.B.P. Methodology, M.F.M., S.T., and N.K. Writing—original draft, M.F.M. and S.T. Writing—review and editing, M.F.M., S.T., N.K., D.B.P., C.C., J.S., C.P. (Charalambos Papageorgiou), J.M.H., D.T., and C.P. (Christos Pitsavos).

References

1. World Population Ageing [Highlights]. Available online: http://www.un.org/en/development/desa/population/publications/pdf/ageing/WPA2017_Highlights.pdf (accessed on 20 January 2019).
2. World Report on Ageing and HeAltH. Available online: www.who.int (accessed on 20 January 2019).
3. Baxter, A.J.; Scott, K.M.; Vos, T.; Whiteford, H.A. Global prevalence of anxiety disorders: A systematic review and meta-regression. *Psychol. Med.* **2013**, *43*, 897–910. [CrossRef] [PubMed]
4. Kasper, S. Anxiety disorders: Under-diagnosed and insufficiently treated. *Int. J. Psychiatry Clin. Pract.* **2006**, *10*, 3–9. [CrossRef] [PubMed]
5. Karanikolos, M.; Mladovsky, P.; Cylus, J.; Thomson, S.; Basu, S.; Stuckler, D.; Mackenbach, J.P.; McKee, M. Financial crisis, austerity, and health in Europe. *Lancet.* **2013**, *381*, 1323–1331. [CrossRef]
6. Foscolou, A.; Tyrovolas, S.; Soulis, G.; Mariolis, A.; Piscopo, S.; Valacchi, G.; Anastasiou, F.; Lionis, C.; Zeimbekis, A.; Tur, J.-A.; et al. The Impact of the Financial Crisis on Lifestyle Health Determinants Among Older Adults Living in the Mediterranean Region: The Multinational MEDIS Study (2005–2015). *J. Prev. Med. Public Health* **2017**, *50*, 1–9. [CrossRef] [PubMed]
7. Tyrovolas, S.; Kassebaum, N.J.; Stergachis, A.; Abraha, H.N.; Alla, F.; Androudi, S.; Car, M.; Chrepa, V.; Fullman, N.; Fürst, T.; et al. The burden of disease in Greece, health loss, risk factors, and health financing, 2000–2016: An analysis of the Global Burden of Disease Study 2016. *Lancet Public Health* **2018**, *3*, e395–e406. [CrossRef]
8. Prina, A.M.; Ferri, C.P.; Guerra, M.; Brayne, C.; Prince, M. Co-occurrence of anxiety and depression amongst older adults in low- and middle-income countries: Findings from the 10/66 study. *Psychol. Med.* **2011**, *41*, 2047–2056. [CrossRef] [PubMed]
9. Jacobson, N.C.; Newman, M.G. Anxiety and depression as bidirectional risk factors for one another: A meta-analysis of longitudinal studies. *Psychol. Bull.* **2017**, *143*, 1155–1200. [CrossRef] [PubMed]
10. Vytal, K.E.; Cornwell, B.R.; Letkiewicz, A.M.; Arkin, N.E.; Grillon, C. The complex interaction between anxiety and cognition: Insight from spatial and verbal working memory. *Front. Hum. Neurosci.* **2013**, *7*, 93. [CrossRef] [PubMed]
11. Gulpers, B.; Ramakers, I.; Hamel, R.; Köhler, S.; Oude Voshaar, R.; Verhey, F. Anxiety as a Predictor for Cognitive Decline and Dementia: A Systematic Review and Meta-Analysis. *Am. J. Geriatr. Psychiatry* **2016**, *24*, 823–842. [CrossRef]
12. Li, X.-X.; Li, Z. The impact of anxiety on the progression of mild cognitive impairment to dementia in Chinese and English data bases: A systematic review and meta-analysis. *Int. J. Geriatr. Psychiatry* **2018**, *33*, 131–140. [CrossRef]
13. Mayer, E.A.; Craske, M.; Naliboff, B.D. Depression, anxiety, and the gastrointestinal system. *J. Clin. Psychiatry* **2001**, *62*, 28–36. [PubMed]
14. Smith, K.J.; Béland, M.; Clyde, M.; Gariépy, G.; Pagé, V.; Badawi, G.; Rabasa-Lhoret, P.; Schmitz, N. Association of diabetes with anxiety: A systematic review and meta-analysis. *J. Psychosom. Res.* **2013**, *74*, 89–99. [CrossRef] [PubMed]
15. Fischer, S.; Ehlert, U. Hypothalamic-pituitary-thyroid (HPT) axis functioning in anxiety disorders. A ystematic review. *Depress. Anxiety* **2018**, *35*, 98–110. [CrossRef] [PubMed]
16. Tully, P.J.; Harrison, N.J.; Cheung, P.; Cosh, S. Anxiety and Cardiovascular Disease Risk: A Review. *Curr. Cardiol. Rep.* **2016**, *18*, 120. [CrossRef] [PubMed]
17. Kyrou, I.; Kollia, N.; Panagiotakos, D.; Georgousopoulou, E.; Chrysohoou, C.; Tsigos, C.; Randeva, H.S.; Yannakoulia, M.; Stefanadis, C.; Papageorgiou, C.; et al. Association of depression and anxiety status with 10-year cardiovascular disease incidence among apparently healthy Greek adults: The ATTICA Study. *Eur. J. Prev. Cardiol.* **2017**, *24*, 145–152. [CrossRef]

18. Boyer, P. Do anxiety and depression have a common pathophysiological mechanism? *Acta Psychiatr. Scand.* **2000**, *102*, 24–29. [CrossRef]
19. Myers, B.; Van Meerveld, B.G. Role of anxiety in the pathophysiology of irritable bowel syndrome: Importance of the amygdala. *Front. Neurosci.* **2009**, *3*, 2. [CrossRef]
20. Olafiranye, O.; Jean-Louis, G.; Zizi, F.; Nunes, J.; Vincent, M. Anxiety and cardiovascular risk: Review of Epidemiological and Clinical Evidence. *Mind Brain* **2011**, *2*, 32–37.
21. Jacka, F.N.; Pasco, J.A.; Mykletun, A.; Williams, L.J.; Hodge, A.M.; O'Reilly, S.L.; Nicholson, G.C.; Kotowicz, M.A.; Berk, M. Association of Western and Traditional Diets with Depression and Anxiety in Women. *Am. J. Psychiatry* **2010**, *167*, 305–311. [CrossRef]
22. Weng, T.-T.; Hao, J.-H.; Qian, Q.-W.; Cao, H.; Fu, J.-L.; Sun, Y.; Huang, L.; Tao, F.-B. Is there any relationship between dietary patterns and depression and anxiety in Chinese adolescents? *Public Health Nutr.* **2012**, *15*, 673–682. [CrossRef]
23. Velten, J.; Lavallee, K.L.; Scholten, S.; Meyer, A.H.; Zhang, X.-C.; Schneider, S.; Margraf, J. Lifestyle choices and mental health: A representative population survey. *BMC Psychol.* **2014**, *2*, 58. [CrossRef] [PubMed]
24. Pitsavos, C.; Panagiotakos, D.B.; Chrysohoou, C.; Stefanadis, C. Epidemiology of cardiovascular risk factors in Greece: Aims, design and baseline characteristics of the ATTICA study. *BMC Public Health* **2003**, *3*, 32. [CrossRef] [PubMed]
25. Papathanasiou, G.; Georgoudis, G.; Papandreou, M.; Spyropoulos, P.; Georgakopoulos, D.; Kalfakakou, V.; Evangelou, A. Reliability measures of the short International Physical Activity Questionnaire (IPAQ) in Greek young adults. *Hellenic J. Cardiol.* **2009**, *50*, 283–294. [PubMed]
26. Friedewald, W.T.; Levy, R.I.; Fredrickson, D.S. Estimation of the concentration of low-density lipoprotein cholesterol in plasma, without use of the preparative ultracentrifuge. *Clin. Chem.* **1972**, *18*, 499–502. [PubMed]
27. Katsouyanni, K.; Rimm, E.B.; Gnardellis, C.; Trichopoulos, D.; Polychronopoulos, E.; Trichopoulou, A. Reproducibility and relative validity of an extensive semi-quantitative food frequency questionnaire using dietary records and biochemical markers among Greek schoolteachers. *Int. J. Epidemiol.* **1997**, *26*, S118–S127. [CrossRef] [PubMed]
28. Willett, W.C.; Sacks, F.; Trichopoulou, A.; Drescher, G.; Ferro-Luzzi, A.; Helsing, E.; Trichopoulos, D. Mediterranean diet pyramid: A cultural model for healthy eating. *Am. J. Clin. Nutr.* **1995**, *61*, 1402S–1406S. [CrossRef]
29. Shivappa, N.; Steck, S.E.; Hurley, T.G.; Hussey, J.R.; Hébert, J.R. Designing and developing a literature-derived, population-based dietary inflammatory index. *Public Health Nutr.* **2014**, *17*, 1689–1696. [CrossRef]
30. Georgousopoulou, E.N.; Kouli, G.-M.; Panagiotakos, D.B.; Kalogeropoulou, A.; Zana, A.; Chrysohoou, C.; Tsigos, C.; Tousoulis, D.; Stefanadis, C.; Pitsavos, C. Anti-inflammatory diet and 10-year (2002–2012) cardiovascular disease incidence: The ATTICA study. *Int. J. Cardiol.* **2016**, 22, 473–478. [CrossRef]
31. Fountoulakis, K.; Papadopoulou, M.; Kleanthous, S.; Papadopoulou, A.; Bizeli, V.; Nimatoudis, I.; Iacovides, A.; Kaprinis, G.S. Reliability and psychometric properties of the Greek translation of the State-Trait Anxiety Inventory form Y: Preliminary data. *Ann. Gen. Psychiatry.* **2006**, *5*, 2. [CrossRef]
32. Zung, W.W.K. A self-rating depression scale. *Arch. Gen. Psychiatry* **1965**, *12*, 63–70. [CrossRef]
33. Briere, J. *Cognitive Distortions Scale (CDS) Professional Manual*; Psychological Assessment Resources: Odessa, FL, USA, 2000.
34. Floyd, F.J.; Widaman, K.F. Factor analysis in the development and refinement of clinical assessment instruments. *Psychol. Assess.* **1995**, *7*, 286–299. [CrossRef]
35. Yannakoulia, M.; Panagiotakos, D.B.; Pitsavos, C.; Tsetsekou, E.; Fappa, E.; Papageorgiou, C.; Stefanadis, C. Eating habits in relations to anxiety symptoms among apparently healthy adults. A pattern analysis from the ATTICA Study. *Appetite* **2008**, *51*, 519–525. [CrossRef] [PubMed]
36. Phillips, C.M.; Shivappa, N.; Hébert, J.R.; Perry, I.J. Dietary inflammatory index and mental health: A cross-sectional analysis of the relationship with depressive symptoms, anxiety and well-being in adults. *Clin. Nutr.* **2018**, *37*, 1485–1491. [CrossRef] [PubMed]
37. Saghafian, F.; Malmir, H.; Saneei, P.; Keshteli, A.H.; Hosseinzadeh-Attar, M.J.; Afshar, H.; Siassi, F.; Esmaillzadeh, A.; Adibi, P. Consumption of fruit and vegetables in relation with psychological disorders in Iranian adults. *Eur. J. Nutr.* **2018**, *57*, 2295–2306. [CrossRef] [PubMed]
38. Vink, D.; Aartsen, M.J.; Schoevers, R.A. Risk factors for anxiety and depression in the elderly: A review. *J. Affect. Disord.* **2008**, *106*, 29–44. [CrossRef]

39. Moylan, S.; Jacka, F.N.; Pasco, J.A.; Berk, M. Cigarette smoking, nicotine dependence and anxiety disorders: A systematic review of population-based, epidemiological studies. *BMC Med.* **2012**, *10*, 123. [CrossRef] [PubMed]
40. Teychenne, M.; Costigan, S.A.; Parker, K. The association between sedentary behaviour and risk of anxiety: A systematic review. *BMC Public Health* **2015**, *15*, 513. [CrossRef]
41. Demmer, R.T.; Gelb, S.; Suglia, S.F.; Keyes, K.M.; Aiello, A.E.; Colombo, P.C.; Galea, S.; Uddin, M.; Koenen, K.C.; Kubzansky, L.D. Sex Differences in the Association Between Depression, Anxiety, and Type 2 Diabetes Mellitus. *Psychosom. Med.* **2015**, *77*, 467–477. [CrossRef]
42. Mwinyi, J.; Pisanu, C.; Castelao, E.; Stringhini, S.; Preisig, M.; Schiöth, H.B. Anxiety Disorders are Associated with Low Socioeconomic Status in Women but Not in Men. *Women's Health Issues* **2017**, *27*, 302–307. [CrossRef]
43. Kang, H.-J.; Bae, K.-Y.; Kim, S.-W.; Shin, I.-S.; Yoon, J.-S.; Kim, J.-M. Anxiety symptoms in Korean elderly individuals: A two-year longitudinal community study. *Int. Psychogeriatr.* **2016**, *28*, 423–433. [CrossRef]
44. Anderson, E.; Shivakumar, G. Effects of exercise and physical activity on anxiety. *Front. Psychiatry* **2013**, *4*, 27. [CrossRef] [PubMed]
45. Rohleder, N.; Kirschbaum, C. The hypothalamic–pituitary–adrenal (HPA) axis in habitual smokers. *Int. J. Psychophysiol.* **2006**, *59*, 236–243. [CrossRef] [PubMed]
46. Vreeburg, S.A.; Zitman, F.G.; van Pelt, J.; DeRijk, R.H.; Verhagen, J.C.M.; van Dyck, R.; Hoogendijk, W.J.G.; Smit, J.H.; Penninx, B.W.J.H. Salivary Cortisol Levels in Persons with and without Different Anxiety Disorders. *Psychosom. Med.* **2010**, *72*, 340–347. [CrossRef] [PubMed]
47. Petkus, A.J.; Reynolds, C.A.; Wetherell, J.L.; Kremen, W.S.; Gatz, M. Temporal dynamics of cognitive performance and anxiety across older adulthood. *Psychol. Aging* **2017**, *32*, 278–292. [CrossRef] [PubMed]
48. Hirschfeld, R.M.A. The Comorbidity of Major Depression and Anxiety Disorders: Recognition and Management in Primary Care. *Prim. Care Companion J. Clin. Psychiatry* **2001**, *3*, 244–254. [CrossRef] [PubMed]
49. Biringer, E.; Mykletun, A.; Dahl, A.A.; Smith, A.D.; Engedal, K.; Nygaard, H.A.; Lund, A. The association between depression, anxiety, and cognitive function in the elderly general population–the Hordaland Health Study. *Int. J. Geriatr. Psychiatry* **2005**, *20*, 989–997. [CrossRef] [PubMed]
50. Hu, F.B. Dietary pattern analysis: A new direction in nutritional epidemiology. *Curr. Opin. Lipidol.* **2002**, *13*, 3–9. [CrossRef]
51. Anderson, A.L.; Harris, T.B.; Tylavsky, F.A.; Perry, S.E.; Houston, D.K.; Hue, T.F.; Strotmeyer, E.S.; Sahyoun, N.R. Dietary patterns and survival of older adults. *J. Am. Diet. Assoc.* **2011**, *111*, 84–91. [CrossRef]
52. Govindaraju, T.; Sahle, B.W.; McCaffrey, T.A.; McNeil, J.J.; Owen, A.J. Dietary Patterns and Quality of Life in Older Adults: A Systematic Review. *Nutrients* **2018**, *10*, 971. [CrossRef]
53. Bakhtiyari, M.; Ehrampoush, E.; Enayati, N.; Joodi, G.; Sadr, S.; Delpisheh, A.; Alihaydari, J.; Homayounfar, R. Anxiety as a consequence of modern dietary pattern in adults in Tehran–Iran. *Eat. Behav.* **2013**, *14*, 107–112. [CrossRef]
54. Dutheil, S.; Ota, K.T.; Wohleb, E.S.; Rasmussen, K.; Duman, R.S. High-Fat Diet Induced Anxiety and Anhedonia: Impact on Brain Homeostasis and Inflammation. *Neuropsychopharmacology* **2016**, *41*, 1874–1887. [CrossRef] [PubMed]
55. Kenny, R.; Dinan, T.; Cai, G.; Spencer, S.J. Effects of mild calorie restriction on anxiety and hypothalamic-pituitary-adrenal axis responses to stress in the male rat. *Physiol. Rep.* **2014**, *2*, e00265. [CrossRef] [PubMed]
56. Willette, A.A.; Coe, C.L.; Birdsill, A.C.; Bendlin, B.B.; Colman, R.J.; Alexander, A.L.; Allison, D.B.; Weindruch, R.H.; Johnson, S.C. Interleukin-8 and interleukin-10, brain volume and microstructure, and the influence of calorie restriction in old rhesus macaques. *Age* **2013**, *35*, 2215–2227. [CrossRef] [PubMed]

4

The Prevalence of Anticholinergic Drugs and Correlation with Pneumonia in Elderly Patients: A Population-Based Study in Taiwan

Chien-Ying Lee [1,2], Yih-Dih Cheng [3,4], Wei-Yuan Cheng [5], Tung-Han Tsai [6] and Kuang-Hua Huang [6,*]

1 Department of Pharmacology, Chung Shan Medical University, Taichung 40201, Taiwan; cshd015@csmu.edu.tw
2 Department of Pharmacy, Chung Shan Medical University Hospital, Taichung 40201, Taiwan
3 School of pharmacy, China Medical University, Taichung 40402, Taiwan; tovis168@gmail.com
4 Department of Pharmacy, China Medical University Hospital, Taichung 40402, Taiwan
5 Taso-Tun Psychiatric Center, Ministry of Health and Welfare, Nantou 54249, Taiwan; continentaln78005@gmail.com
6 Department of Health Services Administration, China Medical University, Taichung 40402, Taiwan; dondon0525@gmail.com
* Correspondence: khhuang@mail.cmu.edu.tw

Abstract: Anticholinergic drugs may increase the risk of serious respiratory infection, especially in the elderly. The study aims to investigate the prevalence of anticholinergic drugs and the correlation of incident pneumonia associated with the use of anticholinergic drugs among the elderly in Taiwan. The study population was 275,005 elderly patients aged ≥65 years old, selected from the longitudinal health insurance database (LHID) in 2016. Among all the elderly patients, about 60% had received anticholinergic medication at least once. Furthermore, the study selected elderly patients who had not been diagnosed with pneumonia and had not received any anticholinergic drugs in the past year in order to evaluate the correlation between pneumonia and anticholinergic drugs. The study excluded elderly patients who died or had received related drugs of incident pneumonia during the study period and selected elderly patients receiving anticholinergic drugs as the case group. Propensity score matching (PSM) on a 1:1 scale was used to match elderly patients that were not receiving any anticholinergic drugs as the control group, resulting in a final sample of 32,215 patients receiving anticholinergic drugs and 32,215 patients not receiving any anticholinergic drugs. Conditional logistic regression was used to estimate the association between anticholinergic drugs and pneumonia after controlling for potential confounders. Compared with patients not receiving anticholinergic drugs, the adjusted odds ratio of patients receiving anticholinergic drugs was 1.33 (95% confidence interval: 1.18 to 1.49). Anticholinergic medication is common among elderly patients in Taiwan. Elderly patients receiving anticholinergic drugs may increase their risk of incident pneumonia. The safety of anticholinergic drugs in the elderly should be of concern in Taiwan.

Keywords: anticholinergic drugs; pneumonia; elderly; potentially inappropriate medication; pharmacoepidemiology

1. Introduction

Anticholinergic drugs act centrally and peripherally on muscarinic acetylcholine receptors. Cimetidine, metoclopramide, and ranitidine are commonly employed in the treatment of the urinary bladder, the respiratory tract, and gastroesophageal disease via the intervention of the muscarinic receptor [1]. The peripheral anticholinergic complaint of dry mouth can promote mucosal damage and increase the risk for serious respiratory infection, secondary to losing the effect of the antimicrobial activity of saliva [2]. Owing to the nonselective nature of this muscarinic receptor antagonist, elderly patients are particularly susceptible to anticholinergic drugs because of age-related changes in pharmacokinetic and pharmacodynamic properties [3].

Anticholinergic drugs are one of the risk factors for pneumonia in elderly patients. It can increase the risk of pneumonia in elderly patients, although the strength of the muscarinic blockade of every anticholinergic drug is different [4,5]. One of the mechanisms for pneumonia is that dry mouth caused by anticholinergic drugs may lead to oropharyngeal and esophageal swallowing impairments and result in aspiration pneumonia [6,7]. The impairment of airway mucociliary transport in patients can prolong bacterial stay in the lungs and eventually contribute to respiratory infections; in addition, lower esophageal sphincter pressure can lead to acid reflux and cause aspiration [8]. The central effects of anticholinergic drugs may increase the risk of pharyngeal aspiration, including sedation and altered mental status, then lead to the incident pneumonia. This can more likely result in bacterial pneumonia when aspirated bacteria are not effectively cleared [9,10]. Sedation and altered mental status have also been associated with poor pulmonary hygiene and may lead to viral respiratory infection. It may also contribute to pneumonia [11]. Another mechanism that could be involved in anticholinergic-induced pneumonia is low levels of mucous secretions, which may increase the risk of incident pneumonia because of bacterial growth [6]. Previous literature suggests that oropharyngeal aspiration is a prominent etiologic factor for pneumonia in elderly adults with swallowing disorders and weak cough reflexes [9–11].

Many elderly patients suffer from multiple chronic diseases and commonly take different prescription medications for multiple conditions. It is known that changes in drug metabolism in the elderly occur with age. There is a common finding in elderly patients, where the use of multiple drugs may cause serious side effects. Many age-related diseases and disease-related conditions may predispose geriatric patients to anticholinergic intoxication [2]. In clinical practice, medications with anticholinergic effects are considered potentially inappropriate when used on the elderly [12,13]. Consequently, anticholinergic rating scales (ARS) are used to express the grade of anticholinergic effect in clinical practice, ranging from limited or none (Level 0), moderate (Level 1), strong (Level 2), and very strong (Level 3) [14,15], while the correlation between anticholinergic gradation and incident pneumonia is inconsistent. Some studies have indicated that the risk of incident pneumonia is not related to high potency anticholinergic drugs (Level 3) [6]. Previous studies have identified several drugs with anticholinergic properties we should be aware of, namely, the possibility of side effects in elderly patients, including respiratory system medicines (cetirizine, loratadine, pseudoephedrine), psychotropic medicines (paroxetine, quetiapine), alimentary tract medicines (cimetidine, ranitidine), and neurological disorder medications (larbidopa–levodopa, levodopa) [15–17].

To date, few studies have been conducted using a nationwide database to evaluate the correlation between pneumonia and anticholinergic drugs in elderly patients, especially in Taiwan [6,18]. It is essential to understand the risk of pneumonia in elderly patients receiving anticholinergic drugs. Therefore, this study was conducted to investigate the prevalence of anticholinergic drugs and the risk factors related to pneumonia and, moreover, estimate the correlation of incident pneumonia associated with the use of anticholinergic drugs among the elderly by using a nationwide database in Taiwan.

2. Materials and Methods

2.1. Data Source

The study is secondary data analysis, from 2015 to 2016, based on the longitudinal health insurance database (LHID) released by the Health and Welfare Data Science Center, Ministry of Health and Welfare (HWDC, MOHW; Registration No. H107175). LHID randomly selected two million beneficiaries from the Taiwan National Health Insurance (NHI) program. The information in LHID included detailed clinical records of the outpatient department and hospitalization, diagnostic codes, and prescribing information. The NHI program is nationwide social insurance that has enrolled up to 99% of citizens since 1995. Hence, the database is a nationally representative health database for Taiwan. HWDC provides scrambled random identification numbers for insured patients to protect the privacy of beneficiaries. This study protocol was approved as a completely ethical review by the Institutional Review Board of China Medical University Hospital, Taiwan (No. CMUH107-REC2-004). The database is anonymous; therefore, the requirement for informed consent was waived.

2.2. Study Subjects

Figure 1 lists the flowchart of the selected patients for inclusion. The study population was 275,005 elderly patients aged ≥65 years old, selected from LHID on 1 January 2016 to investigate the prevalence of anticholinergic drugs. Furthermore, the elderly patients who had not been diagnosed with pneumonia and had not received any anticholinergic drugs in the past year were enrolled in the study to evaluate the correlation between pneumonia and anticholinergic drugs. We also excluded 10,532 patients who died and the 33,189 patients who had received related drugs of incident pneumonia in the study period in order to improve the validity of the study results. The related drugs of incident pneumonia contained amiodarone, angiotensin-converting enzyme inhibitors (ACEIs), amantadine, and steroids [12–17]. Moreover, the study classified elderly patients according to their medication records in 2016 and selected elderly patients who were receiving anticholinergic drugs as the case group. In the study, there were a total of 49 drugs with the potential to cause anticholinergic adverse effects [17], including psychotropic medicines (e.g., paroxetine, quetiapine, trazodone), alimentary tract and metabolism medicines (e.g., cimetidine, metoclopramide, ranitidine, loperamide), respiratory system and allergy medicines (e.g., cetirizine, loratadine, pseudoephedrine), and neurological disorder medications (e.g., carbidopa–levodopa, levodopa) (see Table A1). Furthermore, to reduce the potential confounding caused by unbalanced covariates in nonexperimental settings, we used propensity score matching (PSM) on a 1:1 scale to match elderly patients not receiving any anticholinergic drugs as the control group, resulting in a final sample of 32,215 patients receiving anticholinergic drugs and 32,215 patients not receiving any anticholinergic drugs. The propensity score of the study is the probability of patients receiving anticholinergic drugs, calculated by gender, age, insured salary, urbanization, and the Charlson comorbidity index (CCI).

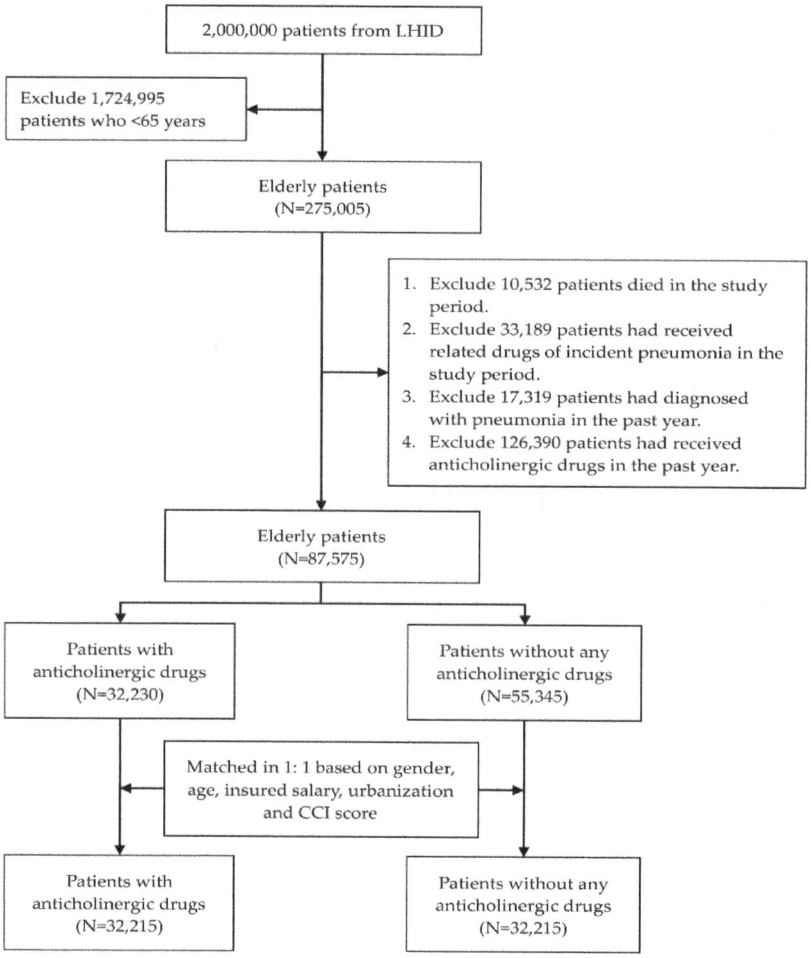

Figure 1. Flowchart of the study subject selection process. (Abbreviations: LHID, longitudinal health insurance database; CCI, Charlson comorbidity index)

2.3. *Study Design*

The study is a retrospective study to investigate the prevalence of anticholinergic drugs among elderly patients in Taiwan. Furthermore, the study design is divided into three phases to assess the correlation between anticholinergic drugs and pneumonia. The first phase was the exclusion period, from 1 January to 31 December 2015, in which to select the study subjects. The second phase was the observation period, from 1 January to 30 November 2016, in which to estimate the correlation between anticholinergic drugs and pneumonia. Patients were followed-up 30 days after anticholinergic drug prescriptions in order to observe the incidence of pneumonia. The third phase was in December 2016 to ensure the follow-up period. Thus, the patients receiving anticholinergic drugs in this phase would not be enrolled as study subjects. The study design diagram is exhibited in Figure 2.

The definition of incident pneumonia in the study was according to the principal diagnosis code in J12–J18, based on the International Classification of Diseases, Tenth Revision, Clinical Modification (ICD-10-CM). The study investigated the association between anticholinergic drugs and pneumonia via conditional logistic regression. Control variables in the study contained gender, age, insured salary, urbanization, CCI scores, and comorbidities related to pneumonia. Comorbidities contained diabetes mellitus (DM; ICD-10-CM: E08-E13), Alzheimer's disease (AD; ICD-10-CM: G30, F00), stroke (ICD-10-CM: I60-I69), Parkinson's disease (PD; ICD-10-CM: G20), major depression disorder (MDD; ICD-10-CM: F32.9, F33.9), chronic kidney disease (CKD; ICD-10-CM: N18), asthma (ICD-10-CM: J45), chronic obstructive pulmonary disease (COPD; ICD-10-CM: J40-J44, J47), heart failure (HF; ICD-10-CM: I50), upper respiratory infection (URI; ICD-10-CM: J00-J06), gastroesophageal reflux disease (GERD; ICD-10-CM: K21), and epilepsy (ICD-10-CM: G40-G41). The definition of comorbidities was with diagnosis at least three times a year, except epileptic seizure. Epileptic seizure was defined by diagnosis once a year.

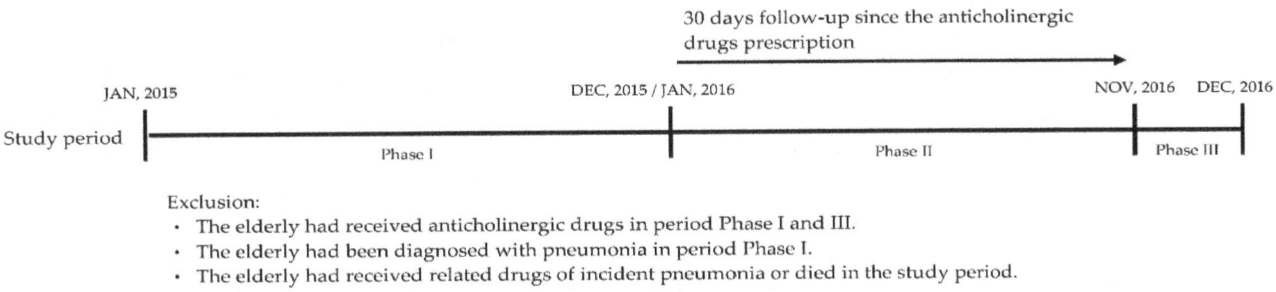

Figure 2. The study design diagram.

2.4. Statistical Analysis

Descriptive statistics were used to summarize distributions of the prevalence of anticholinergic drugs in the elderly in Taiwan. We used the standardized mean difference to examine the balance of case and control groups after matching. We further used conditional logistic regression to estimate the association between anticholinergic drugs and pneumonia after controlling for potential confounders. SAS software version 9.4 (SAS Institute Inc., Cary, NC, USA) was used for statistical analysis in the study, and the statistical significance was defined as p-value < 0.05.

3. Results

3.1. The Prevalence of Anticholinergic Drugs

Table 1 presents the prevalence of anticholinergic drugs in elderly patients. There was a total of 967,887 prescriptions with anticholinergic drugs, about 12.96%, out of all prescriptions. The most frequency anticholinergic prescriptions were cimetidine (2.54%), cetirizine (1.19%), pseudoephedrine (1.15%), metoclopramide (1.13%), ranitidine (0.83%), quetiapine (0.80%), carbidopa–levodopa (0.66%), loratadine (0.65%), trazodone (0.54%), and loperamide (0.51%), sequentially. To elderly patients, there were 165,262 patients (60.09%) who had received anticholinergic medication at least once out of all elderly patients.

Table 1. The distribution of prescriptions in elderly patients.

Prescriptions	No. of Prescriptions		No. of Patients Had Received	
	N	%	N	%
Total	7,467,908	100.00	275,005	100.00
Without anticholinergic drugs	6,500,021	87.04	109,743	39.91
With anticholinergic drugs	967,887	12.96	165,262	60.09
Most frequency anticholinergic drugs				
Cimetidine	189,862	2.54	53,171	19.33
Cetirizine	88,587	1.19	33,987	12.36
Pseudoephedrine	86,201	1.15	36,453	13.26
Metoclopramide	84,483	1.13	30,241	11.00
Ranitidine	61,831	0.83	16,066	5.84
Quetiapine	59,961	0.80	8126	2.95
Carbidopa–Levodopa	49,145	0.66	6371	2.32
Loratadine	48,793	0.65	20,132	7.32
Trazodone	40,079	0.54	6875	2.50
Loperamide	38,237	0.51	20,527	7.46

3.2. *The Baseline Characteristics Distribution of Study Subjects*

After subject selection, there was a total of 64,430 elderly patients in the study, and both groups, with and without anticholinergic drugs, had 32,215 patients. The mean age of patients receiving anticholinergic drugs was 73.58 ± 7.35 years, 51.77% were female, and 72.74% were in highly urbanization areas. As in Table 2, baseline characteristics were well balanced between elderly patients with and without anticholinergic drugs after matching. Among patients receiving anticholinergic drugs, there were 8614 patients (26.74%) with DM, 3457 patients (10.73%) with stroke, 317 patients with Parkinson's disease (0.98%), 3684 patients with CKD (11.43%), 1928 patients with asthma (5.98%), 2781 patients with COPD (8.63%), 1076 patients with HF (3.34%), 18,688 patients with URI (58.01%), 862 patients with GERD (2.68%), and 120 patients with epilepsy (0.37%).

Table 2. The baseline characteristics distribution of study subjects after matching.

Variables	Crude Data						After Matching					
	Anticholinergic Drugs				SMD [3]	*p*-Value [1]	Anticholinergic Drugs				SMD [3]	*p*-Value [1]
	Without		With				Without		With			
	N	%	N	%			N	%	N	%		
Total	55,345	100.00	32,230	100.00			32,215	100.00	32,215	100.00		
Gender [2]					0.08	<0.001					0	0.969
Female	27,610	49.89	17,337	53.79			17,317	53.75	17,322	53.77		
Male	27,735	50.11	14,893	46.21			14,898	46.25	14,893	46.23		
Age (year) [2]	73.28±7.42		73.58±7.35		0.05	<0.001	73.59±7.42		73.58±7.35		0	0.981
65–70	25,432	45.95	14,034	43.54			13,992	43.43	14,034	43.56		
71–75	11,619	20.99	6881	21.35			6878	21.35	6878	21.35		
76–80	8317	15.03	5322	16.51			5344	16.59	5310	16.48		
>80	9977	18.03	5993	18.59			6001	18.63	5993	18.60		
Insured salary [3]					0.06	<0.001					0	0.994
<20,008	18,342	33.14	9070	28.14			9046	28.08	9070	28.15		
20,008–22,800	19,850	35.87	13,174	40.87			13,184	40.93	13,159	40.85		
22,801–50,600	11,176	20.19	6632	20.58			6621	20.55	6632	20.59		
>50,600	5977	10.80	3354	10.41			3364	10.44	3354	10.41		
Urbanization [2]					0.07	<0.001					0	0.903
Urban	42,143	76.15	23,434	72.71			23,480	72.89	23,434	72.74		
Suburban	8781	15.87	5759	17.87			5729	17.78	5747	17.84		
Rural	4421	7.99	3037	9.42			3006	9.33	3034	9.42		
CCI [2, 3]					0.22	<0.001					0	0.989
0	32,820	59.30	15,617	48.45			15,626	48.51	15,617	48.48		
1–2	18,210	32.90	13,155	40.82			13,138	40.78	13,155	40.84		
≥3	4315	7.80	3458	10.73			3451	10.71	3443	10.69		
DM [3]					−0.14	<0.001					−0.02	0.015
No	43,788	79.12	23,605	73.24			23,872	74.10	23,601	73.26		
Yes	11,557	20.88	8625	26.76			8343	25.90	8614	26.74		
AD [3]					−0.04	<0.001					−0.03	<0.001
No	55,148	99.64	32,012	99.32			32,076	99.57	31,997	99.32		
Yes	197	0.36	218	0.68			139	0.43	218	0.68		
Stroke					−0.11	<0.001					−0.04	<0.001
No	51,081	92.30	28,768	89.26			29,131	90.43	28,758	89.27		
Yes	4264	7.70	3462	10.74			3084	9.57	3457	10.73		
PD [3]					−0.08	<0.001					−0.08	<0.001
No	55,175	99.69	31,913	99.02			32,101	99.65	31,898	99.02		
Yes	170	0.31	317	0.98			114	0.35	317	0.98		
MDD [3]					−0.06	<0.001					−0.05	<0.001
No	54,660	98.76	31,579	97.98			31,773	98.63	31,564	97.98		
Yes	685	1.24	651	2.02			442	1.37	651	2.02		
CKD [3]					−0.13	<0.001					−0.08	<0.001
No	51,169	92.45	28,540	88.55			29,312	90.99	28,532	88.57		
Yes	4176	7.55	3690	11.45			2903	9.01	3683	11.43		
Asthma					−0.14	<0.001					−0.11	<0.001
No	53,685	97.00	30,302	94.02			31,048	96.38	30,287	94.02		
Yes	1660	3.00	1928	5.98			1167	3.62	1928	5.98		
COPD [3]					−0.19	<0.001					−0.15	<0.001
No	53,077	95.90	29,448	91.37			30,653	95.15	29,434	91.37		
Yes	2268	4.10	2782	8.63			1562	4.85	2781	8.63		

Table 2. *Cont.*

Variables	Crude Data						After Matching					
	Anticholinergic Drugs				SMD [3]	*p*-Value [1]	Anticholinergic Drugs				SMD [3]	*p*-Value [1]
	Without		With				Without		With			
	N	%	N	%			N	%	N	%		
HF [3]					−0.08	<0.001					−0.05	<0.001
No	54,226	97.98	31,150	96.65			31,429	97.56	31,139	96.66		
Yes	1119	2.02	1080	3.35			786	2.44	1076	3.34		
URI [3]					−0.63	<0.001					−0.59	<0.001
No	39,636	71.62	13,536	42.00			22,565	70.05	13,527	41.99		
Yes	15,709	28.38	18,694	58.00			9650	29.95	18,688	58.01		
GERD [3]					−0.12	<0.001					−0.11	<0.001
No	54,765	98.95	31,368	97.33			31,849	98.86	31,353	97.32		
Yes	580	1.05	862	2.67			366	1.14	862	2.68		
Epilepsy					−0.02	0.004					−0.01	0.075
No	55,199	99.74	32,109	99.62			32,121	99.71	32,095	99.63		
Yes	146	0.26	121	0.38			94	0.29	120	0.37		

[1] Chi-square test. [2] The matching variables and the unit of insured salary are in New Taiwan dollars (NTD). [3] Abbreviations: SMD, Standardized mean difference; CCI, Charlson comorbidity index; DM, diabetes mellitus; AD, Alzheimer's disease; PD, Parkinson's disease; MDD, major depression disorder; CKD, chronic kidney disease; COPD, chronic obstructive pulmonary disease; HF, heart failure; URI, upper respiratory infection; GERD, gastroesophageal reflux disease.

3.3. *The Incidence Rate of Pneumonia in Elderly Patients*

Table 3 indicates that among all participants, 1519 patients had occurred pneumonia, and the incidence rate was 23.58 cases per 1000 elderly patients. The incidence rate of patients receiving anticholinergic drugs was 33.23 cases per 1000 elderly patients. Compared with patients not receiving anticholinergic drugs, the risk ratio was 2.18 times of incident pneumonia. Compared with patients without DM, patients with DM had 1.31 times the risk of incident pneumonia. Additionally, compared with patients without comorbidities, patients with comorbidities had a higher risk of incident pneumonia, including stroke (2.21 times), PD (2.89 times), CKD (1.85 times), asthma (5.54 times), COPD (6.77 times), HF (2.75 times), URI (1.98 times), GERD (2.15 times), and epilepsy (4.61 times).

Table 3. The incidence rate of pneumonia in elderly patients.

Variables	Pneumonia		Risk Ratio
	N	Incident Rate (‰)	
Total	1519	23.58	
Anticholinergic drugs			
Without	529	15.27	
With	990	33.23	2.18
Diabetes mellitus			
No	1036	21.82	
Yes	483	28.48	1.31
Alzheimer's disease			
No	1507	23.52	
Yes	12	33.61	1.43
Stroke			
No	1215	20.99	
Yes	304	46.48	2.21
Parkinson's disease			
No	1490	23.28	
Yes	29	67.29	2.89

Table 3. *Cont.*

Variables	Pneumonia		Risk Ratio
	N	Incident Rate (‰)	
Major depression disorder			
No	1493	23.57	
Yes	26	23.79	1.01
Chronic kidney disease			
No	1255	21.70	
Yes	264	40.09	1.85
Asthma			
No	1187	19.35	
Yes	332	107.27	5.54
Chronic obstructive pulmonary disease			
No	1020	16.98	
Yes	499	114.90	6.77
Heart failure			
No	1404	22.44	
Yes	115	61.76	2.75
Upper respiratory infection			
No	594	16.46	
Yes	925	32.64	1.98
Gastroesophageal reflux disease			
No	1458	23.07	
Yes	61	49.67	2.15
Epilepsy			
No	1496	23.30	
Yes	23	107.48	4.61

3.4. Correlation between Anticholinergic Drugs and Pneumonia

Table 4 points out that patients receiving anticholinergic drugs increased their risk of incident pneumonia (adjusted odds ratio [OR]: 1.33; 95% confidence interval [CI]: 1.18 to 1.49) after controlling for potential confounders. DM increased the risk of incident pneumonia (aOR: 1.44; 95% CI: 1.26 to 1.65). AD also increased the risk of incident pneumonia, but had no statistical significance (aOR: 1.20; 95% CI: 0.66 to 2.17). aORs of incident pneumonia in patients with comorbidities were all significantly higher than patients without, including stroke (aOR: 2.02; 95% CI: 1.75 to 2.33), PD (aOR: 1.94; 95% CI: 1.28 to 2.94), CKD (aOR: 1.57; 95% CI: 1.35 to 1.82), asthma (aOR: 1.57; 95% CI: 1.31 to 1.87), COPD (aOR: 4.93; 95% CI: 4.21 to 5.78), HF (aOR: 1.64; 95% CI: 1.32 to 2.04), URI (aOR: 1.79; 95% CI: 1.60 to 2.00), GERD (aOR: 1.52; 95% CI: 1.15 to 2.01), and epilepsy (aOR: 3.11; 95% CI: 1.92 to 5.03).

Table 4. Comparing the risk of incident pneumonia between elderly patients with and without anticholinergic drugs.

Variables	aOR [1,2]	95% Confidence Interval	*p*-Value
Anticholinergic agent	1.33	1.18–1.49	<0.001
DM [1]	1.44	1.26–1.65	<0.001
AD [1]	1.20	0.66–2.18	0.561
Stroke	2.02	1.75–2.33	<0.001
PD [1]	1.94	1.28–2.94	0.002
MDD [1]	0.74	0.49–1.12	0.158
CKD [1]	1.57	1.35–1.82	<0.001
Asthma	1.57	1.31–1.87	<0.001
COPD [1]	4.93	4.21–5.78	<0.001
HF [1]	1.64	1.32–2.04	<0.001
URI [1]	1.79	1.60–2.00	<0.001
GERD [1]	1.52	1.15–2.01	0.003
Epilepsy	3.11	1.92–5.03	<0.001

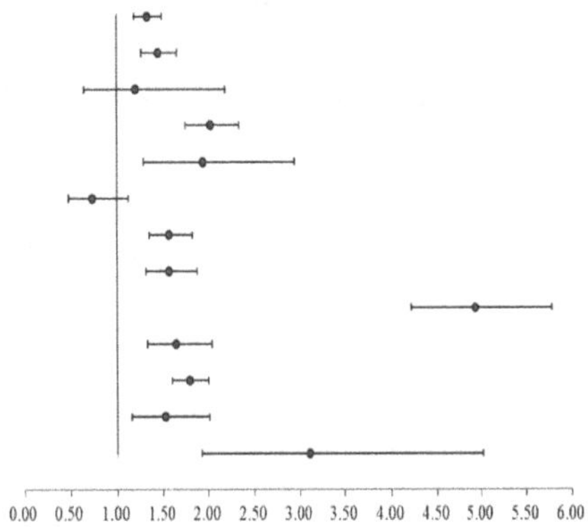

[1] Abbreviations: aOR, adjusted odds ratio; DM, diabetes mellitus; AD, Alzheimer's disease; PD, Parkinson's disease; MDD, major depression disorder; CKD, chronic kidney disease; COPD, chronic obstructive pulmonary disease; HF, heart failure; URI, upper respiratory infection; GERD, gastroesophageal reflux disease. [2] The conditional logistic regression model, stratified by matching variables, was used to estimate the risk.

4. Discussion

Our study results indicate that about 60% of elderly patients had received anticholinergic medication at least once, and the most frequent anticholinergic prescriptions in Taiwan were cimetidine, cetirizine, pseudoephedrine, metoclopramide, and ranitidine. These drugs are used to treat URI and excessive secretions of gastric acid in primary care clinics in Taiwan. A previous study indicated that most frequent anticholinergic drugs were ranitidine, trazodone, paroxetine, oxybutynin, and nortriptyline [19]. Those were used to treat cardiovascular and neurological disorders. This indicates that there is a wide disparity in the prescription pattern of anticholinergic drugs between other countries and Taiwan. It may be related to the difference in medical care-seeking behavior caused by the health care system.

Pneumonia is a life-threatening infectious disease where age is one of the strongest risk factors. Our study demonstrates that anticholinergic drugs are related to incident pneumonia in the elderly. A population-based case–control study by Paul et al. [10] expressed that anticholinergic medication use is associated with pneumonia risk, compared with no use. Moreover, both acute and chronic use of anticholinergic drugs were associated with a higher risk for pneumonia, whereas there was no association with previous use. Another case–control study in America by Chatterjee et al. [6] estimated anticholinergic drug exposure and the risk of pneumonia. The overall use of anticholinergic drugs was associated with the risk of pneumonia, while the effect of anticholinergic drugs was not related to pneumonia. It indicated that even low-potency anticholinergic drugs may cause a significant risk of pneumonia. A nationwide study in Finland had a similar result [18]. Most of the low-potency anticholinergic drugs are cardiovascular drugs, and the risk may be partially explained by comorbidity. The main purpose of our study was to explore the potential relationship between the risk of pneumonia and anticholinergic drug use in the elderly in Taiwan. To enhance the accuracy of the study results, our study used PSM to obtain control groups for each elderly patient receiving anticholinergic drugs. A propensity score is a unit with certain characteristics that is assigned to each elderly patient receiving anticholinergic drugs. The scores can be used to reduce or eliminate selection bias in observational studies by the characteristics of elderly patients with and without anticholinergic drugs [20–23]. Compared with previous studies, our study design and methodology are more rigorous. Our study was inappropriate for further analysis regarding the effect of different levels of anticholinergic drugs due to the elderly subjects in our study being matched based on whether they received anticholinergic drugs rather than different levels of anticholinergic drugs. To our knowledge, there has been no related population-based study to estimate the relationship between incident pneumonia and anticholinergic drug use in Taiwan. Our study was not aimed at exploring the mechanisms between anticholinergic drugs and increased pneumonia risk, but the association between anticholinergic drugs and pneumonia in the elderly was clear. Although the incident rate of pneumonia caused by anticholinergic drugs is relatively rare, future studies should develop more well-designed prospective population trials to be carried out to ascertain the relationship.

The comorbidities may also predispose elderly patients to an increased risk of pneumonia. Our study results were consistent with previous studies that noted that comorbidities, including DM, stroke, PD, CKD, asthma, COPD, HF, URI, and GERD, were risk factors of pneumonia. The elderly with COPD or asthma are a high-risk population of bacterial infection, and one of the major infections is caused by streptococcus pneumoniae bacteria. It can cause many types of illnesses that contained pneumonia, meningitis, and septicemia. Therefore, COPD and asthma are both associated with a greater risk of incident pneumonia in the elderly [24–26]. DM may also increase the pneumonia risk in the elderly due to poor glycemic control. Aging is associated with a progressive decline in respiratory system function, and poor glycemic control can cause microvascular complications of lung capillaries [27–29]. Moreover, previous studies have documented that the elderly with stroke, dementia, or Parkinson's disease have a higher risk of incident pneumonia [26,27,30]. It was possibly attributable to dysphagia, difficulty swallowing, and cough reflexes. Oropharyngeal dysphagia is also one of the risk factors for pneumonia in elderly patients [31–33]. Renal disease in the elderly is clinically important. Previous studies have described that there is a positive direction in the association between predialysis CKD and acute community-acquired infection [34]. Hypoimmunity of the elderly patient with CKD may predispose the patient to acute lower respiratory infections. Another study demonstrated that cardiovascular function declined in elderly patients with heart disease, which would affect the mucociliary clearance functions that trap and remove particulates and pathogens from the airways, leading to an increased risk of incident pneumonia [35]. Furthermore, a population-based cohort study indicated that GERD is associated with a long-term risk of pneumonia, especially in GERD with proton pump inhibitors (PPIs) for a longer treatment than four months [36]. There is a relationship between gastric acid suppressants and an increased risk of pneumonia [37]. Authors have suggested that the inhibition of gastric acid secretion by acid-suppressive therapy allows pathogen colonization from the upper gastrointestinal tract [24].

The major strength of the study is that it is based on a nationwide database, avoiding bias such as selection, nonresponse, and poor recall. Big data analysis is a new trend in modern healthcare research. LHID has completeness in recording prescriptions and clinical diagnosis. Moreover, the study was not only adjusted for potential confounding factors but also used PSM to avoid bias in the selection of study subjects. Therefore, the study indicates the correlation between anticholinergic drugs and pneumonia with a narrower and statistically significant confidence interval.

There were also a few limitations to the study. Some pneumonia-related variables, such as medication adherence, tobacco consumption behavior, and laboratory parameters, cannot be obtained from LHID. Additionally, the study only used the ICD code to define disease without any medical procedure codes. There may be overdiagnosis. Although our study indicated the correlation between anticholinergic drugs and pneumonia, the strength of the anticholinergic effect may also be related to pneumonia. We will explore the risk of incident pneumonia with different anticholinergic drugs in further study. Finally, this study is a type of observational study that analyzes data from a population database. The study result can only provide evidence to demonstrate that anticholinergic drugs are related to incident pneumonia. It is essential to obtain more information from other databases to analyze the cause–effect relation in future research.

5. Conclusions

The use of anticholinergic drugs is common in the elderly in Taiwan because these medications are prescribed for the symptomatic management of medical conditions. Elderly patients receiving anticholinergic drugs may increase their risk of incident pneumonia. Moreover, DM, stroke, PD, CKD, asthma, COPD, HF, URI, and GERD were also associated with incident pneumonia in the elderly. Anticholinergic drugs can have many beneficial effects, but these drugs need to be balanced against potential harm. Drugs with anticholinergic properties can be problematic, especially for the elderly population. Prescribers should consider dose reductions and monitoring when prescribing anticholinergic drugs to elderly patients to reduce the risks of adverse outcomes. Furthermore, randomized clinical trials are warranted to determine the effectiveness and safety of anticholinergic drugs in the elderly.

Author Contributions: Conceptualization, C.-Y.L. and K.-H.H.; formal analysis, W.-Y.C. and T.-H.T.; methodology, C.-Y.L., Y.-D.C., W.-Y.C., and K.-H.H.; validation, K.-H.H.; writing—original draft, C.-Y.L., Y.-D.C., and K.-H.H.; writing—review and editing, K.-H.H. All authors have read and agreed to the published version of the manuscript.

Acknowledgments: We are grateful to Chung Shan Medical University, Taiwan, China Medical University, Taiwan, Asia University, Taiwan, and the Health Data Science Center, China Medical University Hospital, for providing administrative, technical, and funding support that has contributed to the completion of this study. This study is based, in part, on data released by the Health and Welfare Data Science Center, Ministry of Health and Welfare. The interpretation and conclusions contained herein do not represent those of the Ministry of Health and Welfare.

Appendix A

Table A1. The list of anticholinergic drugs.

Anticholinergic Drugs
Amitriptyline hydrochloride
Atropine products
Benztropine mesylate
Carisoprodol
Chlorpheniramine maleate
Chlorpromazine hydrochloride
Cyproheptadine hydrochloride
Dicyclomine hydrochloride
Diphenhydramine hydrochloride
Fluphenazine hydrochloride
Hydroxyzine hydrochloride and hydroxyzine pamoate
Hyoscyamine products
Imipramine hydrochloride
Meclizine hydrochloride
Oxybutynin chloride
Perphenazine
Promethazine hydrochloride
Thioridazine hydrochloride
Thiothixene
Tizanidine hydrochloride
Trifluoperazine hydrochloride
Amantadine hydrochloride
Baclofen
Cetirizine hydrochloride
Cimetidine
Clozapine
Cyclobenzaprine hydrochloride
Desipramine hydrochloride
Loperamide hydrochloride

Table A1. *Cont.*

Anticholinergic Drugs
Loratadine
Nortriptyline hydrochloride
Olanzapine
Prochlorperazine maleate
Pseudoephedrine hydrochloride-triprolidine hydrochloride
Tolterodine tartrate
Carbidopa-levodopa
Entacapone
Haloperidol
Metocarbamol
Metoclopramide hydrochloride
Mirtazapine
Paroxetine hydrochloride
Pramipexole dihydrochloride
Quetiapine fumarate
Ranitidine hydrochloride
Risperidone
Selegiline hydrochloride
Trazodone hydrochloride
Ziprasidone hydrochloride

Source: Rudolph, J.L.; Salow, M.J.; Angelini, M.C.; McGlinchey, R.E. The anticholinergic risk scale and anticholinergic adverse effects in older persons. *Arch. Intern. Med.* **2008**, *168*, 508–513.

References

1. Soukup, O.; Winder, M.; Killi, U.K.; Wsol, V.; Jun, D.; Ramalho, T.D.C.; Tobin, G. Acetylcholinesterase Inhibitors and Drugs Acting on Muscarinic Receptors-Potential Crosstalk of Cholinergic Mechanisms during Pharmacological Treatment. *Curr. Neuropharmacol.* **2017**, *15*, 637–653. [CrossRef] [PubMed]
2. Feinberg, M. The Problems of Anticholinergic Adverse Effects in Older Patients. *Drugs Aging* **1993**, *3*, 335–348. [CrossRef]
3. Tune, L.E. Anticholinergic effects of medication in elderly patients. *J. Clin. Psychiatry* **2001**, *62*, 11–14. [PubMed]
4. Gutiérrez, F.; Masiá, M. Improving Outcomes of Elderly Patients with Community-Acquired Pneumonia. *Drugs Aging* **2008**, *25*, 585–610. [CrossRef] [PubMed]
5. Stupka, J.E.; Mortensen, E.M.; Anzueto, A.; Restrepo, M.I. Community-acquired pneumonia in elderly patients. *Aging Health* **2009**, *5*, 763–774. [CrossRef] [PubMed]
6. Chatterjee, S.; Carnahan, R.M.; Chen, H.; Holmes, H.M.; Johnson, M.L.; Aparasu, R.R. Anticholinergic Medication Use and Risk of Pneumonia in Elderly Adults: A Nested Case-Control Study. *J. Am. Geriatr. Soc.* **2016**, *64*, 394–400. [CrossRef]
7. Venkatesan, P.; Gladman, J.R.F.; Macfarlane, J.T.; Barer, D.; Berman, P.; Kinnear, W.; Finch, R.G. A hospital study of community acquired pneumonia in the elderly. *Thorax* **1990**, *45*, 254–258. [CrossRef] [PubMed]
8. Riquelme, R.; Torres, A.; El-Ebiary, M.; De La Bellacasa, J.P.; Estruch, R.; Mensa, J.; Fernández-Solà, J.; Hernández, C.; Rodriguez-Roisin, R. Community-acquired pneumonia in the elderly: A multivariate analysis of risk and prognostic factors. *Am. J. Respir. Crit. Care Med.* **1996**, *154*, 1450–1455. [CrossRef]
9. Huxley, E.J.; Viroslav, J.; Gray, W.R.; Pierce, A.K. Pharyngeal aspiration in normal adults and patients with depressed consciousness. *Am. J. Med.* **1978**, *64*, 564–568. [CrossRef]
10. Paul, K.J.; Walker, R.L.; Dublin, S. Anticholinergic Medications and Risk of Community-Acquired Pneumonia in Elderly Adults: A Population-Based Case-Control Study. *J. Am. Geriatr. Soc.* **2015**, *63*, 476–485. [CrossRef]
11. Marik, P.E.; Kaplan, D. Aspiration Pneumonia and Dysphagia in the Elderly. *Chest* **2003**, *124*, 328–336. [CrossRef]
12. Fick, D.M.; Cooper, J.W.; Wade, W.E.; Waller, J.L.; MacLean, J.R.; Beers, M.H. Updating the Beers criteria for potentially inappropriate medication use in older adults: Results of a US consensus panel of experts. *Arch. Intern. Med.* **2003**, *163*, 2716–2724. [CrossRef] [PubMed]

13. Shrank, W.; Polinski, J.M.; Avorn, J. Quality Indicators for Medication Use in Vulnerable Elders. *J. Am. Geriatr. Soc.* **2007**, *55*, S373–S382. [CrossRef] [PubMed]
14. Gorup, E.; Rifel, J.; Šter, M.P. Anticholinergic burden and most common anticholinergic-acting medicines in older general practice patients. *Slov. J. Public Health* **2018**, *57*, 140–147. [CrossRef] [PubMed]
15. Salahudeen, M.; Duffull, S.B.; Nishtala, P. Anticholinergic burden quantified by anticholinergic risk scales and adverse outcomes in older people: A systematic review. *BMC Geriatr.* **2015**, *15*, 31. [CrossRef]
16. Sittironnarit, G.; Ames, D.; Bush, A.I.; Faux, N.G.; Flicker, L.; Foster, J.; Hilmer, S.N.; Lautenschlager, N.T.; Maruff, P.; Masters, C.L.; et al. Effects of Anticholinergic Drugs on Cognitive Function in Older Australians: Results from the AIBL Study. *Dement. Geriatr. Cogn. Disord.* **2011**, *31*, 173–178. [CrossRef]
17. Rudolph, J.L.; Salow, M.J.; Angelini, M.C.; McGlinchey, R.E. The Anticholinergic Risk Scale and Anticholinergic Adverse Effects in Older Persons. *Arch. Intern. Med.* **2008**, *168*, 508. [CrossRef]
18. Lampela, P.; Tolppanen, A.; Tanskanen, A.; Tiihonen, J.; Hartikainen, S.; Taipale, H. Anticholinergic Exposure and Risk of Pneumonia in Persons with Alzheimer's Disease: A Nested Case-Control Study. *J. Alzheimer Dis.* **2017**, *56*, 119–128. [CrossRef]
19. Miyashita, N.; Yamauchi, Y. Bacterial Pneumonia in Elderly Japanese Populations. *Jpn. Clin. Med.* **2018**, *9*, 1179670717751433. [CrossRef]
20. Lee, T.-Y.; Hsu, Y.-C.; Tseng, H.-C.; Yu, S.-H.; Lin, J.-T.; Wu, M.-S.; Wu, C.-Y. Association of Daily Aspirin Therapy With Risk of Hepatocellular Carcinoma in Patients With Chronic Hepatitis B. *JAMA Intern. Med.* **2019**, *179*, 633–640. [CrossRef]
21. Cheng, Y.-T.; Cheng, C.-T.; Wang, S.-Y.; Wu, V.C.-C.; Chu, P.-H.; Chou, A.-H.; Chen, C.-C.; Ko, P.-J.; Liu, K.-S.; Chen, S.-W. Long-term Outcomes of Endovascular and Open Repair for Traumatic Thoracic Aortic Injury. *JAMA Netw. Open* **2019**, *2*, e187861. [CrossRef]
22. Wang, C.J.; Cheng, S.H.; Wu, J.-Y.; Lin, Y.-P.; Kao, W.-H.; Lin, C.-L.; Chen, Y.-J.; Tsai, S.-L.; Kao, F.-Y.; Huang, A.T. Association of a Bundled-Payment Program With Cost and Outcomes in Full-Cycle Breast Cancer Care. *JAMA Oncol.* **2017**, *3*, 327–334. [CrossRef] [PubMed]
23. Wei, K.-C.; Bee, Y.-S.; Wang, W.-H.; Huang, Y.-T.; Lu, T.-H. Incidence of Cataract Surgery in Patients After Percutaneous Cardiac Intervention in Taiwan. *JAMA Intern. Med.* **2016**, *176*, 710. [CrossRef] [PubMed]
24. Woodhead, M. Inhaled corticosteroids cause pneumonia or do they? *Am. J. Respir. Crit. Care Med.* **2007**, *176*, 111–112. [CrossRef]
25. Farr, B.; Woodhead, M.; Macfarlane, J.; Bartlett, C.; McCracken, J.; Wadsworth, J.; Miller, D. Risk factors for community-acquired pneumonia diagnosed by general practitioners in the community. *Respir. Med.* **2000**, *94*, 422–427. [CrossRef] [PubMed]
26. Almirall, J.; Bolíbar, I.; Serra-Prat, M.; Roig, J.; Hospital, I.; Carandell, E.; Agustí, M.; Ayuso, P.; Estela, A.; Torres, A.; et al. New evidence of risk factors for community-acquired pneumonia: A population-based study. *Eur. Respir. J.* **2008**, *31*, 1274–1284. [CrossRef] [PubMed]
27. Jackson, M.L.; Neuzil, K.M.; Thompson, W.W.; Shay, D.; Yu, O.; Hanson, C.A.; Jackson, L.A. The Burden of Community-Acquired Pneumonia in Seniors: Results of a Population-Based Study. *Clin. Infect. Dis.* **2004**, *39*, 1642–1650. [CrossRef]
28. Bouter, K.; Diepersloot, R.J.; Van Romunde, L.K.; Uitslager, R.; Masurel, N.; Hoekstra, J.B.; Erkelens, D.W. Effect of epidemic influenza on ketoacidosis, pneumonia and death in diabetes mellitus: A hospital register survey of 1976–1979 in The Netherlands. *Diabetes Res. Clin. Pract.* **1991**, *12*, 61–68. [CrossRef]
29. Martin, J.-J.; Boavida, J.M.; Raposo, J.F.; Froes, F.; Nunes, B.; Ribeiro, R.T.; Macedo, M.; Penha-Gonçalves, C. Diabetes hinders community-acquired pneumonia outcomes in hospitalized patients. *BMJ Open Diabetes Res. Care* **2016**, *4*, e000181. [CrossRef]
30. Kalf, J.; De Swart, B.; Bloem, B.R.; Munneke, M. Prevalence of oropharyngeal dysphagia in Parkinson's disease: A meta-analysis. *Park. Relat. Disord.* **2012**, *18*, 311–315. [CrossRef]
31. Loeb, M.; Neupane, B.; Walter, S.D.; Hanning, R.; Carusone, S.C.; Lewis, D.; Krueger, P.; Simor, A.E.; Nicolle, L.; Marrie, T.J. Environmental Risk Factors for Community-Acquired Pneumonia Hospitalization in Older Adults. *J. Am. Geriatr. Soc.* **2009**, *57*, 1036–1040. [CrossRef] [PubMed]
32. Almirall, J.; Rofes, L.; Serra-Prat, M.; Icart, R.; Palomera, E.; Arreola, V.; Clavé, P. Oropharyngeal dysphagia is a risk factor for community-acquired pneumonia in the elderly. *Eur. Respir. J.* **2012**, *41*, 923–928. [CrossRef] [PubMed]

33. Chang, Y.-P.; Yang, C.-J.; Hu, K.-F.; Chao, A.-C.; Chang, Y.-H.; Hsieh, K.-P.; Tsai, J.-H.; Ho, P.-S.; Lim, S.-Y. Risk factors for pneumonia among patients with Parkinson's disease: A Taiwan nationwide population-based study. *Neuropsychiatr. Dis. Treat.* **2016**, *12*, 1037–1046. [CrossRef]
34. McDonald, H.; Thomas, S.L.; Nitsch, R. Chronic kidney disease as a risk factor for acute community-acquired infections in high-income countries: A systematic review. *BMJ Open* **2014**, *4*, e004100. [CrossRef]
35. Bornheimer, R.; Shea, K.M.; Sato, R.; Weycker, D.; Pelton, S.I. Risk of exacerbation following pneumonia in adults with heart failure or chronic obstructive pulmonary disease. *PLoS ONE* **2017**, *12*, e0184877. [CrossRef]
36. Hsu, W.-T.; Lai, C.-C.; Wang, Y.-H.; Tseng, P.-H.; Wang, K.; Wang, C.-Y.; Chen, L. Risk of pneumonia in patients with gastroesophageal reflux disease: A population-based cohort study. *PLoS ONE* **2017**, *12*, e0183808. [CrossRef]
37. Laheij, R.J.; Sturkenboom, M.C.J.M.; Hassing, R.-J.; Dieleman, J.; Stricker, B.H.C.; Jansen, J.B.M.J. Risk of Community-Acquired Pneumonia and Use of Gastric Acid–Suppressive Drugs. *JAMA* **2004**, *292*, 1955–1960. [CrossRef]

5

Food Insecurity is Associated with Mild Cognitive Impairment among Middle-Aged and Older Adults in South Africa: Findings from a Nationally Representative Survey

Ai Koyanagi [1,2,3,*], Nicola Veronese [4,5], Brendon Stubbs [6,7,8], Davy Vancampfort [9,10], Andrew Stickley [11,12], Hans Oh [13], Jae Il Shin [14,15,16], Sarah Jackson [17], Lee Smith [18] and Elvira Lara [2,19]

1 Research and Development Unit, Parc Sanitari Sant Joan de Déu, Universitat de Barcelona, Fundació Sant Joan de Déu, 08830 Barcelona, Spain
2 Instituto de Salud Carlos III, Centro de Investigación Biomédica en Red de Salud Mental, CIBERSAM, 28029 Madrid, Spain; elvira.lara@uam.es
3 ICREA, Pg. Lluis Companys 23, 08010 Barcelona, Spain
4 Aging Branch, Neuroscience Institute, National Research Council, 35128 Padova, Italy; ilmannato@gmail.com
5 National Institute of Gastroenterology "S. De Bellis" Research Hospital, Castellana Grotte, 70013 Bari, Italy
6 Physiotherapy Department, South London and Maudsley NHS Foundation Trust, Denmark Hill, London SE5 8AZ, UK; brendon.stubbs@kcl.ac.uk
7 Department of Psychological Medicine, Institute of Psychiatry, Psychology and Neuroscience, King's College London, London WC2R 2LS, UK
8 Faculty of Health, Social Care and Education, Anglia Ruskin University, Chelmsford CM1 1SQ, UK
9 Department of Rehabilitation Sciences, KU Leuven, 3001 Leuven, Belgium; davy.vancampfort@kuleuven.be
10 University Psychiatric Center KU Leuven, KU Leuven, 3000 Leuven, Belgium
11 Department of Preventive Intervention for Psychiatric Disorders, National Institute of Mental Health, National Center of Neurology and Psychiatry, Kodaira, Tokyo 187-8553, Japan; amstick66@gmail.com
12 The Stockholm Center for Health and Social Change (SCOHOST), Södertörn University, 141 89 Huddinge, Sweden
13 School of Social Work, University of Southern California, CA 90015, USA; hansoh@usc.edu
14 Department of Pediatrics, Yonsei University College of Medicine, Yonsei-ro 50, Seodaemun-gu, C.P.O. Box 8044, Seoul 03722, Korea; SHINJI@yuhs.ac
15 Division of Pediatric Nephrology, Severance Children's Hospital, Seoul 03722, Korea
16 Institute of Kidney Disease Research, Yonsei University College of Medicine, Seoul 03722, Korea
17 Department of Behavioural Science and Health, University College London, London WC1E 7HB, UK; s.e.jackson@ucl.ac.uk
18 The Cambridge Centre for Sport and Exercise Sciences, Anglia Ruskin University, Cambridge CB1 1PT, UK; Lee.Smith@anglia.ac.uk
19 Department of Psychiatry, Hospital Universitario de La Princesa, Instituto de Investigación Sanitaria Princesa (IIS-Princesa), 28006 Madrid, Spain
* Correspondence: a.koyanagi@pssjd.org

Abstract: There are no studies on the association between food insecurity and mild cognitive impairment (MCI). Thus, cross-sectional, community-based data on individuals aged ≥50 years from the World Health Organization's Study on Global AGEing and Adult Health (SAGE) conducted in South Africa (2007–2008) were analyzed to assess this association. The definition of MCI was based on the National Institute on Ageing-Alzheimer's Association criteria. Past 12-month food insecurity was assessed with two questions on frequency of eating less and hunger due to lack of food. Multivariable logistic regression analysis was conducted. The sample consisted of 3,672 individuals aged ≥50 years [mean (SD) age 61.4 (18.3); 56% females]. The prevalence of MCI was

8.5%, while 11.0% and 20.8% experienced moderate and severe food insecurity, respectively. After adjustment for potential confounders, moderate and severe food insecurity were associated with 2.82 (95%CI = 1.65–4.84) and 2.51 (95%CI = 1.63–3.87) times higher odds for MCI compared with no food insecurity, respectively. The OR for those aged ≥65 years with severe food insecurity was particularly high (OR = 3.87; 95%CI = 2.20–6.81). In conclusion, food insecurity was strongly associated with MCI among South African older adults. Future longitudinal research is required to assess whether addressing food insecurity may reduce risk of MCI and subsequent dementia.

Keywords: mild cognitive impairment; food insecurity; South Africa; epidemiology

---

1. Introduction

Dementia is a debilitating syndrome that results in the deterioration of memory, thinking, behavior, and the ability to conduct daily activities. It is one of the main causes of disability and dependency among the older adult population globally [1]. The 2016 Global Burden of Disease (GBD) study showed that 28.8 million disability-adjusted life years (DALYs) are attributed to dementia, and that dementia is the fifth leading cause of death globally [2]. Worldwide, it has been estimated that approximately 50 million people have dementia, of which about 60% live in low- and middle-income countries (LMICs), while there are nearly 10 million new cases each year [3]. As a consequence of global aging, the total number of people with dementia is expected to triple from its current figure by 2050 and reach 152 million, with this increase being largely attributable to rising numbers in LMICs [3]. Despite the overwhelming burden of dementia, especially in the years to come, there are no truly disease-modifying treatments for dementia [4]. Thus, there is a crucial need to identify modifiable risk factors for the preclinical transitional stages of dementia such as mild cognitive impairment (MCI). MCI has a high progression rate to dementia (12%, 20%, and 50% at 1, 3, and 5 years, respectively [5]), and is increasingly being considered as an important stage for intervention to prevent or delay the onset of dementia.

Currently, there is increasing evidence that food insecurity is associated with cognitive decline [6–8]. Food insecurity is defined as "limited or uncertain availability of nutritionally adequate and safe foods or limited or uncertain ability to acquire food in socially acceptable ways" [9]. It has been hypothesized that food insecurity may increase risk of cognitive decline via stress, depression, or poor nutritional intake [8]. However, there are no studies specifically on the association between food insecurity and MCI, or studies on food insecurity and any form of cognitive impairment from LMICs despite the fact that food insecurity is more common in this setting [10].

South Africa is an apposite setting in which to examine the association between food insecurity and MCI as the level of food insecurity has been reported to be high in this country [11], which may be attributable to the extremely high levels of absolute poverty compared with other middle-income countries [12]. Furthermore, rapid urbanization, the HIV epidemic, and increasing food prices are also likely to be implicated in the high rate of food insecurity in South Africa [11–13]. Finally, an extremely high prevalence of obesity and hypertension have been reported in South Africa [14], and these factors can potentially contribute to an upward trend in dementia in the future as these conditions are known to be risk factors for dementia [15]. Thus, the aim of the current study was to assess whether food insecurity is associated with MCI using data from a nationally representative sample of older adults in South Africa collected as part of the Study on Global AGEing and Adult Health (SAGE).

2. Materials and Methods

Data from the SAGE survey conducted in South Africa between 2007–2008 were analyzed. This dataset is publically available to all interested researchers via the WHO website (http://www.who.int/healthinfo/sage/en/) upon request. Detailed sampling information can be found in the above-mentioned WHO website. Briefly, a stratified multistage cluster sampling design was used to obtain a nationally representative sample. Strata were defined by the nine provinces (Eastern Cape, Free State, Gauteng, Kwa-Zulu Natal, Limpopo, Mpumalanga, North West, Northern Cape and Western Cape), locality (urban or rural), and predominant racial group (African/Black, White, Colored and Indian/Asian). Enumeration areas (EAs) constituted the primary sampling units (PSUs) and were selected with probability proportional to size: the measure of size being the number of individuals aged 50 or over in the EA. A different questionnaire was administered to a proxy respondent if the selected individual could not participate in the survey due to limited cognitive function. Information from proxies was not used in the current study. The survey response rate was 75%. Household weights were post-stratified by province and locality according to the South African Community Survey 2007. Individual weights were post-stratified by province, sex and age groups according to the 2009 Medium Mid-Year population estimates from Statistics South Africa. Ethical approval was obtained from the WHO Ethical Review Committee and Human Sciences Research Council, Pretoria, South Africa. All participants provided written informed consent.

2.1. *Mild Cognitive Impairment (MCI)*

We used the recommendations of the National Institute on Aging-Alzheimer's Association to define MCI [16]. The exact same algorithms used in past SAGE publications were applied [17,18]. Briefly, MCI was defined as fulfilling all of the following conditions:

(a) Concern regarding cognitive changes: This condition referred to replying 'bad' or 'very bad' to the question "How would you best describe your memory at present?" and/or answering 'worse' to the question "Compared to 12 months ago, would you say your memory is now better, the same or worse than it was then?"

(b) Objective evidence of impairment in at least one cognitive domain: The following performance tests were used to assess cognitive function: word list immediate and delayed verbal recall based on the Consortium to Establish a Registry for Alzheimer's Disease [19], which evaluated learning and episodic memory; digit span forward and backwards based on the Weschler Adult Intelligence Scale [20], that assessed working and attention memory; and the animal naming task [19], which evaluated verbal fluency. Individuals with a level of performance that was below -1 SD after adjustment for education and age on at least one of these tests were considered to have this condition.

(c) Preserved independence in functional abilities: Questions on self-reported past-30-day difficulties with basic activities of daily living (ADL) were used to assess this condition [21]. Specifically, the questions were: "How much difficulty did you have in getting dressed?" and "How much difficulty did you have with eating (including cutting up your food)?" The response options included none, mild, moderate, severe, and extreme (cannot do). Independence in functional activities was considered to be preserved if the participant answered either none, mild, or moderate to both of these questions. All other participants were omitted from the analysis (83 individuals aged $\geq$50 years).

(d) Absence of dementia: Individuals who could not participate in the survey due to severe cognitive impairment were excluded from the current study.

2.2. *Food Insecurity*

Food insecurity was defined with the use of the two following questions: "In the last 12 months, how often did you ever eat less than you felt you should because there wasn't enough food?" and "In the last 12 months, were you ever hungry, but didn't eat because you couldn't afford enough food?" Both of these questions had as response options: every month (coded = 1); almost every month (coded = 2); some months, but not every month (coded = 3); only in 1 or 2 months (coded = 4); never (coded = 5). These items were based on similar items found in food security questionnaires such as the US Household Food Security Survey Module and National Health and Nutrition Examination Survey (NHANES) Food Security module. As in a previous SAGE study, those who answered 1 through 3 to both questions or answered 1 to either item were categorized as severely food insecure. Those who did not fulfill the criteria for severe food insecurity but answered 2 through 4 for either question were coded as moderately food insecure. Those who answered 5 to both items were categorized as food secure [22].

2.3. Control Variables

Past literature was used as a guide to select the control variables [7]. Specifically, these included sex, age (years), years of education, wealth quintiles based on income, race (Black, White, other), low physical activity, smoking (never, past, current), alcohol use in the past 30 days, past 12 month DSM-IV depression, body mass index (BMI) based on measured weight and height [<18.5 (underweight), 18.5–24.9 (normal), 25.0–29.9 (overweight), $\geq$30 kg/m^2 (obese)], and chronic physical conditions (diabetes, hypertension, stroke). Stroke and diabetes were based only on lifetime self-reported diagnosis. Hypertension referred to having self-reported diagnosis, systolic blood pressure $\geq$140 mmHg, or diastolic blood pressure $\geq$90 mmHg. The Global Physical Activity Questionnaire was used to assess the level of physical activity [23]. Low physical activity was defined as <150 minutes of moderate-to-vigorous physical activity in a typical week [24]. The endorsement of DSM-IV depression was based on the World Mental Health Survey version of the Composite International Diagnostic Interview [25].

2.4. Statistical Analysis

The statistical analysis was done with Stata 14.1 (Stata Corp LP, College station, TX, USA). The analysis was limited to those aged $\geq$50 years. Middle-aged individuals were also included in the current study because cognitive dysfunction can appear up to 10 years prior to dementia diagnosis [26], and intervening in mid-life is now considered crucial [27]. The difference in sample characteristics by level of food insecurity was tested by Chi-squared tests and Student's *t*-tests for categorical and continuous variables, respectively.

We conducted multivariable logistic regression analysis to assess the association between food insecurity (exposure) and MCI (outcome) in the overall sample (i.e., age $\geq$50 years) and by age group (50–64 and $\geq$65 years) as the risk factors for MCI may differ between mid-life and late-life [28]. The regression analysis was adjusted for age, sex, education, wealth, race, physical activity, smoking, alcohol use, BMI, diabetes, stroke, hypertension, and depression. Given that some authors have suggested that depression may be an important mediator in the association between food insecurity and cognitive decline [8], we also constructed a model without adjustment for depression using the overall sample to assess the degree to which the association between food insecurity and MCI is explained by depression. All variables were included in the regression analysis as categorical variables with the exception of age and years of education (continuous variables). The sample weighting and the complex study design were taken into account in the analyses. Results from the regression analyses are presented as odds ratios (ORs) with 95% confidence intervals (CIs). The level of statistical significance was set at $p < 0.05$.

3. Results

The final analytical sample comprised 3,672 individuals aged $\geq$50 years [mean (SD) age 61.4 (18.3) years; 56% females]. The proportion of those aged 50–64 and $\geq$65 years was 66.8% and 33.2%, respectively. Overall, the prevalence of MCI was 8.5% (95%CI = 6.9–10.3), while the prevalence of moderate (unweighted n = 332) and severe (unweighted n = 677) food insecurity was 11.0% (95%CI = 9.0–13.4) and 20.8% (95%CI = 17.9–23.9), respectively. The sample characteristics are shown in Table 1. Compared to respondents without food insecurity, those who were food insecure were significantly more likely to have less education and wealth, and lower levels of physical activity, and be of Black race.

Table 1. Sample characteristics (overall and by food insecurity).

Characteristic		Overall	Food Insecurity			p-Value [a]
			None	Moderate	Severe	
Sex	Female	56.0	54.4	56.5	62.8	0.047
	Male	44.0	43.5	37.2	43.6	
Age (years)	Mean (SD)	61.4 (18.3)	61.7 (18.9)	62.5 (17.4)	60.1 (17.1)	0.074
Education (years)	Mean (SD)	6.1 (10.1)	6.8 (11.0)	4.5 (8.1)	4.7 (7.3)	<0.001
Wealth	Poorest	20.7	14.7	27.7	32.7	<0.001
	Poorer	19.9	17.9	20.8	26.4	
	Middle	18.5	17.7	25.1	19.8	
	Richer	19.8	22.1	20.3	13.2	
	Richest	21.1	27.6	6.0	7.9	
Race	Black	74.3	68.2	80.1	88.9	<0.001
	White	9.2	12.9	2.0	1.5	
	Other	16.5	19.0	17.9	9.6	
Low physical activity	No	50.0	54.1	39.5	41.9	0.002
	Yes	50.0	45.9	60.5	58.1	
Smoking	Never	66.6	66.1	69.0	66.7	0.162
	Past	23.8	23.3	20.2	27.3	
	Current	9.7	10.7	10.8	6.0	
Alcohol consumption	No	86.0	86.8	91.1	80.7	0.007
	Yes	14.0	13.2	8.9	19.3	
BMI (kg/m^2)	Normal	24.0	23.3	21.5	25.8	0.382
	Overweight	26.5	27.8	22.1	25.5	
	Obese	46.6	46.4	51.9	45.1	
	Underweight	2.9	2.5	4.5	3.6	
Diabetes	No	90.9	91.3	88.1	90.5	0.465
	Yes	9.1	8.7	11.9	9.5	
Stroke	No	96.6	96.6	96.7	96.3	0.951
	Yes	3.4	3.4	3.3	3.7	
Hypertension	No	21.4	21.8	16.7	20.5	0.278
	Yes	78.6	78.2	83.3	79.5	
Depression	No	97.1	97.7	97.6	95.0	0.064
	Yes	2.9	2.3	2.4	5.0	

Abbreviation: SD Standard deviation; BMI Body mass index; Data are percentage unless otherwise stated. [a] p-value was calculated by Chi-squared tests and Student's t-tests for categorical and continuous variables, respectively.

The prevalence of MCI was higher among those with food insecurity than in those without food insecurity (Figure 1). For example, overall, the prevalence of MCI among those without food insecurity was 5.9% but this increased to 14.8% and 13.5% among those with moderate and severe food insecurity, respectively.

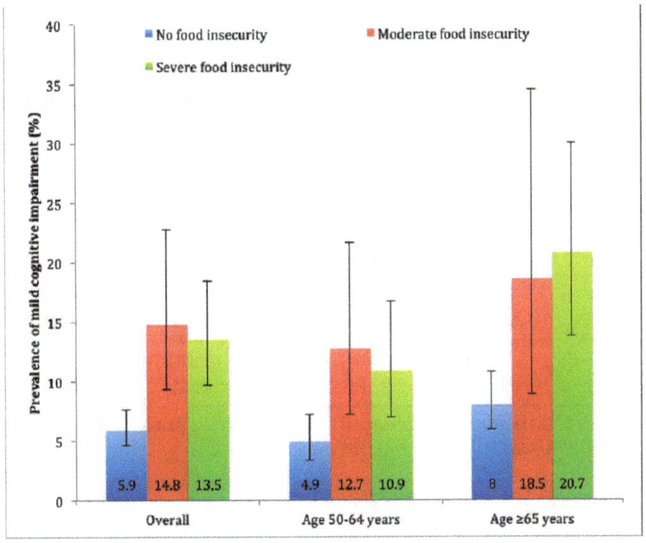

Figure 1. Prevalence of mild cognitive impairment by food insecurity status. Estimates are based on weighted sample. Bars denote 95% confidence interval.

The association between food insecurity and MCI estimated by multivariable logistic regression is shown in Table 2. After adjustment for a variety of sociodemographic and behavioral factors as well as physical health conditions and depression, compared to no food insecurity, moderate and severe food insecurity were associated with 2.82 (95%CI = 1.65–4.84) and 2.51 (95%CI = 1.63–3.87) times higher odds for MCI, respectively, in the overall sample. These estimates were not substantially different from the model that did not include depression with the corresponding figures being 2.83 (95%CI = 1.65–4.85) and 2.58 (95%CI = 1.68–3.97), respectively (data shown only in text). The OR among those aged ≥65 years with severe food insecurity was particularly elevated (OR = 3.87; 95%CI = 2.20–6.81).

Table 2. Association of food insecurity and other covariates with mild cognitive impairment (outcome) estimated by multivariable logistic regression.

Characteristic	Category	Age					
		Overall		50–64 years		≥65 years	
		OR	95%CI	OR	95%CI	OR	95%CI
Food insecurity	None	1.00		1.00		1.00	
	Moderate	2.82 ***	[1.65,4.84]	2.84 **	[1.41,5.69]	2.76 *	[1.19,6.41]
	Severe	2.51 ***	[1.63,3.87]	1.98 *	[1.06,3.72]	3.87 ***	[2.20,6.81]
Sex	Female	1.00		1.00		1.00	
	Male	0.56 **	[0.37,0.85]	0.59	[0.32,1.06]	0.54	[0.26,1.10]
Age (years)		1.05 ***	[1.03,1.07]	1.05	[0.99,1.11]	1.04 *	[1.01,1.08]
Education (years)		0.98	[0.93,1.03]	0.95	[0.89,1.02]	1.01	[0.94,1.09]
Wealth	Poorest	1.00		1.00		1.00	
	Poorer	1.08	[0.64,1.83]	0.68	[0.34,1.36]	2.32	[0.99,5.40]
	Middle	1.51	[0.82,2.80]	1.06	[0.52,2.16]	2.95	[0.98,8.87]
	Richer	1.82	[0.96,3.46]	1.54	[0.73,3.27]	2.45	[0.87,6.93]
	Richest	1.35	[0.60,3.04]	1.12	[0.37,3.42]	2.11	[0.63,7.09]
Race	Black	1.00		1.00		1.00	
	White	0.23 *	[0.07,0.74]	0.18	[0.03,1.02]	0.24 *	[0.06,0.96]
	Other	0.87	[0.50,1.50]	0.92	[0.46,1.80]	0.58	[0.25,1.34]
Low physical activity	No	1.00		1.00		1.00	
	Yes	0.79	[0.52,1.20]	0.72	[0.40,1.31]	0.75	[0.45,1.23]
Smoking	Never	1.00		1.00		1.00	
	Past	1.11	[0.67,1.82]	1.45	[0.76,2.77]	0.71	[0.36,1.37]
	Current	1.15	[0.63,2.11]	1.16	[0.54,2.48]	1.1	[0.41,2.93]
Alcohol consumption	No	1.00		1.00		1.00	
	Yes	2.44 **	[1.39,4.28]	2.90 **	[1.49,5.64]	1.57	[0.71,3.48]
BMI (kg/m^2)	Normal	1.00		1.00		1.00	
	Overweight	0.95	[0.53,1.69]	1.69	[0.82,3.49]	0.40 *	[0.18,0.89]
	Obese	1.17	[0.74,1.85]	1.63	[0.85,3.11]	0.61	[0.31,1.21]
	Underweight	0.89	[0.40,2.01]	0.92	[0.30,2.84]	0.76	[0.20,2.80]
Diabetes	No	1.00		1.00		1.00	
	Yes	0.9	[0.46,1.76]	0.97	[0.39,2.43]	0.87	[0.33,2.29]
Stroke	No	1.00		1.00		1.00	
	Yes	4.64 ***	[1.91,11.29]	5.02 **	[1.81,13.91]	2.92 *	[1.02,8.39]
Hypertension	No	1.00		1.00		1.00	
	Yes	0.9	[0.55,1.46]	1.17	[0.58,2.34]	0.56	[0.30,1.03]
Depression	No	1.00		1.00		1.00	
	Yes	1.77	[0.68,4.58]	2.41	[0.92,6.31]	0.58	[0.06,6.00]

Abbreviation: OR Odds ratio; CI Confidence interval; BMI Body mass index. Models are mutually adjusted for all variables in the Table. * $p < 0.05$, ** $p < 0.01$, *** $p < 0.001$.

4. Discussion

In our study on community-dwelling adults aged ≥50 years in South Africa, we found a high prevalence of food insecurity (31.8%). After adjustment for potential confounders, moderate and severe food insecurity were associated with significant 2.82 and 2.51 times higher odds for MCI, while the OR was particularly elevated for severe food insecurity among those aged ≥65 years (OR = 3.87). Depression was not a major explanatory factor in this association.

To the best of our knowledge, this is the first study to specifically examine the relationship between food insecurity and MCI. Our findings are in line with previous studies that have examined the association between food insecurity and cognitive function in the USA although these studies were on general cognitive function and not MCI. One community-based cross-sectional study conducted among a representative sample of 1358 Puerto Ricans aged 45–75 years living in Massachusetts found that the adjusted difference in the Mini-Mental State Examination (MMSE) score was 0.90 lower among those with very low food security as compared to those who were food secure [8]. A longitudinal follow-up study among 597 participants aged 40–75 years based on the same study population found that food insecurity at baseline was associated with lower global cognitive function after two years of follow-up [7]. Finally, one cross-sectional US study using data from the NHANES found that among 1851 adults between 60 and 85 years, food insecurity was associated with poor cognitive function [6].

The exact mechanisms linking food insecurity and MCI are unknown, but there are several hypotheses. It is possible that stress resulting from food insecurity may increase the risk of MCI. For example, prolonged elevation of cortisol (an HPA axis response to chronic stress) can lead to alterations in brain structure and function (e.g., in the hippocampus) and subsequent cognitive decline [29]. Also, increases in pro-inflammatory cytokines induced by stress [30] may lead to an increased risk of dementia [31]. Furthermore, food insecurity often compromises diet quality, as people tend to switch to more affordable but less nutritious food when food is scarce (e.g., high fat and carbohydrates, low vitamins and micronutrients) [32]. Poor diet has been associated with increased risk of cognitive decline. For example, vitamin B, C, and E have all been shown to have a protective effect against dementia [33]. Furthermore, randomized clinical trials have shown that supplementation of n-3 polyunsaturated fatty acids [34] and folic acid [35] may improve cognitive function in older people with MCI. Finally, high carbohydrate intake has been associated with higher risk of MCI [36].

Our finding that a particularly strong association was observed among older individuals concurs with that of the study by Gao and colleagues [8], which found that the difference in MMSE scores between very low food insecurity and food secure were −1.75 and −0.48 for those aged ≥60 and <60 years, respectively [8]. This age difference may be related to increased vulnerability of the brain among the older population. For example, older adults have smaller hippocampal volumes and this may increase susceptibility to cognitive deficits when exposed to stress [37]. The fact that people aged ≥65 years had 3.87 times higher odds for MCI compared with those without food insecurity is an important finding as the risk of dementia is particularly elevated in this age group [38].

Strengths of the study include the large sample size and the use of nationally representative data. However, some limitations should be taken into consideration when interpreting the findings. First, participants with mild forms of dementia could have been included in our study sample as the study did not include a clinical assessment of dementia. Second, there is no consensus regarding the acceptable level of functional impairment in MCI [39]. The definition of preservation of independence in functional abilities used in our study, which has been used in previous publications [17,18,28,40], was rather conservative. This was done to avoid the omission of MCI cases with disability not related to their cognitive ability. Despite these potential limitations, it is worth noting that the prevalence of MCI in our study was consistent with previously reported figures [41]. Third, data on biomarkers such as cerebrospinal fluid Aβ and tau were not available. These data could have provided a better understanding on how food insecurity affects brain pathology [4]. Fourth, the estimates in the analyses stratified by age should be interpreted with caution as the sample size was small and some estimates had wide confidence intervals. Next, we lacked information on HIV infection, which has been reported to be associated with a higher risk of food insecurity [42] and impaired cognitive function [43]. However, given that the link between food insecurity and HIV infection is likely to be mainly explained by poverty [42], we believe that the adjustment for wealth in our study is likely to have minimized the potential for residual confounding due to HIV infection. Furthermore, our measure of food insecurity was based on two questions and did not constitute a comprehensive food insecurity measure. Finally, because this was a cross-sectional study, causality cannot be inferred. For example, it is possible that people with cognitive impairments have difficulty in utilizing social safety net services, and this might have led to food insecurity.

5. Conclusions

In conclusion, we found that the prevalence of food insecurity is high in South African older adults, and that food insecurity is associated with MCI, with this association being particularly pronounced among individuals aged ≥65 years. Although biological plausibility suggests that food insecurity may lead to MCI, future studies with a longitudinal and experimental design are warranted to assess causality and the utility of addressing food insecurity as a preventive strategy for MCI and subsequent dementia.

Author Contributions: Conceptualization, A.K. and E.L.; methodology, A.K., N.V.; formal analysis, A.K., N.V., E.L; writing—original draft preparation, A.K.; writing—review and editing, all authors.

Acknowledgments: Ai Koyanagi's work is supported by the PI15/00862 project, integrated into the National R + D + I and funded by the ISCIII - General Branch Evaluation and Promotion of Health Research - and the European Regional Development Fund (ERDF-FEDER).

References

1. Wimo, A.; Guerchet, M.; Ali, G.C.; Wu, Y.T.; Prina, A.M.; Winblad, B.; Jonsson, L.; Liu, Z.; Prince, M. The worldwide costs of dementia 2015 and comparisons with 2010. *Alzheimers Dement.* **2017**, *13*, 1–7. [CrossRef] [PubMed]
2. GBD 2016 Dementia Collaborators. Global, regional, and national burden of Alzheimer's disease and other dementias, 1990–2016: A systematic analysis for the Global Burden of Disease Study 2016. *Lancet Neurol.* **2019**, *18*, 88–106. [CrossRef]
3. World Health Organization. Available online: https://www.who.int/news-room/fact-sheets/detail/dementia (accessed on 20 February 2019).
4. Livingston, G.; Sommerlad, A.; Orgeta, V.; Costafreda, S.G.; Huntley, J.; Ames, D.; Ballard, C.; Banerjee, S.; Burns, A.; Cohen-Mansfield, J.; et al. Dementia prevention, intervention, and care. *Lancet* **2017**, *390*, 2673–2734. [CrossRef]
5. Solfrizzi, V.; Panza, F.; Colacicco, A.M.; D'Introno, A.; Capurso, C.; Torres, F.; Grigoletto, F.; Maggi, S.; Del Parigi, A.; Reiman, E.M.; et al. Vascular risk factors, incidence of MCI, and rates of progression to dementia. *Neurology* **2004**, *63*, 1882–1891. [CrossRef]
6. Frith, E.; Loprinzi, P.D. Food insecurity and cognitive function in older adults: Brief report. *Clin. Nutr.* **2017**. [CrossRef]
7. Wong, J.C.; Scott, T.; Wilde, P.; Li, Y.G.; Tucker, K.L.; Gao, X. Food Insecurity Is Associated with Subsequent Cognitive Decline in the Boston Puerto Rican Health Study. *J. Nutr.* **2016**, *146*, 1740–1745. [CrossRef] [PubMed]
8. Gao, X.; Scott, T.; Falcon, L.M.; Wilde, P.E.; Tucker, K.L. Food insecurity and cognitive function in Puerto Rican adults. *Am. J. Clin. Nutr.* **2009**, *89*, 1197–1203. [CrossRef] [PubMed]
9. Bickel, G.; Nord, M.; Price, C.; Hamilton, W.; Cook, J. *Guide to Measuring Household Food Security*; Department of Agriculture, Food and Nutrition Service: Alexandria, VA, USA, 2000.
10. FAO; IFAD; UNICEF; WFP; WHO. *The State of Food Security and Nutrition in the World 2017*; Building Resilience for Peace and Food Security; FAO: Rome, Italy, 2017.
11. Misselhorn, A.; Hendriks, S.L. A systematic review of sub-national food insecurity research in South Africa: Missed opportunities for policy insights. *PLoS ONE* **2017**, *12*, e0182399. [CrossRef]

12. Altman, M.; Hart, T.G.; Jacobs, P.T. Household food security status in South Africa. *Agrekon* **2009**, *48*, 345–361. [CrossRef]
13. Misselhorn, A.A. What drives food insecurity in southern Africa? A meta-analysis of household economy studies. *Glob. Environ. Chang.* **2005**, *15*, 33–43. [CrossRef]
14. Stubbs, B.; Vancampfort, D.; Veronese, N.; Schofield, P.; Lin, P.Y.; Tseng, P.T.; Solmi, M.; Thompson, T.; Carvalho, A.F.; Koyanagi, A. Multimorbidity and perceived stress: A population-based cross-sectional study among older adults across six low- and middle-income countries. *Maturitas* **2018**, *107*, 84–91. [CrossRef]
15. World Alzheimer Report 2015. Available online: https://www.alz.co.uk/research/world-report-2015 (accessed on 31 January 2019).
16. Albert, M.S.; DeKosky, S.T.; Dickson, D.; Dubois, B.; Feldman, H.H.; Fox, N.C.; Gamst, A.; Holtzman, D.M.; Jagust, W.J.; Petersen, R.C.; et al. The diagnosis of mild cognitive impairment due to Alzheimer's disease: Recommendations from the National Institute on Aging-Alzheimer's Association workgroups on diagnostic guidelines for Alzheimer's disease. *Alzheimers Dement.* **2011**, *7*, 270–279. [CrossRef]
17. Koyanagi, A.; Lara, E.; Stubbs, B.; Carvalho, A.F.; Oh, H.; Stickley, A.; Veronese, N.; Vancampfort, D. Chronic Physical Conditions, Multimorbidity, and Mild Cognitive Impairment in Low- and Middle-Income Countries. *J. Am. Geriatr. Soc.* **2018**. [CrossRef] [PubMed]
18. Koyanagi, A.; Oh, H.; Vancampfort, D.; Carvalho, A.F.; Veronese, N.; Stubbs, B.; Lara, E. Perceived Stress and Mild Cognitive Impairment among 32,715 Community-Dwelling Older Adults across Six Low- and Middle-Income Countries. *Gerontology* **2019**, *65*, 155–163. [CrossRef]
19. Morris, J.C.; Heyman, A.; Mohs, R.C.; Hughes, J.P.; van Belle, G.; Fillenbaum, G.; Mellits, E.D.; Clark, C. The Consortium to Establish a Registry for Alzheimer's Disease (CERAD). Part I. Clinical and neuropsychological assessment of Alzheimer's disease. *Neurology* **1989**, *39*, 1159–1165.
20. The Psychological Corporation. *The Psychological Corporation: The WAIS III-WMS III Updated Technical Manual*; The Psychological Corporation: San Antonio, TX, USA, 2002.
21. Katz, S.; Ford, A.B.; Moskowitz, R.W.; Jackson, B.A.; Jaffe, M.W. Studies of illness in the aged. The index of ADL: A standardized measure of biological and psychosocial function. *JAMA* **1963**, *185*, 914–919. [CrossRef]
22. Schrock, J.M.; McClure, H.H.; Snodgrass, J.J.; Liebert, M.A.; Charlton, K.E.; Arokiasamy, P.; Naidoo, N.; Kowal, P. Food insecurity partially mediates associations between social disadvantage and body composition among older adults in india: Results from the study on global AGEing and adult health (SAGE). *Am. J. Hum. Biol.* **2017**, *29*. [CrossRef] [PubMed]
23. Bull, F.C.; Maslin, T.S.; Armstrong, T. Global physical activity questionnaire (GPAQ): Nine country reliability and validity study. *J. Phys. Act. Health* **2009**, *6*, 790–804. [CrossRef] [PubMed]
24. Vancampfort, D.; Stubbs, B.; Lara, E.; Vandenbulcke, M.; Swinnen, N.; Koyanagi, A. Mild cognitive impairment and physical activity in the general population: Findings from six low- and middle-income countries. *Exp. Gerontol.* **2017**, *100*, 100–105. [CrossRef] [PubMed]
25. Vancampfort, D.; Stubbs, B.; Mugisha, J.; Firth, J.; Schuch, F.B.; Koyanagi, A. Correlates of sedentary behavior in 2,375 people with depression from 6 low- and middle-income countries. *J. Affect. Disord.* **2018**, *234*, 97–104. [CrossRef]
26. Amieva, H.; Jacqmin-Gadda, H.; Orgogozo, J.M.; Le Carret, N.; Helmer, C.; Letenneur, L.; Barberger-Gateau, P.; Fabrigoule, C.; Dartigues, J.F. The 9 year cognitive decline before dementia of the Alzheimer type: A prospective population-based study. *Brain* **2005**, *128 Pt 5*, 1093–1101. [CrossRef]
27. World Alzheimer Report 2014. Available online: https://www.alz.co.uk/research/world-report-2014 (accessed on 29 January 2019).
28. Lara, E.; Koyanagi, A.; Olaya, B.; Lobo, A.; Miret, M.; Tyrovolas, S.; Ayuso-Mateos, J.L.; Haro, J.M. Mild cognitive impairment in a Spanish representative sample: Prevalence and associated factors. *Int. J. Geriatr. Psychiatry* **2016**, *31*, 858–867. [CrossRef]
29. Pruessner, J.C.; Dedovic, K.; Pruessner, M.; Lord, C.; Buss, C.; Collins, L.; Dagher, A.; Lupien, S.J. Stress regulation in the central nervous system: Evidence from structural and functional neuroimaging studies in human populations—2008 Curt Richter Award Winner. *Psychoneuroendocrinology* **2010**, *35*, 179–191. [CrossRef]
30. Leonard, B.E. The HPA and immune axes in stress: The involvement of the serotonergic system. *Eur. Psychiatry* **2005**, *20* (Suppl. 3), S302–S306. [CrossRef]

31. Lai, K.S.P.; Liu, C.S.; Rau, A.; Lanctot, K.L.; Kohler, C.A.; Pakosh, M.; Carvalho, A.F.; Herrmann, N. Peripheral inflammatory markers in Alzheimer's disease: A systematic review and meta-analysis of 175 studies. *J. Neurol. Neurosurg. Psychiatry* **2017**. [CrossRef] [PubMed]
32. Pilgrim, A.; Barker, M.; Jackson, A.; Ntani, G.; Crozier, S.; Inskip, H.; Godfrey, K.; Cooper, C.; Robinson, S. Does living in a food insecure household impact on the diets and body composition of young children? Findings from the Southampton Women's Survey. *J. Epidemiol. Community Health* **2012**, *66*, e6. [CrossRef]
33. Fenech, M. Vitamins Associated with Brain Aging, Mild Cognitive Impairment, and Alzheimer Disease: Biomarkers, Epidemiological and Experimental Evidence, Plausible Mechanisms, and Knowledge Gaps. *Adv. Nutr.* **2017**, *8*, 958–970. [CrossRef] [PubMed]
34. Bo, Y.; Zhang, X.; Wang, Y.; You, J.; Cui, H.; Zhu, Y.; Pang, W.; Liu, W.; Jiang, Y.; Lu, Q. The n-3 Polyunsaturated Fatty Acids Supplementation Improved the Cognitive Function in the Chinese Elderly with Mild Cognitive Impairment: A Double-Blind Randomized Controlled Trial. *Nutrients* **2017**, *9*, 54. [CrossRef] [PubMed]
35. Ma, F.; Li, Q.; Zhou, X.; Zhao, J.; Song, A.; Li, W.; Liu, H.; Xu, W.; Huang, G. Effects of folic acid supplementation on cognitive function and Abeta-related biomarkers in mild cognitive impairment: A randomized controlled trial. *Eur. J. Nutr.* **2017**. [CrossRef]
36. Roberts, R.O.; Roberts, L.A.; Geda, Y.E.; Cha, R.H.; Pankratz, V.S.; O'Connor, H.M.; Knopman, D.S.; Petersen, R.C. Relative intake of macronutrients impacts risk of mild cognitive impairment or dementia. *J. Alzheimers Dis.* **2012**, *32*, 329–339. [CrossRef] [PubMed]
37. Lupien, S.J.; Maheu, F.; Tu, M.; Fiocco, A.; Schramek, T.E. The effects of stress and stress hormones on human cognition: Implications for the field of brain and cognition. *Brain Cogn.* **2007**, *65*, 209–237. [CrossRef]
38. Jorm, A.F.; Jolley, D. The incidence of dementia: A meta-analysis. *Neurology* **1998**, *51*, 728–733. [CrossRef] [PubMed]
39. Lindbergh, C.A.; Dishman, R.K.; Miller, L.S. Functional Disability in Mild Cognitive Impairment: A Systematic Review and Meta-Analysis. *Neuropsychol. Rev.* **2016**, *26*, 129–159. [CrossRef]
40. Lara, E.; Koyanagi, A.; Domenech-Abella, J.; Miret, M.; Ayuso-Mateos, J.L.; Haro, J.M. The Impact of Depression on the Development of Mild Cognitive Impairment over 3 Years of Follow-Up: A Population-Based Study. *Dement. Geriatr. Cogn. Disord.* **2017**, *43*, 155–169. [CrossRef]
41. Petersen, R.C. Mild Cognitive Impairment. *Continuum (Minneap Minn)* **2016**, *22*, 404–418. [CrossRef]
42. Masa, R.; Chowa, G.; Nyirenda, V. Prevalence and Predictors of Food Insecurity among People Living with HIV Enrolled in Antiretroviral Therapy and Livelihood Programs in Two Rural Zambian Hospitals. *Ecol. Food Nutr.* **2017**, *56*, 256–276. [CrossRef] [PubMed]
43. Kanmogne, G.D.; Fonsah, J.Y.; Tang, B.; Doh, R.F.; Kengne, A.M.; Umlauf, A.; Tagny, C.T.; Nchindap, E.; Kenmogne, L.; Franklin, D.; et al. Effects of HIV on executive function and verbal fluency in Cameroon. *Sci. Rep.* **2018**, *8*, 17794. [CrossRef] [PubMed]

6

Evaluation of a Combined HIV and Geriatrics Clinic for Older People Living with HIV

Tom Levett [1,2], Katie Alford [3], Jonathan Roberts [1], Zoe Adler [1], Juliet Wright [1,4] and Jaime H. Vera [1,3,*]

1 Division of Medicine, Brighton and Sussex University Hospitals NHS Trust, UK; t.levett@nhs.net (T.L.); jonathan.roberts10@nhs.net (J.R.); zoe.adler@nhs.net (Z.A.); juliet.wright6@nhs.net (J.W.)
2 Department of Clinical and Experimental Medicine, Brighton and Sussex Medical School, Falmer, Brighton BN1 9PX, UK
3 Department of Global Health and Infection, Brighton and Sussex Medical School, Falmer, Brighton BN1 9PX, UK; K.Alford2@bsms.ac.uk
4 Department of Medical Education, Brighton and Sussex Medical School, Falmer, Brighton BN1 9PX, UK
* Correspondence: j.vera@bsms.ac.uk

Abstract: As life expectancy in people living with HIV (PLWH) has increased, the focus of management has shifted to preventing and treating chronic illnesses, but few services exist for the assessment and management of these individuals. Here, we provide an initial description of a geriatric service for people living with HIV and present data from a service evaluation undertaken in the clinic. We conducted an evaluation of the first 52 patients seen in the clinic between 2016 and 2019. We present patient demographic data, assessment outcomes, diagnoses given, and interventions delivered to those seen in the clinic. The average age of attendees was 67. Primary reasons for referral to the clinic included management of complex comorbidities, polypharmacy, and suspected geriatric syndrome (falls, frailty, poor mobility, or cognitive decline). The median (range) number of comorbidities and comedications (non-antiretrovirals) was 7 (2–19) and 9 (1–15), respectively. All attendees had an undetectable viral load. Geriatric syndromes were observed in 26 (50%) patients reviewed in the clinic, with frailty and mental health disease being the most common syndromes. Interventions offered to patients included combination antiretroviral therapy modification, further health investigations, signposting to rehabilitation or social care services, and in-clinic advice. High levels of acceptability among patients and healthcare professionals were reported. The evaluation suggests that specialist geriatric HIV services might play a role in the management of older people with HIV with geriatric syndromes.

Keywords: HIV; geriatrics; comprehensive geriatric assessment

---

1. Introduction

Increased life expectancy in people living with HIV (PLWH) has brought the challenges of ageing and age-related issues to HIV clinical care [1]. In the UK, 39% of those accessing HIV services are now aged 50 and over, representing over 36,000 individuals considered "older" with HIV [2]. Cohort ageing is set to continue, with modelling work based on PLWH in the Netherlands predicting that, by 2030, 73% will be aged over 50 [3]. Importantly, as PLWH grow older, they appear to be experiencing disproportionally more age-related comorbidities than age-matched HIV-negative populations [4–6]. This is accompanied by greater polypharmacy, as well as issues of functional and cognitive decline, frailty, and falls [7,8]. These issues may be grouped as "geriatric syndromes", highlighting a role for geriatric/elderly medicine within current HIV care [8–10].

How best to deliver geriatric care to PLWH remains unclear. Some service providers advocate for dedicated HIV-ageing services, and a small number of such services have developed or are developing around the world [11]. Joint HIV/speciality clinics have been effective within other specialties [12,13], therefore opening the door to the possibility of HIV-ageing clinics. However, outside of single-organ specialties, the clinical need and criteria for referral are harder to define. One approach is to clinically assess patients at a set age, such as 50 [14], though with the median age of HIV services users in the UK at 46, demand may be excessively high. An alternative could be the use of frailty or frailty syndromes in a "needs-based approach". Tools to identify patients at risk of frailty using scoring methods are increasingly used internationally and have recently been integrated into UK primary care [15]. In October 2019, the European AIDS Clinical Society (EACS) published the first HIV guidance that advocates for frailty screening in older PLWH.

Frailty represents a reduction in physiological reserve that makes one vulnerable to adverse health outcomes [16]. It is prevalent in PLWH and has been associated with falls, incident multi-morbidity, hospitalisation, and death [17–19]. Frailty may present non-specifically (fatigue, weight loss) or as frailty syndromes such as falls, functional decline, and immobility. Additionally, frailty may contribute to medical complexity (polypharmacy and multi-morbidity) and has been associated with low mood and cognitive decline [20,21]. The recommended approach to the assessment and management of frailty is through Comprehensive Geriatric Assessment (CGA) [22]. Proactive identification of frailty and the introduction of CGA can enable early intervention to help PLWH to remain independent. CGA is a multidimensional, interdisciplinary diagnostic process used to determine the medical, psychosocial, and functional capabilities of older adults. Evidence suggests that CGA-based care can improve functional capacity and reduce the risk of institutionalisation when applied to other chronic conditions such as cancer, renal disease, and cardiovascular disease [23–25].

Older PLWH may face a complicated healthcare landscape [26], with HIV-specific management falling down the list of health priorities in favour of age-related issues, which HIV services may be ill-equipped to deal with due to lack of time, resources, or geriatric expertise.

In order to address the issues facing this ageing cohort, the Silver Clinic was established in the Brighton and Sussex University Hospitals Trust. This multi-disciplinary HIV-ageing clinic utilises a CGA approach to assess and manage age-related problems in PLWH. This paper aims to describe the service and results of an initial service evaluation of the clinic.

2. Methods

The Silver Clinic team consists of an (i) HIV consultant physician, (ii) Geriatrics consultant physician, (iii) HIV nurse specialist, and (iv) HIV pharmacist. The clinic operates monthly within the HIV outpatient (Lawson) unit. Clinic referrals come from any HIV healthcare professional (HCP) involved in the care of the patient. The Silver Clinic team is blinded to the process of referral. Current referral criteria are age (>50 years), presence of complex comorbidities and/or polypharmacy, or geriatric syndromes including frailty, falls, and difficulties with activities of daily living. All patients attending the clinic up until October 2019 were included in this evaluation. No exclusion criteria were applied. As this was a service evaluation, ethical approval was not obtained following assessment by the UK Health Research Authority (http://www.hra-decisiontools.org.uk/research/). Written inform consent was provided for the case study.

2.1. Clinic Process

Before attending, new patients are asked to complete a number of screening questionnaires focussed around physical, functional, mood, and cognitive status. The questionnaires are patient-reported outcome measure (PROM) tools that serve two purposes. Firstly, they help practitioners to identify medical, social, or mental health issues that patients have before they are seen in the clinic. Secondly, they can be used to monitor the impact of the service. Prior to first clinic attendance, a multidisciplinary case-based discussion of each patient is organised. This includes: background and PROM review, evaluation of current clinical problems, and anticipated need of further investigations. All patients then receive a dual consultation with the HIV and elderly medicine physician focused on CGA. This explores patient demographics; social characteristics; comorbidity (including medications); functional, physical, mental health, and frailty status (Table 1). All assessments are triangulated by the multidisciplinary (MDT) to generate a comprehensive individualised management plan that is overseen by the Silver Clinic team and communicated to the referring clinician and the GP where the patient consents. The clinic process for the service is shown in Figure 1.

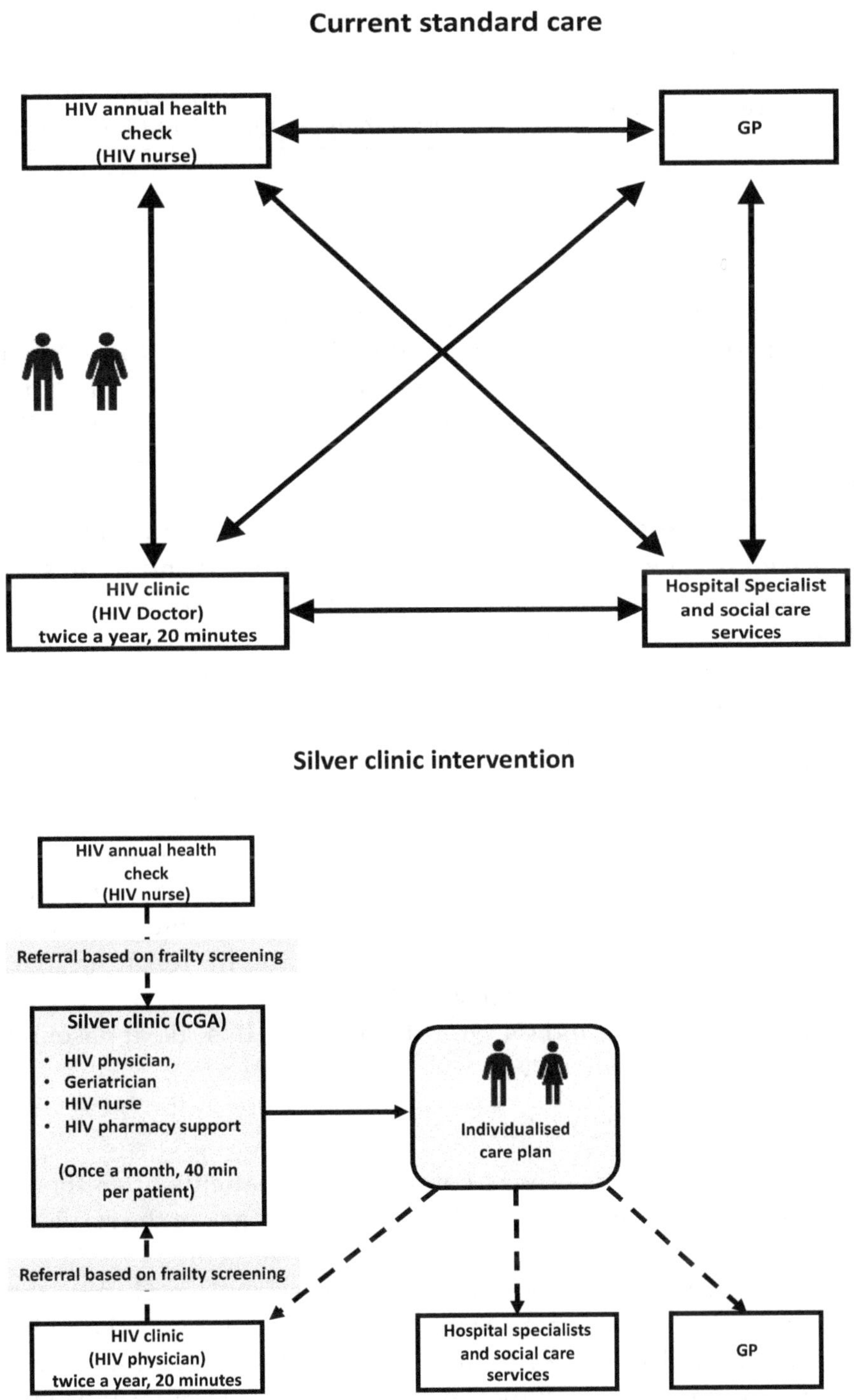

Figure 1. Silver Clinic process and position alongside standard care.

Table 1. Clinical assessments performed within the Silver Clinic.

Test Category	
Blood Tests	Calcium, TFTs, PSA, HbA1c, B12/Folate, Vitamin D
HIV clinical data	Year of diagnosis, nadir and current CD4 cell count, current CD8 cell count, CD4:CD8 ratio, antiretroviral history
Other clinical data	Urinalysis, height, weight, body mass index, blood pressure (lying and standing)
Mood assessment	Hospital Anxiety and Depression Scale
Frailty assessment	FRAIL scale
Patient reported outcome measures	Euroqol-5D-5L Older Peoples' Quality of Life Questionnaire

TFTs, thyroid function tests; PSA, prostate-specific antigens; HbA1c, Haemoglobin A1c.

2.2. Clinical Assessments

Clinical data are drawn from patient notes and most recent routine HIV health checks. Baseline observations, including postural blood pressure and body mass index (BMI), are performed. Blood tests are taken to exclude issues contributing to age-related comorbidities, including vitamin B12 and folate deficiency, associated with neuropsychiatric issues, depression, and demyelinating myelopathy; calcium and 25-OH-Vitamin-D for bone health, falls, and mobility. The full assessment strategy is shown in Error! Reference source not found.

Mood symptoms are assessed using the Hospital Anxiety and Depression Scale (HADS), a short, self-report screening questionnaire for generalised anxiety and depression among patients in non-psychiatric settings. The questionnaire is split into two sub-scales for anxiety (HADS-A) and depression (HADS-D), in which a score ≥11 is considered diagnostic [27].

Patient-reported outcome measures (PROM) include the Older Peoples' Quality of Life Questionnaire (OPQL-brief), a 13-item validated tool for assessing quality of life (QoL) in older people. Scores range from 13 to 65, indicating lowest to highest QoL [28,29]. EuroQol five-dimension descriptive system (EQ-5D-5L) is a brief self-reported measure of generic health and perceived health status that has been used across a number of health conditions and populations [30,31]. The tool includes a visual analogue scale on which individuals indicate their current health state in relation to best and worst imaginable health (100–0, respectively). FRAIL Scale is a clinical screening tool for the identification of frailty. It comprises five self-reported components of fatigue—resistance, ambulation, illnesses, and weight loss—which are scored as present or absent, resulting in a score from 0 to 5. Those scoring 0 are robust, 1–2 prefrail and ≥3 frail [32].

Changes in scores for EQ-5D-5L and OPQL-brief and FRAIL scale at baseline (first assessment) and discharge (12 months) were calculated.

2.3. Patient and Healthcare Professional Satisfaction

A voluntary self-completed survey was completed by patients after the clinic appointment. The survey asked patients to provide qualitative "free-text" feedback of the service, including whether and how it benefitted them and suggestions for service improvement.

An 8-question online questionnaire for healthcare professionals, excluding those working in the Silver Clinic, was accessible from January to March 2018. This was created and hosted using Bristol Online Surveys and distributed via email to all HIV staff. Job role, clinic awareness and referral experience, perceived importance of the clinic, and improvement to older PLWH care were assessed. Partially completed questionnaires were omitted from analysis.

2.4. Statistical Analysis

Descriptive statistics using frequency, mean, or median with respective corresponding percentages, standard deviation, and interquartile range were used to summarize the data. Paired sample *t*-tests were used to evaluate the impact of the Silver Clinic intervention on scores for each PROM (EQ-5D-5L and OPQL-brief and FRAIL scale) from baseline to discharge from the clinic. A framework method of analysis was employed for qualitative data, with frequencies and percentages reported for qualitative variables where grouping was possible [33].

3. Results

From January 2015 to October 2019, the Silver clinic assessed 52 patients. Demographic characteristics, HIV, and other clinical data of clinic attendees are presented in Table 2. The median (range) age of attendees was 67 years (53–87), and the majority were white males identifying as men that have sex with men (MSM), reflecting the clinic population. Attendees had well-controlled chronic HIV, with 100% virally suppressed. Primary referral reason for patients attending the clinic was 67% (35) multimorbidity optimisation, 13% (7) problematic polypharmacy, and 17% (10) suspected geriatric syndrome (falls, frailty, mobility issues, cognitive decline).

Table 2. Summary of patient characteristics.

Clinical Characteristics (n = 52)	Median (IQR) Otherwise Stated
Age (years)	67 (53–87)
Male, n (%)	47 (90)
White ethnicity, n (%)	50 (96)
Identified sexuality, n (%)	
MSM	41 (78)
Heterosexual	9 (17)
Other	2 (4)
Current smoker, n (%)	17 (32)
Alcohol use, n (%)	
Less than 10 units per week	41(77)
Between 10 and 20 units per week	5 (9)
>20 units per week	3 (4)
Recreational drug use n (%)	6 (11)
Comorbidities	7 (2–19)
Comedications	9 (1–15)
QRISK3 *	25 (6–52)
Bone densitometry, n (%)	
Osteoporosis	15 (28)
Osteopenia	33 (63)
Normal BMD	4 (7)
HIV Clinical Parameters	
Time since HIV diagnosis: years (median; range)	17 (6–34)
Duration of cART: years (median; range)	17 (5–30)
cART-based regimen n (%)	
Protease inhibitor	28 (53)
NNRTI	12 (23)
INSTI	12 (23)
HIV RNA < 50 copies/mL, n (%)	52 (100)
Nadir CD4 (cells/µL)	287 (223)
Current CD4 (cells/µL)	563 (368)
CD4:CD8 ratio	0.60 (0.1)

MSM, men who have sex with men; cART, antiretroviral therapy; QRISK®3-2018 cardiovascular risk calculator.

Geriatric syndromes were observed in all patients reviewed in the clinic, with frailty and mental health disease being the most common syndromes, as shown in Figure 2. Patients had a median (IQR) of 7 (2–19) comorbidities. Cardiovascular disease was the most common, reported by 36 patients (70%), followed by neurological disorder (63%), chronic pain syndrome (44%), and mental health conditions (42%). Polypharmacy defined as more than five non-antiretroviral drugs was common, with a median of nine (1–15) medications in addition to their ARVs. The most common comedications at first assessment were cardiovascular medications, followed by analgesics (61%), mental health drugs (40%), and supplements such as vitamins, etc. (53%). Notably, 30% were taking opioid medications for pain and 19% taking benzodiazepines to manage insomnia.

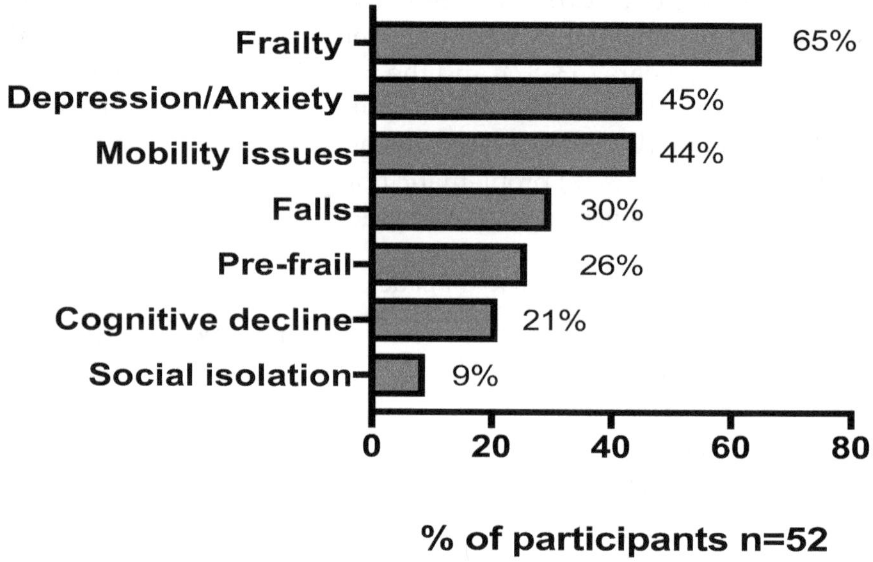

Figure 2. Frequencies of geriatric syndromes.

3.1. Patient-Reported Outcomes

Perceived health-related QoL at first assessment was poor on both the EQ-5D-5L and OPQOL, with mean scores (SD) for the visual scale on the EQ-5D-5L 56.76 (21.2) and 32.76 (8.48) for the OPQOL, respectively. Thirty-four (65%) patients were classified as frail; 14 (26%) were deemed prefrail and 4 (4%) robust using the FRAIL scale. Mental health was assessed using the HADS: 46% (23) had depression or anxiety symptoms at first assessment. No significant changes in EQ-5D-5L and OPQOL-Brief scores were observed at discharge compared to baseline ($p = 0.885$ and $p = 0.218$, respectively). Moreover, no changes in frailty status were observed at discharge using the FRAIL scale ($p = 0.495$)

3.2. Clinic Outcomes

At the point of data analysis, most patients had attended the clinic at least twice, with the median number of visits being two (2–8). The greatest number of visits was eight (two patients). ARV switch recommendations were made in six patients due to toxicities or drug–drug interactions (DDI). Twenty-seven specialist referrals were made, including to the broader multidisciplinary team including physiotherapy and occupational therapy. The clinic has now discharged 42 patients, 4 await follow-up appointment and 6 patients remain open to the service "as needed.

Case Study

To better understand that type of patients we see in the service we described the case of Mr X, a 69-year-old male who was diagnosed with HIV in 1999. He attended the Silver Clinic with complaints of feeling "fed up" and intermittent faecal incontinence. He has multiple comorbidities with associated polypharmacy, as shown in Table 3. He is an ex-smoker who drinks less than 4 units/week, with no recreational drug use. He lives alone and reports feeling socially isolated. He has poor mobility but dislikes using a recommended walking stick and reports three falls during the last 3 months. He relies heavily on his car as he lives in a rural village. His social benefits were reduced last year. His HIV is well controlled, with a current CD4 count of 750 cell/mL and undetectable viral load on a regimen of Darunavir, Ritonavir, and Lamivudine (3TC). His Q-Risk score was 16.5%.

Table 3. Mr X comorbidities and medications.

Medical Comorbidities	Comedications
Type 2 diabetes	1. Paroxetine 40 mg daily
Depression	2. Gabapentin 400 mg twice daily
Osteopenia	3. Aspirin 75 mg daily
Dyslipidaemia	4. Zopiclone 7.5 mg at night
Chronic back pain secondary to (degenerative disease and C-spine injury)	5. Pravastatin 10 mg at night 6. Zomorph MR 60 mg twice daily
Peripheral neuropathy (ART-related)	7. Metformin 1 g twice daily
Chronic inflammatory demyelinating polyneuropathy unresponsive to immunoglobulin	8. Folic Acid 5 mg daily 9. Oramorph 5–10 mg as needed

1. Proactive treatment of constipation (causing overflow incontinence) and opioid reduction.
2. Fall prevention through occupational and physiotherapy referral and bone scan with subsequent osteoporosis treatment to reduce fracture risk.
3. Medicines rationalisation with ART modification to a one tablet regimen (Rezolsta: Darunavir/Cobistat), which in turn allowed Zopiclone withdrawal.
4. Signposting to community peer services aimed at increasing socialisation and an application for a disabled parking "Blue Badge" was supported.
5. Referral to Cognitive Behavioural Therapy with the hope that improvements in mental health may also stem from comorbidity optimisation.

At follow-up, despite subjectively his symptoms persisting, QOL based on the EQ-5D-5L and OPQOL had improved.

3.3. Patient Satisfaction

All patients were asked to provide their views of the clinic. Fourteen responses (35%) were received, with 13 (93%) stating that they were "very satisfied" with the service they received, and one respondent was "somewhat satisfied". Qualitative feedback themes identified among respondents were "friendliness/kindness" (28%), "felt listened to" (14%), professional/helpful service (43%). Additional comments referred to the opportunity for in-depth explanation and care coordination.

3.4. Healthcare Professionals' Views of the Silver Clinic

Fourteen (63%) staff responded to our invitation to provide views on the clinic; this included six (43%) doctors, six (43%) nurses, and two (14%) pharmacists. All participants were aware of the clinic, and six (42%) had made referrals. Twelve (85%) believed the Silver Clinic was "very important" for the management of older PLWH and the other two (14%) believed it was "quite important". All respondents felt that the clinic improved the management of older PLWH.

4. Discussion

HIV services have a history of being proactive in their innovation of care models to address the changing needs of their patients. Clear trajectories towards HIV cohort ageing exists in the UK with accompanying age-related medical and psychosocial issues [34]. The Silver Clinic was created to address this emerging need—by employing multidisciplinary working and principles of geriatric care, it has sought to improve the care management of this complex cohort. This service evaluation demonstrates that the average age of Silver Clinic attendees was 67 years old, with the majority referred for management of multimorbidity, polypharmacy, and geriatric/frailty syndromes, which one might anticipate within general elderly medical services.

Classical geriatric syndromes have been demonstrated in older adults, with HIV at higher frequency and earlier age than one might expect for the general population. In one US study of 155 PLWH, median age 57, the prevalence of falls was 26%, and 54% described two or more geriatric syndromes, which were associated with greater comorbidity and lower nadir CD4 count [8]. In our clinic, cohort geriatric syndromes were common, with 44% complaining of mobility issues and 30% experiencing falls. These may be linked to other observed findings of mood disorder in 45% and social isolation in 9%. Social isolation was shown to be more common in older adults with HIV compared to those without (59% vs. 51%, $p < 0.001$) in the Veterans Aging Cohort Study and was associated with increased hospitalisation and mortality [35].

The majority of clinic attendees were frail (65%) based on the FRAIL scale, with a further 26% deemed prefrail. This is considerably higher than frailty prevalence seen in previous studies of PLWH, where frailty based on the Fried Phenotype (FP) ranged from 3 to 28% [36]; using this same measure, prevalence was 3% for frailty and 38% prefrailty in a large UK community study of adults aged 37–73 years [37]. The larger proportion with frailty in our group is reflective of the service model and its remit as a needs-based service, with frailty syndromes within the referral criteria. Targeting of frail and prefrail individuals is vital, however, as both are associated with an increased risk of incident disability in both personal and instrumental activities of daily living and mortality compared to robust individuals [32,38]. Though the natural trajectory of frailty is progressive, studies have demonstrated stability in frail state at one year, as was demonstrated in this non-interventional evaluation of the service [39]. The ongoing presence of frailty in this selected cohort suggests that they may have the most to gain from ongoing geriatric medical input.

The clinic users had a high burden of comorbidity and polypharmacy, particularly mood disorder (45%) and chronic pain, with 30% on regular opiates. High levels of comorbidity and polypharmacy have been noted in cohorts of PLWH [14,40], with both related to greater duration of HIV rather than older age [40]. Chronic opiate use for non-cancer pain is higher in PLWH and is associated with greater comorbidity, and it is an independent risk factor for falls, along with other medications such as benzodiazepines, in this group [41,42]. Comorbidity and polypharmacy, including chronic pain, combined with both frailty and broader geriatric syndromes, would support a multimorbidity-based approach as advocated by the National Institute of Health and Care Excellence. The use of patient-centred care focused around how one's comorbidities and their treatments impact on quality of life and how they align with their life priorities, emphasising strong care coordination [43]. These models are compatible with geriatric principles of care that have been advocated within the HIV literature [11,44,45]. Patient-reported QoL was poor at baseline, with no significant change at one year. This likely reflects the level of comorbidity and functional limitation, alongside unmeasured psychosocial factors [46]. Whilst the former were addressed from a diagnostic perspective, service users could benefit from broader MDT intervention, care coordination, and community-based intervention centred on social prescribing and peer support [47].

It was gratifying to see that the survey of HCPs indicated appropriate awareness of the Silver Clinic, with many reporting the positive improvement to the management of older PLWH as a consequence of the clinic. However, a recent UK survey identified the existence of only two dedicated HIV-ageing services nationwide, with two-thirds of respondents citing insufficient population as the reason for no perceived need for such a service [48], yet we know that a predominantly older adult HIV population is predicted in the near future [3]. HIV-ageing services are now being reported more widely, mainly in high income settings, which are either based on geriatric syndromes or metabolic comorbidities in PLWH [49]. Attendees reported high levels of satisfaction with the clinic, though it should be noted that the number providing feedback was self-selecting and small (35%). However, service user feedback is vital in both the development and evaluation of any new ageing services, with respondents in one survey favouring the maintenance of care within HIV settings, alongside enhanced communication and care coordination [50].

To our knowledge, this represents the first evaluation of a UK-based joint HIV-ageing service run on a needs- rather than age-based approach that utilises CGA principles. It is limited in its presentation of single-site data that are purely descriptive in nature. Other limitations include the small sample size, which also limits the generalizability and reproducibility of the data. Data presented here are not able to define the longer-term benefit regarding preservation of function, admission avoidance, and mortality, as well as the cost-effectiveness of attending the Silver Clinic. However, this is the case for many new services, which are not, at present, being driven by a supporting evidence base. The role of such a clinic, and in particular the role of CGA applied to individuals living with HIV, represents areas of research need within HIV and ageing, which is supported by a nationwide service evaluation on HIV-ageing services that identified a lack of evidence base as a barrier for service development [48]. However, the Silver Clinic is a trail-blazer for other services, with a model that, since conception, meets the recommendations from both the 2019 EACS guidance on frailty screening in PLWH [51] and the 2018 British HIV Association Standards of Care document, which advocates the involvement of a geriatrician with HIV knowledge in the care of service users requiring complex HIV care [52].

5. Conclusions

We have operationalised a dedicated HIV-ageing service founded on geriatric medicine principles that is acceptable to both service users and referrers within HIV medicine. Referral pathways have identified a clinic cohort with high burden of frailty, comorbidity, and geriatric syndromes that might benefit from comprehensive geriatric assessment. Ongoing evaluation and research in this area is crucial to demonstrate the effectiveness of this model of care and/or help in building an evidence base to support other models of care for those ageing with HIV.

Author Contributions: J.H.V., K.A., J.W. and T.L. contributed to the study concept and design, analysis and interpretation of data and drafting of manuscript. J.R., Z.A., contributed to the acquisition of data and revision of the manuscript. All authors have read and agreed to the published version of the manuscript.

References

1. Harris, T.G.; Rabkin, M.; El-Sadr, W.M. Achieving the fourth 90. *AIDS* **2018**, *32*, 1563–1569. [CrossRef] [PubMed]
2. Nash, S.; Desai, S.; Croxford, S.; Guerra, L.; Lowndes, C.; Connor, N.; Gill, O.N. *Progress towards Ending the HIV Epidemic in the United Kingdom: 2018 Report*; Public Health England: London, UK, 2018.
3. Smit, M.; Brinkman, K.; Geerlings, S.; Smit, C.; Thyagarajan, K.; Van Sighem, A.; De Wolf, F.; Hallett, T.B. Future challenges for clinical care of an ageing population infected with HIV: A modelling study. *Lancet Infect. Dis.* **2015**, *15*, 810–818. [CrossRef]
4. Schouten, J.; Wit, F.W.; Stolte, I.G.; Kootstra, N.A.; Van Der Valk, M.; Geerlings, S.E.; Prins, M.; Reiss, P.; Kooij, K.W.; Van Zoest, R.A.; et al. Cross-sectional comparison of the prevalence of age-associated comorbidities and their risk factors between HIV-infected and uninfected individuals: The AGEhIV cohort study. *Clin. Infect. Dis.* **2014**, *59*, 1787–1797. [CrossRef] [PubMed]
5. Althoff, K.N.; Jacobson, L.P.; Cranston, R.D.; Detels, R.; Phair, J.P.; Li, X.; Margolick, J.B.; for the Multicenter AIDS cohort study (MACS). Age, comorbidities, and AIDS predict a frailty phenotype in men who have sex with men. *J. Gerontol. Ser. A Biol. Sci. Med. Sci.* **2013**, *69*, 189–198. [CrossRef]
6. Guaraldi, G.; Orlando, G.; Zona, S.; Menozzi, M.; Carli, F.; Garlassi, E.; Berti, A.; Rossi, E.; Roverato, A.; Palella, F. Premature age-related comorbidities among HIV-infected persons compared with the general population. *Clin. Infect. Dis.* **2011**, *53*, 1120–1126. [CrossRef] [PubMed]
7. Halloran, M.; Boyle, C.; Kehoe, B.; Bagkeris, E.; Mallon, P.; A Post, F.; Vera, J.; Williams, I.; Anderson, J.; Winston, A.; et al. Polypharmacy and drug–drug interactions in older and younger people living with HIV: The POPPY study. *Antivir. Ther.* **2019**, *24*, 193–201. [CrossRef]

8. Greene, M.; Covinsky, K.E.; Valcour, V.; Miao, Y.; Madamba, J.; Lampiris, H.; Cenzer, I.S.; Martin, J.; Deeks, S.G. Geriatric syndromes in older HIV-infected adults. *J. Acquir. Immune Defic. Syndr.* **2015**, *69*, 161–167. [CrossRef] [PubMed]
9. Guaraldi, G.; Rockwood, K. Geriatric-HIV medicine is born. *Clin. Infect. Dis.* **2017**, *65*, 507–509. [CrossRef] [PubMed]
10. Hawkins, K.L.; Brown, T.T.; Margolick, J.B.; Erlandson, K.M. Geriatric syndromes: New frontiers in HIV and sarcopenia. *AIDS* **2017**, *31*, S137–S146. [CrossRef]
11. Singh, H.K.; Del Carmen, T.; Freeman, R.; Glesby, M.J.; Siegler, E.L. From one syndrome to many: Incorporating geriatric consultation into HIV care. *Clin. Infect. Dis.* **2017**, *65*, 501–506. [CrossRef]
12. McClure, M.; Singh, G.J.; Rayment, M.; Jones, R.; Levy, J.B. Clinical outcomes of a combined HIV and renal clinic. *Clin. Kidney J.* **2012**, *5*, 530–534. [CrossRef] [PubMed]
13. Koganti, S.; Loes, S.K.-D.; Hutchinson, S.; Johnson, M.; Rakhit, R.D. Management of cardiovascular conditions in a cohort of patients with HIV: Experience from a joint HIV/cardiology clinic. *Clin. Med.* **2015**, *15*, 442–446. [CrossRef] [PubMed]
14. Waters, L.; Patterson, B.; Scourfield, A.; Hughes, A.; De Silva, S.; Gazzard, B.; Barton, S.; Asboe, D.; Pozniak, A.; Boffito, M. A dedicated clinic for HIV-positive individuals over 50 years of age: A multidisciplinary experience. *Int. J. STD AIDS* **2012**, *23*, 546–552. [CrossRef]
15. NHS England; LTC Team. *Toolkit for General Practice in Supporting Older People Living with Frailty*; NHS England: London, UK, 2017.
16. Clegg, A.; Young, J.; Iliffe, S.; Rikkert, M.O.; Rockwood, K. Frailty in elderly people. *Lancet* **2013**, *381*, 752–762. [CrossRef]
17. Tassiopoulos, K.; Abdo, M.; Wu, K.; Koletar, S.L.; Palella, F.J.; Kalayjian, R.; Taiwo, B.; Erlandson, K.M. Frailty is strongly associated with increased risk of recurrent falls among older HIV-infected adults. *AIDS* **2017**, *31*, 2287–2294. [CrossRef]
18. Guaraldi, G.; Brothers, T.D.; Zona, S.; Stentarelli, C.; Carli, F.; Malagoli, A.; Santoro, A.; Menozzi, M.; Mussi, C.; Mussini, C.; et al. A frailty index predicts survival and incident multimorbidity independent of markers of HIV disease severity. *AIDS* **2015**, *29*, 1633–1641. [CrossRef] [PubMed]
19. Akgun, K.M.; Tate, J.P.; Crothers, K.; Crystal, S.; Leaf, D.A.; Womack, J.; Brown, T.T.; Justice, A.C.; Oursler, K.K. An adapted frailty-related phenotype and the VACS index as predictors of hospitalization and mortality in HIV-infected and uninfected individuals. *J. Acquir. Immune Defic. Syndr.* **2014**, *67*, 397–404. [CrossRef]
20. Collard, R.M.; Comijs, H.C.; Naarding, P.; Penninx, B.W.; Milaneschi, Y.; Ferrucci, L.; Voshaar, R.C.O. Frailty as a predictor of the incidence and course of depressed mood. *J. Am. Med. Dir. Assoc.* **2015**, *16*, 509–514. [CrossRef]
21. Underwood, J.; Robertson, K.R.; Winston, A. Could antiretroviral neurotoxicity play a role in the pathogenesis of cognitive impairment in treated HIV disease? *AIDS* **2015**, *29*, 253–261. [CrossRef]
22. British Geriatric Society, Fit for Frailty. 2017. Available online: https://www.bgs.org.uk/sites/default/files/content/resources/files/2018-05-14/fff2_short.pdf (accessed on 1 June 2019).
23. Ellis, G.; Gardner, M.; Tsiachristas, A.; Langhorne, P.; Burke, O.; Harwood, R.H.; Conroy, S.P.; Kircher, T.; Somme, D.; Saltvedt, I.; et al. Comprehensive geriatric assessment for older adults admitted to hospital. *Cochrane Database Syst. Rev.* 2017. [CrossRef]
24. Stuck, A.E.; Iliffe, S. Comprehensive geriatric assessment for older adults. *BMJ* **2011**, *343*, d6799. [CrossRef]
25. Garrard, J.W.; Cox, N.J.; Dodds, R.M.; Roberts, H.C.; Sayer, A.A. Comprehensive geriatric assessment in primary care: A systematic review. *Aging Clin. Exp. Res.* **2019**, *32*, 197–205. [CrossRef] [PubMed]
26. Terrence Higgins Trust, Uncharted Territory: A Report into the First Generation Growing Older with HIV. 2017. Available online: https://www.tht.org.uk/sites/default/files/2018-03/uncharted_territory_final_low-res.pdf (accessed on 13 October 2020).
27. Zigmond, A.S.; Snaith, R.P. The hospital anxiety and depression scale. *Acta Psychiatr. Scand.* **1983**, *67*, 361–370. [CrossRef] [PubMed]
28. Bowling, A.; Hankins, M.; Windle, G.; Bilotta, C.; Grant, R. A short measure of quality of life in older age: The performance of the brief older people's quality of life questionnaire (OPQOL-brief). *Arch. Gerontol. Geriatr.* **2013**, *56*, 181–187. [CrossRef]

29. Kaambwa, B.; Gill, L.; McCaffrey, N.; Lancsar, E.; Cameron, I.D.; Crotty, M.; Gray, L.; Ratcliffe, J. An empirical comparison of the OPQoL-Brief, EQ-5D-3 L and ASCOT in a community dwelling population of older people. *Health Qual. Life Outcomes* **2015**, *13*, 164. [CrossRef] [PubMed]
30. Herdman, M.; Gudex, C.; Lloyd, A.; Janssen, M.; Kind, P.; Parkin, D.; Bonsel, G.; Badia, X. Development and preliminary testing of the new five-level version of EQ-5D (EQ-5D-5L). *Qual. Life Res.* **2011**, *20*, 1727–1736. [CrossRef]
31. Dyer, M.T.D.; A Goldsmith, K.; Sharples, L.S.; Buxton, M.J. A review of health utilities using the EQ-5D in studies of cardiovascular disease. *Health Qual. Life Outcomes* **2010**, *8*, 13. [CrossRef]
32. Kojima, G. Quick and Simple FRAIL Scale predicts incident activities of daily living (ADL) and instrumental ADL (IADL) disabilities: A systematic review and meta-analysis. *J. Am. Med. Dir. Assoc.* **2018**, *19*, 1063–1068. [CrossRef]
33. Gale, N.K.; Heath, G.; Cameron, E.; Rashid, S.; Redwood, S. Using the framework method for the analysis of qualitative data in multi-disciplinary health research. *BMC Med. Res. Methodol.* **2013**, *13*, 117. [CrossRef]
34. Bagkeris, E.; Burgess, L.; Mallon, P.W.; Post, F.A.; Boffito, M.; Sachikonye, M.; Anderson, J.; Asboe, D.; Garvey, L.; Vera, J.; et al. Cohort profile: The Pharmacokinetic and clinical observations in PeoPle over fiftY (POPPY) study. *Int. J. Epidemiol.* **2018**, *47*, 1391–1392e. [CrossRef]
35. Greysen, S.R.; Horwitz, L.I.; Covinsky, K.E.; Gordon, K.; Ohl, M.; Justice, A.C. Does social isolation predict hospitalization and mortality among HIV+ and uninfected older veterans? *J. Am. Geriatr. Soc.* **2013**, *61*, 1456–1463. [CrossRef] [PubMed]
36. Levett, T.J.; Cresswell, F.V.; Malik, M.A.; Fisher, M.; Wright, J. Systematic Review of Prevalence and predictors of frailty in individuals with human immunodeficiency virus. *J. Am. Geriatr. Soc.* **2016**, *64*, 1006–1014. [CrossRef] [PubMed]
37. Hanlon, P.; I Nicholl, B.; Jani, B.D.; Lee, D.; McQueenie, R.; Mair, F.S. Frailty and pre-frailty in middle-aged and older adults and its association with multimorbidity and mortality: A prospective analysis of 493 737 UK Biobank participants. *Lancet Public Health* **2018**, *3*, e323–e332. [CrossRef]
38. Kojima, G. Frailty Defined by FRAIL Scale as a predictor of mortality: A systematic review and meta-analysis. *J. Am. Med. Dir. Assoc.* **2018**, *19*, 480–483. [CrossRef]
39. Gill, T.M.; Gahbauer, E.A.; Allore, H.G.; Han, L. Transitions between frailty states among community-living older persons. *Arch. Intern. Med.* **2006**, *166*, 418–423. [CrossRef] [PubMed]
40. Guaraldi, G.; Malagoli, A.; Calcagno, A.; Mussi, C.; Celesia, B.M.; Carli, F.; Piconi, S.; De Socio, G.V.; Cattelan, A.M.; Orofino, G.; et al. The increasing burden and complexity of multi-morbidity and polypharmacy in geriatric HIV patients: A cross sectional study of people aged 65–74 years and more than 75 years. *BMC Geriatr.* **2018**, *18*, 99. [CrossRef]
41. Silverberg, M.J.; Ray, G.T.; Saunders, K.; Rutter, C.M.; Campbell, C.I.; Merrill, J.O.; Sullivan, M.D.; Banta-Green, C.J.; Von Korff, M.; Weisner, C. Prescription long-term opioid use in HIV-infected patients. *Clin. J. Pain* **2012**, *28*, 39–46. [CrossRef]
42. Erlandson, K.M.; Allshouse, A.A.; Jankowski, C.M.; Duong, S.; Mawhinney, S.; Kohrt, W.M.; Campbell, T.B. Risk factors for falls in HIV-infected persons. *J. Acquir. Immune Defic. Syndr.* **2012**, *61*, 484–489. [CrossRef]
43. NICE, Multimorbidity: Clinical Assessment and Management. National Institute of Health Research Guidelines. 2016. Available online: https://www.nice.org.uk/guidance/ng56 (accessed on 13 October 2020).
44. Greene, M.; Justice, A.C.; Covinsky, K.E. Assessment of geriatric syndromes and physical function in people living with HIV. *Virulence* **2016**, *8*, 586–598. [CrossRef] [PubMed]
45. Levett, T.; Wright, J. How to assess and manage frailty in patients with HIV. *Sex. Transm. Infect.* **2017**, *93*, 476–477. [CrossRef] [PubMed]
46. Langebeek, N.; Kooij, K.W.; Wit, F.W.; Stolte, I.G.; Sprangers, M.A.G.; Reiss, P.; Nieuwkerk, P.T. Impact of comorbidity and ageing on health-related quality of life in HIV-positive and HIV-negative individuals. *AIDS* **2017**, *31*, 1471–1481. [CrossRef] [PubMed]
47. Vargas, R.B.; Cunningham, W.E. Evolving trends in medical care-coordination for patients with HIV and AIDS. *Curr. HIV/AIDS Rep.* **2006**, *3*, 149–153. [CrossRef] [PubMed]
48. Cresswell, F.; Levett, T. Specialist care of older adults with HIV infection in the UK: A service evaluation. *HIV Med.* **2017**, *18*, 519–524. [CrossRef] [PubMed]
49. Siegler, E.L.; O Burchett, C.; Glesby, M.J. Older people with HIV are an essential part of the continuum of HIV care. *J. Int. AIDS Soc.* **2018**, *21*, e25188. [CrossRef]

50. Pollard, A.; Llewellyn, C.; Cooper, V.; Sachikonye, M.; Perry, N.; Nixon, E.; Miners, A.; Youssef, E.; Sabin, C. Patients' perspectives on the development of HIV services to accommodate ageing with HIV: A qualitative study. *Int. J. STD AIDS* **2017**, *29*, 483–490. [CrossRef]
51. European AIDS Clinical Society EACS. Available online: https://www.eacsociety.org/files/2019_guidelines-10.0_final.pdf (accessed on 13 October 2020).
52. BHIVA, Standards of Care for People Living with HIV. 2018. Available online: https://www.bhiva.org/file/KrfaFqLZRlBhg/BHIVA-Standards-of-Care-2018.pdf (accessed on 13 October 2020).

7

Active Navigation in Virtual Environments Benefits Spatial Memory in Older Adults

Melissa E. Meade [1,*], John G. Meade [1], Hélène Sauzeon [2,3] and Myra A. Fernandes [1]

1 Department of Psychology, University of Waterloo, Waterloo, ON N2L 3G1, Canada; jon.meadee@gmail.com (J.G.M.); mafernan@uwaterloo.ca (M.A.F.)
2 Lab EA413-Handicap, Activité, Cognition & Santé, Université de Bordeaux, F-33000 Bordeaux, France; helene.sauzeon@u-bordeaux.fr
3 Flowers Team-INRIA Center, F-33405 Talence, France
* Correspondence: mmeade@uwaterloo.ca

Abstract: We investigated age differences in memory for spatial routes that were either actively or passively encoded. A series of virtual environments were created and presented to 20 younger (Mean age = 19.71) and 20 older (Mean age = 74.55) adults, through a cardboard viewer. During encoding, participants explored routes presented within city, park, and mall virtual environments, and were later asked to re-trace their travelled routes. Critically, participants encoded half the virtual environments by passively viewing a guided tour along a pre-selected route, and half through active exploration with volitional control of their movements by using a button press on the viewer. During retrieval, participants were placed in the same starting location and asked to retrace the previously traveled route. We calculated the percentage overlap in the paths travelled at encoding and retrieval, as an indicator of spatial memory accuracy, and examined various measures indexing individual differences in their cognitive approach and visuo-spatial processing abilities. Results showed that active navigation, compared to passive viewing during encoding, resulted in a higher accuracy in spatial memory, with the magnitude of this memory enhancement being significantly larger in older than in younger adults. Regression analyses showed that age and score on the Hooper Visual Organizational test predicted spatial memory accuracy, following the passive and active encoding of routes. The model predicting accuracy following active encoding additionally included the distance of stops from an intersection as a significant predictor, illuminating a cognitive approach that specifically contributes to memory benefits in following active navigation. Results suggest that age-related deficits in spatial memory can be reduced by active encoding.

Keywords: aging; spatial memory; active exploration; virtual reality

---

1. Active Navigation in Virtual Environments Benefits Older Adults' Spatial Memory

Spatial navigation deficits are frequently experienced in the older adult population [1–3]. For example, age-related deficits are commonly observed in the memory for locations, landmarks, routes, and maps [2,4]. Such declines in navigation and spatial memory are critical, because they pose a potential threat to independent living for older adults [5–9], prompting the need to find ways to lessen these age-related deficits. The assessment of age-related impairments in spatial cognition has been facilitated by recent advancements in virtual reality (VR) technology [10], allowing for the efficient examination of navigation performance in virtual environments. In the current study, we took advantage of VR methodology to investigate ways for improving spatial memory performance in a navigation task, in older and younger adults. Specifically, the goal of the current study was to determine whether age-related differences in memory for virtual routes are reduced following active exploration, compared to passive guidance. Additionally, we examined whether individual differences in visuo-spatial ability, and cognitive indices during route exploration, meaningfully contributed to spatial memory performance.

2. Active vs. Passive Encoding of Spatial Information

The term active navigation refers to a condition wherein the participant has motor and/or volitional control of their movement through an environment, whereas passive navigation generally consists of a guided tour [11]. Active navigation has been described to contain both cognitive (mental manipulation of spatial information, allocation of attention, and decision-making) and physical (motor control for locomotion and proprioceptive and vestibular sensory information) components [11], which combine to create rich multi-modal associations that benefit subsequent memory performance [12]. A variety of past studies in young adults suggest significant spatial memorial benefits when encoding is active, rather than passive [13–16].

The memory benefit from active, relative to passive, navigation can be conceptualized as a subject-performed task effect (SPT effect) [17,18]. The SPT effect describes a pattern of superior memory performance when encoding involves the direct engagement of the participant, such as when performing rather than watching an action that is associated with a to-be-remembered word [19]. Importantly, the SPT effect remains unchanged with aging, enhancing memory performance in older adults [20–22]. The encoding tasks that involve an SPT have been described to have a high degree of environmental support, accounting for a boost in memory in seniors [23,24]. With regard to encoding manipulations, the environmental support refers to a situation in which older adults do not need to self-initiate encoding operations. By this account, active navigation should provide a good form of environmental support, as it involves the SPT of physically and cognitively engaging with the to-be-remembered spatial information. Past studies, however, have reported inconsistent results regarding the benefits of active relative to passive navigation in older adults. Specifically, benefits from active navigation are sometimes observed in older adults [15,25,26], but there is also evidence showing that active encoding hinders memory performance in seniors [2,27].

The degree of involvement of both decision-making processes and motor processing in active exploration conditions could be critical for explaining the inconsistencies regarding age differences in active/passive manipulation. It is well-known that older adults have to allocate additional cognitive resources to control their locomotion [28,29], suggesting that the physical components of active navigation are unlikely to be the reason for any memory benefit in seniors. Indeed, active navigation with low levels of motor control benefits spatial memory, whereas a high degree of motoric requirement creates an additional cognitive load that impairs memory in older adults [27].

Some have suggested that the cognitive components of active navigation benefit the memory (for directions and the locations of landmarks), more so than physical motor processing [29–31]. Decision-making in particular has been shown to be beneficial in older adults for episodic memory of landmarks and objects [15] and it may elicit a self-reference effect that is known to benefit older adults' spatial memory [32–34]. In other words, the engagement of cognitive and decision-making processes during active navigation conditions could be particularly beneficial for older adults. Likewise, factors related to decision-making, such as intrinsic motivation or curiosity [35,36] may also contribute to the memory benefit from active exploration. As recently claimed by [37], momentary feelings of curiosity can help older adults' memories and executive functions, because the phasic activation of the noradrenergic and dopaminergic systems modulate hippocampal activity [38], facilitating memory and learning. As such, it may be that the cognitive components of active navigation drive the observed active encoding memory benefits in older adults.

Related to this, it is possible that the cognitive processes engaged by the active exploration of an environment allow for more unique associations to be formed with landmarks, and thus enhance the memory for the links between certain environments and paths travelled. Others have suggested that such relational knowledge is critical, as retrieval becomes more likely when the target is part of a rich network of associations, as opposed to being encoding in isolation [12]. This relational encoding can take the form of distinctive sensorimotor associations, and increased elaboration during encoding, due to goal-directed exploration. By actively encoding an experience, and thereby increasing the amount of associations that are credited to an episodic memory, later memory recall can be expected to be improved [12].

3. Using Virtual Reality to Examine Spatial Memory

In recent years, VR technology has become widely used for studying spatial cognition and navigation performance in both younger [39–42], and older adults [10,12,43]. One of the major advantages of VR is the high degree of experimental control that is afforded, to investigate the cognitive and behavioral components that are involved in spatial navigation. For example, VR provides the ability to control for variables that differ between age groups, such as physical fatigue and mobility issues during navigation. Furthermore, the use of VR in the current study allowed for the creation of a series of environments with controlled parameters, including environment size, number of intersections, and visual content, as well as the novel approach of examining spatial memory following trials of either active or passive encoding. Additionally, we developed a means to precisely measure the overlaps in the routes travelled at encoding and retrieval, to provide a measure of memory accuracy in re-tracing a previously travelled route.

Research into the effects of aging on route navigation have largely focused on differences in learning performance and the assessment of knowledge for a highly familiar environment. However, it is not the case that we will only ever need to navigate through familiar environments; rather we frequently encounter new spaces by we need to successfully navigate after brief encounters. As such, in the present study, we took the novel approach of investigating the age difference in memory for routes that were previously travelled on only one occasion. We created a set of virtual environments in which participants traveled routes, and then later re-traced those routes to assess spatial memory performance. During the encoding, participants either traveled routes by actively exploring through volitional control of their own movements, by passively viewing a guided tour. This paradigm was analogous to drivers and passengers in a car, with active trials affording the control that a driver has in deciding on the route and manipulating movement, whereas the passive trials are akin to a passenger simply viewing the route travelled within the environment. We expected that our active encoding manipulation would provide a higher degree of environmental support, as it constitutes a SPT; given that environmental support is particularly helpful to seniors [23,24], active versus passive encoding should benefit older adults' memories more so than younger adults.

4. Method

4.1. Participants

Twenty-two younger (M_{age} = 19.71, SD = 2.19, 11 females) and 22 older (M_{age} = 74.55, SD = 7.82, 10 females) adults participated in our study. Younger adults were undergraduate students at the University of Waterloo who signed up for the study and received partial course credit for their participation. Older adults were recruited from the Waterloo Research in Aging Participant (WRAP) database, and received $10.00 remuneration for their participation. WRAP is a database of healthy seniors residing in the Kitchener–Waterloo area recruited by means of newspaper ads, flyers, and local television segments to participate in research studies taking place on campus at the University of Waterloo. All older adults completed the Montreal Cognitive Assessment (MoCA) to assess cognitive decline [44]. The average MoCA score was 26.95 out of 30 (SD = 2.29), with a range of 20 to 30. Two participants fell below the cut-off a score of 26 (obtaining scores of 24 and 20); which was generally used to indicate normal healthy aging; however, we opted to include all older adults who were tested, as we are not aiming to make a distinction between normal healthy aging and MCI in the current study.

4.2. Materials

VR equipment. The VR program was run on an Asus© Zenfone 3 Laser ™ (see specificities on www.asus.com, Asus, Taipei, Taiwan) and a lightweight hand-held cardboard VR headset for viewing. The VR application run on the Android phone was designed using the 3D engine Unity© (ver. 2017.2.0.f3, Unity Technologies ApS, San Francisco, CA, USA). Twelve virtual environments (VE) were built according to three styles of: city streets, mall hallways, and park trails (see Figure 1 for samples). The virtual environments were topographically similar, with an average area of 234 square meters. Additionally, each environment had six intersections, which is a point where 3+ roads converge.

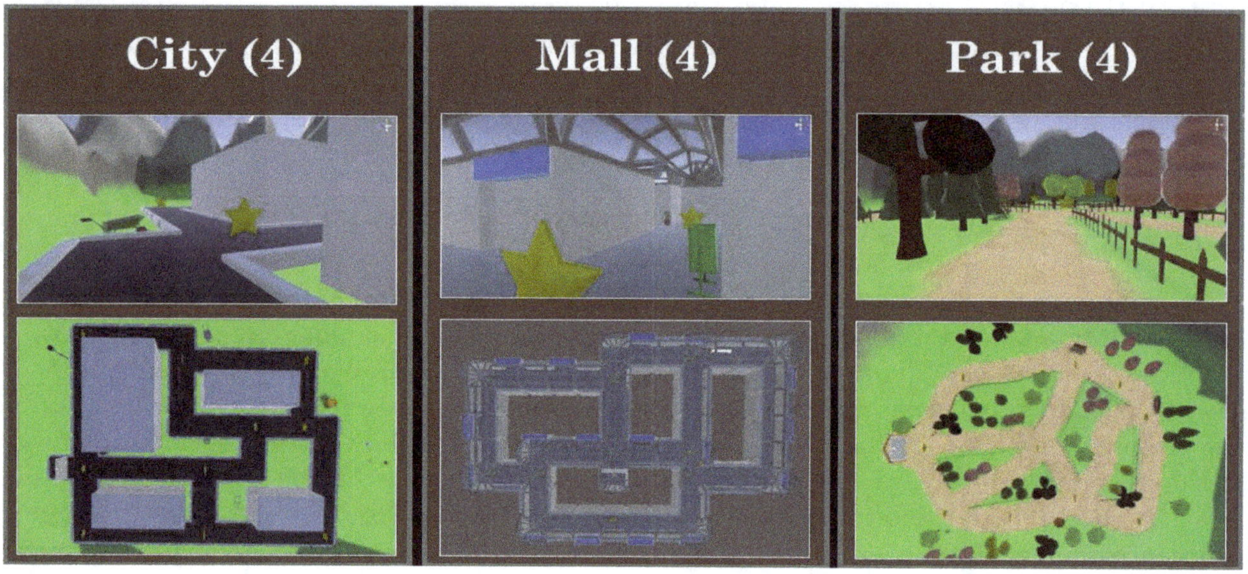

Figure 1. First-person view and bird's-eye view of the three virtual environment styles. For each style, we created 4 exemplars, though only one from each is shown here. The Stars are visible in the environments during encoding, but not during retrieval. Participants only experienced the environments from a first-person perspective.

Neuropsychological assessments. Spatial visualization ability was evaluated with the Hooper Visual Orientation test [45], which had good internal reliability, as indicated by a coefficient α of 0.88 [46]. This test is scored out of 30; it contains 30 line drawings of common objects that are portrayed as having been cut up and misaligned; participants had to mentally rotate and piece together the visual information, to identify the depicted object. Performance on the Hooper test was included to determine whether spatial visualization abilities were related to, and predictive of, spatial memory performance following active and passive encoding.

The spatial orientation ability was measured with the Santa Barbara Sense-of-Direction scale, which has good internal reliability, as indicated by a coefficient α of 0.88 [47]. For this, the test participants rated their endorsement of 15 statements about spatial orientation abilities, such as "I am good at giving directions', indicating whether they strongly agreed or disagreed, using a 7-point scale. After reverse scoring the necessary items, the responses were summed and divided by 15 to provide an average score of between 1–7 [47]. This measure was included to determine whether the perceived spatial orientation abilities were related to spatial memory performance following active and passive encoding.

5. Procedure

The study received clearance from the ethics review board at the University of Waterloo; all participants gave their written informed consent prior to beginning the experiment. Throughout the entire experiment, participants were seated in comfortable chairs that could turn a full 360° circle, which was placed in the center of a testing room. Following a verbal explanation of how to use the VR headset, participants were given unlimited time to complete a training phase with the VR equipment designed to help them learn how to move in the virtual space. Specifically, they were told that to move forward in VR, they should press a button on the headset, and to change their direction within VR, they were to physically rotate in the spinning chair with their legs. Participants were advised to take as much time as needed in the training phase, to become comfortable with the environment and the movement mechanism. Immediately following the training phase, the experimental session began.

In the experimental session, participants completed 12 cycles of encoding-filler-retrieval phases. The encoding phase was 30 seconds in duration. Once 30 seconds elapsed, the screen turned black and the participant immediately performed a filler task which involved counting backwards by 7's from 100, for 20 seconds, in order to reduce recency effects [48]. In the retrieval phase, participants were placed within the VR environment at the same starting point as the environment they had just experienced. Participants were told that they had 30 seconds to re-trace the exact path just previously travelled in the environment. Participants were given a 1- to 5-min break halfway through the experimental session (i.e., after completing six encoding-filler-retrieval cycles), resuming when they indicated they were ready.

Active vs. passive manipulation. The within-subjects active/passive navigation manipulation was implemented during the encoding phase. Of the 12 virtual environments, six were actively encoded, and six were passively encoded. The order of active and passive trials was mixed, with an instruction appearing at the beginning of each new encoding-filler-retrieval cycle, indicating whether the participant was to explore the environment (active) or watch a guided tour (passive). Participants knew that they would subsequently be asked to retrace the travelled route. In the active trials, the participant had full volitional control of their movement along the paths in the environment, and they were free to choose the route they traveled. To motivate participants to continue to move and explore the environment in the active condition (and not to simply walk back and forth so that their route was later easier to remember) they were told to 'collect' as many star icons along the path as possible, by walking over the stars. Each environment had 10 stars dispersed throughout the environment, along the paths (as shown in Figure 1). On the passive trials, the participant did not control their movement, or route, in the environment, and instead experienced a recording from the active exploration of a previous participant. Using a previous participant's active exploration for the passive trials, in this yoked control manner, was purposely done to equate route length, pauses along the path, and the number of turns, across the active and passive trials.

6. Results

Participant Characteristics. While age differences in spatial abilities were of primary interest in the current study, we also wanted to determine whether any sex differences that we presented in our data, given the previous work, suggested that males perform better than females on a variety of spatial processing measures [49]. To determine whether there were differences between the age groups and sexes, on the neuropsychological assessments included in the study, we ran two 2 (Age: younger, older) × 2 (Sex: male, female) ANOVAS separately, for the performance on the Hooper Visual Orientation test [45] and on the Santa Barbara Sense-of-Direction scale [47]. The analysis on the Hooper Visual Organization performance revealed a main effect of Age, $F(1, 40) = 26.12$, $MSE = 0.26$, $p < 0.001$, and $\eta^2 = 0.40$, such that the scores were higher for younger than for older adults, but there was no effect of Sex, $F(1, 40) = 2.09$, $MSE = 0.02$, $p = 0.16$, $\eta^2 = 0.05$. There were no main effects of Age, $F(1, 40) = 0.06$, $MSE = 0.14$, $p = 0.80$, $\eta^2 = 0.002$, or Sex, $F(1, 40) = 0.48$, $MSE = 1.07$, $p = 0.50$, $\eta^2 = 0.01$ on the Santa Barbara Sense-of-Direction scale, and no interactions on either measure.

Calculation of Route Overlap. The dependent variable of interest was the accuracy in re-tracing the same route at retrieval that had been traveled during encoding. To obtain this measure of spatial memory performance, the overlap between the routes travelled by each participant at encoding and retrieval, for each trial type, was calculated, to produce a 'percent overlap' value for each environment. The percent overlap values were computed by using the Python programming language (https://www.python.org/), Python Software Foundation, Wilmington, DE, USA), to first normalize the routes travelled (during both encoding and retrieval) against the established paths in the environments, and then to compare those normalized routes. The process of normalizing the participant's paths involved removing positional data points that corresponded to the subject travelling between specified points on the pathways in the environments. The normalized path that this process produced is a distilled representation of the position data, which allowed us to measure the overlap values that were not obscured by other effects (such as a participant travelling in a straight line during encoding, versus a sinusoidal path in retrieval). See Figure 2 for a visual representation of the normalized paths used in the calculation of the Route Overlap values. This process resulted in 12 values for percent overlap scores per person, 6 of which corresponded to active trials, and six to passive trials. For each participant, the averages were calculated for the active and passive trials separately, resulting in one measure representing performance following active encoding, and another following passive encoding. See the example in Figure 2.

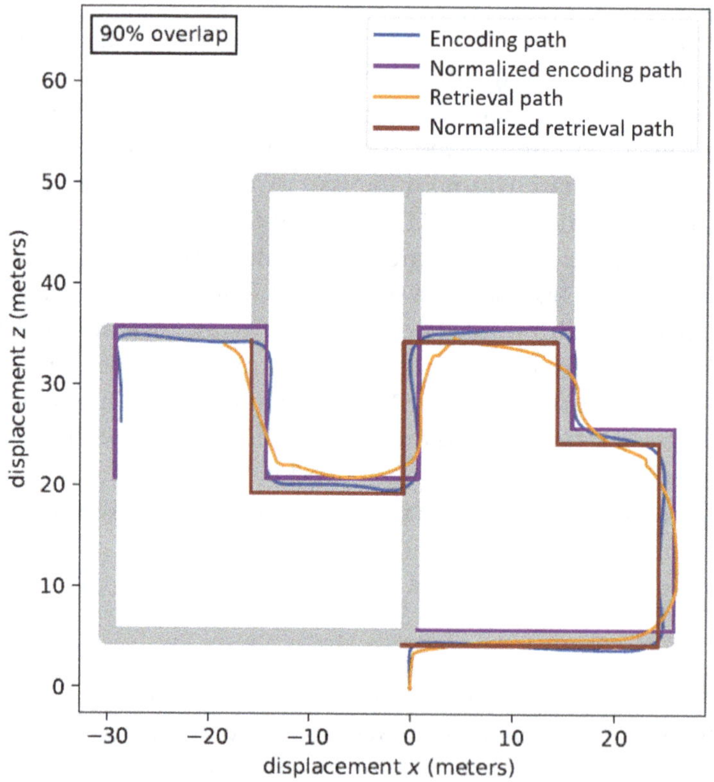

Figure 2. Example of the paths travelled in one of the virtual environments at encoding and retrieval before and after normalization.

Route overlap analyses. A mixed measures ANOVA (Analysis of variance) (2 (Age: younger, older) $\times$ 2 (Trial type: active, passive) $\times$ 2 (Sex: male, female)) was conducted on the Route Overlap values, with the Trial type as a within-subjects factor, and Age and Sex as between-subjects factors. The analysis revealed a significant main effect of Trial type, $F(1, 40) = 23.07$, $MSE = 0.27$, $p < 0.001$, $\eta^2 = 0.37$, such that the Route Overlap was more accurate for active than passive encoding. A main effect was also found for Age, $F(1, 40) = 83.44$, $MSE = 1.99$, $p < 0.001$, $\eta^2 = 0.68$, such that the Route Overlap was higher for younger than for older adults. No main effect was found for Sex, $F(1, 40) = 0.03$, $MSE = 0.001$, $p = 0.86$, $\eta^2 = 0.06$. There was a significant two-way interaction between Trial type and

Age $F(1, 40) = 5.65$, $MSE = 0.07$, $p = 0.03$, $\eta^2 = 0.12$. The Age × Sex interactions was non-significant, $F(1, 40) = 2.42$, $MSE = 0.06$, $p = 0.13$, $\eta^2 = 0.06$, as was the Trial type × Sex, $F(1, 40) = 1.38$, $MSE = 0.02$, $p = 0.25$, $\eta^2 = 0.03$. The 3-way interaction was also non-significant, $F(1, 40) = 0.38$, $MSE = 0.005$, $p = 0.54$, $\eta^2 = 0.01$.

To better understand the interaction between Age and Trial type, two paired-sample t-tests were conducted on with Route Overlap accuracy, separately for younger and older adults. For younger adults, there was a marginally significant difference, $t(21) = 1.98$, $p = 0.06$, $d = 0.35$, such that the Route Overlap was higher following active encoding, compared to passive encoding. For older adults, the Route Overlap was significantly higher following active encoding, compared to passive encoding, $t(21) = 4.55$, $p < 0.001$, $d = 0.61$. See Figure 3 for the mean values.

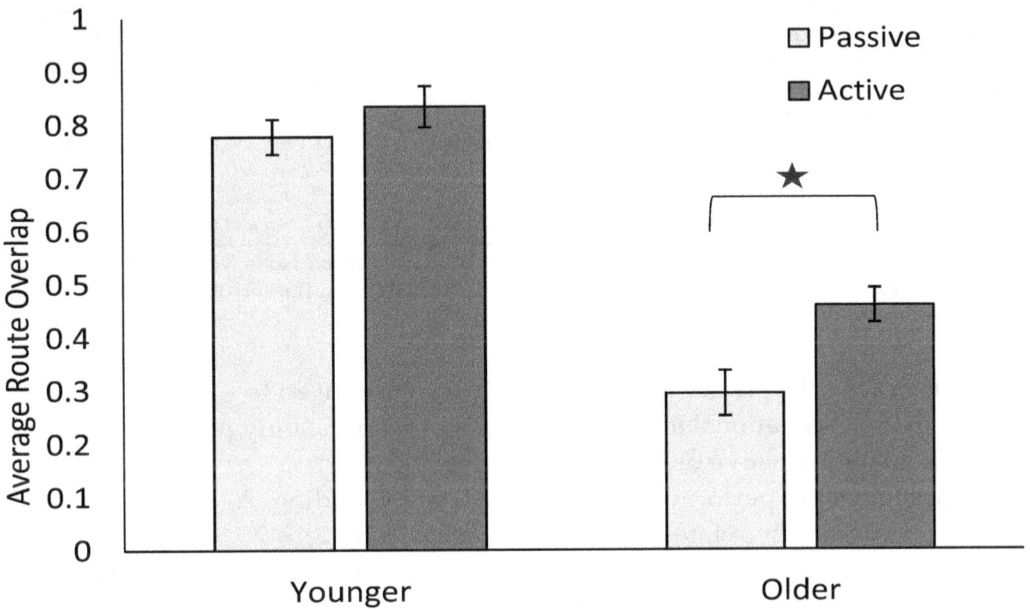

Figure 3. Average percent Route Overlap values for active and passive encoding in younger and older adults. Error bars represent the standard error. The star represents significant differences between active and passive conditions for older adults.

Correlations with neuropsychological assessments. To determine whether spatial memory performance was related to performance in the Hooper Visual Orientation test [45] and the Santa Barbara Sense-of-Direction scale [47], we ran a series of partial correlations separately, for active and passive encoding, while controlling for age. A significant and positive relationship was found between Route Overlap accuracy and the Hooper Visual Orientation test, for both active ($r = 0.51$, $p = 0.001$) and passive ($r = 0.42$, $p = 0.005$) Trial types, suggesting, as expected, that better spatial visualization abilities are related to superior spatial memory performance, regardless of whether one actively or passively encodes a route. Correlations with the Santa Barbara Sense-of-Direction scale were non-significant.

Correlations with cognitive indices. Given our goal of determining the factors underlying the benefits of Active encoding, we conducted exploratory analyses on a number of measures obtained from our virtual reality program. Specifically, a number of partial correlations were analyzed. Table 1 shows the factors considered, along with the correlation and the statistical significance values. Given the large number of correlations, we applied both the Bonferroni [50] and Benjamini–Hochberg corrections [51], the latter of which was included as an alternative to the highly conservative Bonferroni correction. Three correlations remained significant after the Benjamini–Hochberg correction. As the number of stars collected during the active trials increased, so did memory accuracy ($r = 0.39$, $p = 0.009$); this relationship held only for active but not passive encoding trials. During encoding, there were occasions where the participant stopped along the route (during both active and passive trial types); we measured the distance of a stop from the nearest intersection, and found that as this distance got smaller, memory accuracy increased ($r = -0.39$, $p = 0.01$). Similarly, we measured this distance during the retrieval phase (when a participant was re-tracing their route), and found the same relationship ($r = -0.38$, $p = 0.01$). The relationships the distances of the stops from the intersections and Route Overlap held only for the active, and not the passive encoding trials.

Table 1. Correlations between memory accuracy (percent overlap values) following active and passive encoding, and various neuropsychological factors, as well as task performance measures.

	Active	Passive
SBSD	$r = -0.07$, $p = 0.62$	$r = 0.11$, $p = 0.48$
Hooper	$r = 0.51$, $p = 0.001$ [a,b]	$r = 0.42$, $p = 0.005$ [b]
Number of stars passed during encoding	$r = 0.39$, $p = 0.009$ [b]	$r = 0.09$, $p = 0.57$
Number of intersections passed during encoding	$r = -0.006$, $p = 0.97$	$r = 0.10$, $p = 0.52$
Length of the path travelled at encoding	$r = -0.09$, $p = 0.57$	$r = 0.03$, $p = 0.83$
Length of the path travelled at retrieval	$r = -0.004$, $p = 0.98$	$r = -0.13$, $p = 0.41$
Total duration of stopped movement during encoding	$r = 0.06$, $p = 0.72$	$r = 0.03$, $p = 0.86$
Number of stops during encoding	$r = 0.14$, $p = 0.36$	$r = -0.03$, $p = 0.85$
Distance of stops from the nearest intersection during encoding	$r = -0.39$, $p = 0.01$ [b]	$r = -0.01$, $p = 0.96$
Total duration of stopped movement during retrieval	$r = -0.23$, $p = 0.13$	$r = 0.06$, $p = 0.70$
Number of stops during retrieval	$r = 0.04$, $p = 0.82$	$r = 0.01$, $p = 0.95$
Distance of stops from the nearest intersection during retrieval	$r = -0.38$, $p = 0.01$ [b]	$r = -0.25$, $p = 0.11$

Both the Bonferroni and Benjamini–Hochberg corrections for multiple comparisons were conducted; SBSD = Santa Barbara Sense of Direction scale; [a] Correlations were significant following Bonferroni correction; [b] Correlations were significant following Benjamini–Hochberg correction.

Regression analyses. Step-wise regression analyses were used to examine whether any of the factors considered in the correlational analyses (see Table 1) significantly predicted participants' Route Overlap accuracies following active or passive encoding.

In Step 1 of the analysis of performance following active encoding, Age entered into the regression equation, and was significantly related to Route Overlap, $F(1,42) = 75.86$, $p < 0.001$. At Step 2, the Hooper Visual Orientation test performance was entered into the equation, $t = 3.05$, $p = 0.004$, and at Step 3, the distance of participants' stops from the nearest intersection during encoding was entered, $t = -2.18$, $p = 0.035$. At Step 4, the number of stars collected failed to be entered into the equation, $t = 1.94$, $p = 0.06$. The final model significantly predicted Route Overlap, $F(3, 40) = 38.00$, $p < 0.001$, with an R^2 of 0.740, decreasing with Age ($\beta = -0.56$) and distance from the nearest decision point ($\beta = -0.19$), and increasing with the Hooper performance ($\beta = 0.27$).

In Step 1 of the passive encoding analysis, Age entered into the regression equation and was significantly related to Route Overlap, $F(1,42) = 101.82$, $p < 0.001$. At Step 2, the Hooper Visual Orientation test performance was entered into the equation, $t = 2.24$, $p = 0.031$, and at Step 3, the length of the path travelled at retrieval failed to be entered into the equation, $t = -1.60$, $p = 0.12$. The final model significantly predicted Route Overlap, $F(2, 41) = 58.26$, $p < 0.001$, with an R^2 of 0.74, decreasing with Age ($\beta = -0.68$) and increasing with Hooper performance ($\beta = 0.24$).

7. Discussion

In this study we created a series of virtual environments in which younger and older adult participants travelled routes and then later re-traced those routes, allowing us to assess spatial memory performance. Critically, participants either traveled routes during encoding by active exploration through the volitional control of their movements, or by passively viewing a guided tour. As expected, we found that actively navigating through virtual environments resulted in more accurate performances in re-tracing the travelled routes, than passively viewing a recorded navigation during encoding. As expected, those with higher scores on the Hooper Visual Organizational test had more accurate spatial memories, regardless of how the routes were encoded. Importantly, we showed that the memory enhancement from active encoding was larger for older than younger adults, indicating that age-related deficits in spatial memory can be reduced by active encoding. Our analysis also revealed that the cognitive approach of stopping close to an intersection benefitted later spatial memory following active encoding. We suggest that active encoding provides a high degree of environmental support for older adults, by prompting cognitive engagement with the route information, which can serve to improve encoding and subsequent retrieval of that information.

The positive relationship found between memory accuracy and scores on the Hooper Visual Orientation test suggests that individuals who can create better mental visualizations are better at creating a mental image of the travelled routes, which benefits performance when retracing those routes. The Hooper Visual Orientation test measures one's ability to mentally rotate and piece together misarranged visual information to identify the depicted object [45,46]. As such, it may be the case that individuals with higher scores on this test are better at mentally translating and combining the visual components of travelled sections of the route, to create a survey representation of the environment. Indeed, this relationship emerged for both active and passive encoding, which indicates that regardless of how one interacts with an environment, the ability to visualize a mental map supports the memory retrieval of route information.

The finding that older adults' spatial memory performance was enhanced following active relative to passive encoding, is consistent with other findings in the literature [15,25,26]. For example, Sauzéon and colleagues [26] demonstrated that older adults had better memories for objects in a virtual apartment following active exploration rather than a passively guided tour. Additionally, active encoding has been found to benefit older adults' memory for spatial information [15,25] showing that when participants are active 'drivers', their memory is better than when they act as passive 'passengers' in virtual environments. Our findings build on this previous work, by demonstrating that when attempting to retrace a route that is encountered on only one previous occasion, having actively been in control of the initial navigation benefitted memory more than passive guidance. These findings contribute to the literature, suggesting that age-related deficits in spatial memory abilities can be ameliorated through the use of active encoding strategies for navigation.

The finding that memory accuracy was related to the number of stars collected following active, but not passive encoding suggests that during active navigation, attention is indeed oriented towards information that is relevant to the traveled route. Notably, no relationship was found between memory accuracy and the length of the path traveled, meaning that the collection of stars must have provided a unique benefit towards encoding. One possibility is that a memory benefit was obtained through intrinsic motivation or curiosity [35,36] associated with collecting the stars. As described in the introduction, it has been suggested that momentary feelings of curiosity boost memory and executive functions [37], because phasic activation of the noradrenergic and dopaminergic systems modulate hippocampal activity [38]. Regardless of the potential mechanism, it is clear from our results that having a larger number of interesting or notable targets in the environment during encoding enhanced memory recall.

We also found a relationships between mental accuracy and the distance of stops from the nearest intersection during encoding and retrieval, such that stopping near an intersection was related to better performance in retracing the route. Furthermore, in the regression analysis, stopping near an intersection during active encoding was found to be predictive of the accuracy in route overlap. When participants stopped moving near an intersection within the environment during encoding, it facilitated their later memory in recalling the spatial route travelled. It may also be the case that the intersections, or decision points, are critical components of the overall spatial representation of the route. Enhanced encoding of these points likely led to a better spatial representation of the details of the route. When the participants stopped moving in the environment during retrieval, they were possibly attempting to remember the decisions that were previously made at the intersection during encoding, and correcting their planned route if necessary. However, it is important to note that only stopping near an intersection during active encoding, and not retrieval, was a significant predictor of route overlap accuracy. This finding suggests that stopping to focus attention on decision points during exploration in the environment aids spatial memory performance.

In older adults, links have been found between poor spatial representation abilities and declines in both executive functioning [52,53] and episodic memory [27]. The effortfulness hypothesis [54], which states that, because of age-related sensory limitations, there are more cognitive resources that are allocated to the identification of perceptual information, rather than to the encoding of meaningful content, could explain why spatial memory deficits occur in older adults. For example, if limited cognitive resources are directed towards the identification or perceptual processing of a landmark, encoding of the spatial location of the landmark or of the route travelled would be hindered. Indeed, navigational strategies are effortful and cognitively demanding, requiring executive functioning, spatial abilities, and memory [43], which are well-documented as being in decline in older adults. Critically, however, it should be possible to reduce age-related differences in spatial memory performance by implementing encoding strategies that direct cognitive resources specifically to the encoding of spatial information. While our task involved physical components (motor control for locomotion, proprioceptive, and vestibular sensory information) from pressing the movement button and spinning the chair to change directions, it was likely not difficult or demanding enough to create a cognitive burden on the older adults. It would be interesting for future work, to include a divided attention condition, in which participants need to respond to a secondary task while simultaneously navigating during encoding, to determine if heavily taxing their available cognitive resources results in a diminished effect of active encoding.

Notably, we found that older adults had significantly poorer spatial visualization abilities than younger adults, which may be linked to a common deficit that is associated with the poorer spatial memory performance observed in this age group. Older adults have been found to rely more on egocentric rather than allocentric representations during navigation [55,56], the latter of which involves a more highly developed survey representation of space [57], and this is possibly supported by processes that are similar to those supporting general spatial visualization functions. Evidence suggests that degradation in the hippocampal region is related to declines in survey abilities in older adults [58,59] and also to visual perceptual processing [60], which may be involved in spatial scene construction abilities that are supported by the hippocampus [61,62]. Indeed, older adults have been shown to have worse performances than younger adults in both spatial and scene construction tasks that involve imagining an event [63]. An interesting avenue for future work would be to investigate the links between visual imagery abilities, scene construction, and spatial representations, and how these change in the aging brain.

8. Conclusions

The results from this study demonstrate that actively navigating, rather than passively encoding environments results in a more accurate performance when re-tracing a travelled route. Importantly, the magnitude of the memory enhancement from active relative to passive encoding was larger for older than younger adults, reducing the commonly observed age-related deficit in spatial memory performance. Additionally, our findings demonstrate that higher scores on the Hooper Visual Organizational test, and pausing near intersections during active encoding are related to, and predictive of, route overlap accuracy, illuminating the cognitive components that contribute to the benefits of active navigation memory. Overall, our findings suggest that older adults can improve their spatial memory performance for travelled routes by actively controlling their exploration of new environments.

Author Contributions: Conceptualization, M.E.M., M.A.F., and H.S.; methodology, M.E.M., J.G.M., and M.A.F.; software, J.G.M.; validation, M.E.M., J.G.M., and M.A.F.; formal analysis, M.E.M.; investigation, M.E.M.; resources, M.A.F., and H.S.; data curation, M.E.M., and J.G.M.; writing—original draft preparation, M.E.M.; writing—review and editing, M.E.M., J.G.M., M.A.F., and H.S.; visualization, M.E.M. and J.G.M.; supervision, M.A.F.; project administration, M.E.M. and M.A.F.; funding acquisition, M.A.F. and H.S.

References

1. Kirasic, K.C. Spatial cognition and behavior in young and elderly adults: Implications for learning new environments. *Psychol. Aging* **1991**, *6*, 10–18. [CrossRef] [PubMed]
2. Wilkniss, S.M.; Jones, M.G.; Korol, D.L.; Gold, P.E.; Manning, C.A. Age-related differences in an ecologically based study of route learning. *Psychol. Aging* **1997**, *12*, 372–375. [CrossRef] [PubMed]
3. De Beni, R.; Pazzaglia, F.; Gardini, S. The role of mental rotation and age in spatial perspective-taking tasks: When age does not impair perspective-taking performance. *Appl. Cognit. Psychol.* **2006**, *20*, 807–821. [CrossRef]
4. Jonker, C.; Launer, L.J.; Hooijer, C.; Lindeboom, J. Memory Complaints and Memory Impairment in Older Individuals. *J. Am. Geriatr. Soc.* **1996**, *44*, 44–49. [CrossRef] [PubMed]
5. Leitsch, S.; Algase, D.L.; Hong, G.-R.; Beattie, E.; Song, J.-A.; Yao, L. The Interrelatedness of Wandering and Wayfinding in a Community Sample of Persons with Dementia. *Dement. Geriatr. Cogn. Disord.* **2004**, *17*, 231–239.
6. Henderson, V.W.; Mack, W.; Williams, B.W. Spatial Disorientation in Alzheimer's Disease. *Arch. Neurol.* **1989**, *46*, 391–394. [CrossRef] [PubMed]
7. Kavcic, V.; Duffy, C.J. Attentional dynamics and visual perception: mechanisms of spatial disorientation in Alzheimer's disease. *Brain* **2003**, *126*, 1173–1181. [CrossRef] [PubMed]
8. Monacelli, A.M.; Cushman, L.A.; Kavcic, V.; Duffy, C.J. Spatial disorientation in Alzheimer's disease: The remembrance of things passed. *Neurology* **2003**, *61*, 1491–1497. [CrossRef] [PubMed]
9. Pai, M.-C.; Pai, M.; Jacobs, W.J. Topographical disorientation in community-residing patients with Alzheimer's disease. *Int. J. Geriatr. Psychiatry* **2004**, *19*, 250–255. [CrossRef] [PubMed]
10. Cogné, M.; Taillade, M.; N'Kaoua, B.; Tarruella, A.; Klinger, E.; Larrue, F.; Sauzéon, H.; Joseph, P.-A.; Sorita, E. The contribution of virtual reality to the diagnosis of spatial navigation disorders and to the study of the role of navigational aids: A systematic literature review. *Ann. Phys. Rehabil. Med.* **2017**, *60*, 164–176. [CrossRef] [PubMed]
11. Chrastil, E.R.; Warren, W.H. Active and passive contributions to spatial learning. *Psychon. Bull. Rev.* **2011**, *19*, 1–23. [CrossRef] [PubMed]
12. Markant, D.B.; Ruggeri, A.; Gureckis, T.M.; Xu, F. Enhanced Memory as a Common Effect of Active Learning. *Mind Brain Educ.* **2016**, *10*, 142–152. [CrossRef]
13. Chrastil, E.R.; Warren, W.H. Active and passive spatial learning in human navigation: Acquisition of survey knowledge. *J. Exp. Psychol. Learn. Mem. Cognit.* **2013**, *39*, 1520–1537. [CrossRef] [PubMed]
14. Vidal, M.; Kemeny, A.; Gaunet, F.; Berthoz, A. Active, passive and snapshot exploration in a virtual environment: influence on scene memory, reorientation and path memory. *Cogn. Brain Res.* **2001**, *11*, 409–420.
15. Jebara, N.; Orriols, E.; Zaoui, M.; Berthoz, A.; Piolino, P. Effects of Enactment in Episodic Memory: A Pilot Virtual Reality Study with Young and Elderly Adults. *Front. Neuroinform.* **2014**, *6*, 338. [CrossRef] [PubMed]
16. Sandamas, G.; Foreman, N. Active Versus Passive Acquisition of Spatial Knowledge While Controlling a Vehicle in a Virtual Urban Space in Drivers and Non-Drivers. *SAGE Open* **2015**, *5*, 215824401559544. [CrossRef]
17. Brooks, B.M. The Specificity of Memory Enhancement During Interaction with a Virtual Environment. *Memory* **1999**, *7*, 65–78. [CrossRef] [PubMed]
18. Sauzéon, H.; Pala, P.A.; Larrue, F.; Wallet, G.; Déjos, M.; Zheng, X.; Guitton, P.; N'Kaoua, B. The Use of Virtual Reality for Episodic Memory Assessment. *Exp. Psychol.* **2012**, *59*, 99–108. [CrossRef] [PubMed]
19. Zimmer, H.D.; Engelkamp, J. Levels-of-processing effects in subject-performed tasks. *Mem. Cogn.* **1999**, *27*, 907–914. [CrossRef]
20. Karlsson, T.; Backman, L.; Herlitz, A.; Nilsson, L.G.; Winblad, B.; Osterlind, P.O. Memory improvement at different stages of Alzheimer's disease. *Neuropsychologia* **1989**, *27*, 737–742. [CrossRef]
21. Silva, A.R.; Pinho, M.S.; Souchay, C.; Moulin, C.J.A. Evaluating the subject-performed task effect in healthy older adults: Relationship with neuropsychological tests. *Socioaffect. Neurosci. Psychol.* **2015**, *5*, 53. [CrossRef] [PubMed]

22. Essen, J.D.; Von Essen, J.D.; Nilsson, L.-G. Memory effects of motor activation in subject-performed tasks and sign language. *Psychon. Bull. Rev.* **2003**, *10*, 445–449. [CrossRef]
23. Craik, F.I.M.; Routh, D.A.; Broadbent, D.E. On the Transfer of Information from Temporary to Permanent Memory [and Discussion]. *Philos. Trans. R. Soc. B* **1983**, *302*, 341–359. [CrossRef]
24. Craik, F.I.M.; Jennings, J.M. Human memory. In *The Handbook of Aging and Cognition*; Craik, F.I.M., Salthouse, T.A., Eds.; Lawrence Erlbaum Associates: Hillsdale, NJ, USA, 1992; pp. 51–110.
25. Plancher, G.; Tirard, A.; Gyselinck, V.; Nicolas, S.; Piolino, P. Using virtual reality to characterize episodic memory profiles in amnestic mild cognitive impairment and Alzheimer's disease: Influence of active and passive encoding. *Neuropsychologia* **2012**, *50*, 592–602. [CrossRef] [PubMed]
26. Sauzéon, H.; N'Kaoua, B.; Pala, P.A.; Taillade, M.; Guitton, P. Age and active navigation effects on episodic memory: A virtual reality study. *Br. J. Psychol.* **2015**, *107*, 72–94. [CrossRef] [PubMed]
27. Taillade, M.; Sauzéon, H.; Dejos, M.; Pala, P.A.; Larrue, F.; Wallet, G.; Gross, C.; N'Kaoua, B. Executive and memory correlates of age-related differences in wayfinding performances using a virtual reality application. *Aging Neuropsychol. Cognit.* **2013**, *20*, 298–319. [CrossRef] [PubMed]
28. Li, K.Z.; Lindenberger, U.; Freund, A.M.; Baltes, P.B. Walking While Memorizing: Age-Related Differences in Compensatory Behavior. *Psychol. Sci.* **2001**, *12*, 230–237. [CrossRef] [PubMed]
29. Hausdorff, J.M.; Yogev, G.; Springer, S.; Simon, E.S.; Giladi, N. Walking is more like catching than tapping: Gait in the elderly as a complex cognitive task. *Exp. Brain Res.* **2005**, *164*, 541–548. [CrossRef] [PubMed]
30. Bakdash, J.Z.; Linkenauger, S.A.; Proffitt, D. Comparing Decision-Making and Control for Learning a Virtual Environment: Backseat Drivers Learn Where They are Going. *Proc. Hum. Factors Ergon. Soc. Ann. Meet.* **2008**, *52*, 2117–2121. [CrossRef]
31. Bakdash, J.; Linkenauger, S.; Stefanucci, J.; Witt, J.; Banton, T.; Proffitt, D. Perceived distance influences simulated walking time. *J. Vis.* **2010**, *8*, 1151. [CrossRef]
32. Feyereisen, P. Enactment effects and integration processes in younger and older adults' memory for actions. *Memory* **2009**, *17*, 374–385. [CrossRef] [PubMed]
33. Gutchess, A.H.; Kensinger, E.A.; Yoon, C.; Schacter, D.L. Ageing and the self-reference effect in memory. *Memory* **2007**, *15*, 822–837. [CrossRef] [PubMed]
34. Lalanne, J.; Rozenberg, J.; Grolleau, P.; Piolino, P. The Self-Reference Effect on Episodic Memory Recollection in Young and Older Adults and Alzheimer's Disease. *Curr. Alzheimer Res.* **2013**, *10*, 1107–1117. [CrossRef] [PubMed]
35. Ryan, R.M.; Deci, E.L. Intrinsic and Extrinsic Motivations: Classic Definitions and New Directions. *Contemp. Educ. Psychol.* **2000**, *25*, 54–67. [CrossRef] [PubMed]
36. Kashdan, T.B.; Silvia, P.J. Curiosity and Interest: The Benefits of Thriving on Novelty and Challenge. *Curiosit. Interest Benefits Thriving Nov. Chall.* **2012**, *2*, 367–374.
37. Sakaki, M.; Yagi, A.; Murayama, K. Curiosity in old age: A possible key to achieving adaptive aging. *Neurosci. Biobehav. Rev.* **2018**, *88*, 106–116. [CrossRef] [PubMed]
38. Oudeyer, P.Y.; Gottlieb, J.; Lopes, M. Intrinsic motivation, curiosity, and learning: Theory and applications in educational technologies. In *Progress in Brain Research*; Elsevier: Amsterdam, The Netherlands, 2016; Volume 229, pp. 257–284.
39. Hegarty, M.; Montello, D.R.; Richardson, A.E.; Ishikawa, T.; Lovelace, K. Spatial abilities at different scales: Individual differences in aptitude-test performance and spatial-layout learning. *Intelligence* **2006**, *34*, 151–176. [CrossRef]
40. Moffat, S. Age differences in spatial memory in a virtual environment navigation task. *Neurobiol. Aging* **2001**, *22*, 787–796. [CrossRef]
41. Moffat, S.D.; Resnick, S.M. Effects of age on virtual environment place navigation and allocentric cognitive mapping. *Behav. Neurosci.* **2002**, *116*, 851–859. [CrossRef] [PubMed]
42. Cushman, L.A.; Stein, K.; Duffy, C.J. Detecting navigational deficits in cognitive aging and Alzheimer disease using virtual reality. *Neurology* **2008**, *71*, 888–895. [CrossRef] [PubMed]
43. Taillade, M.; N'Kaoua, B.; Sauzéon, H. Age-Related Differences and Cognitive Correlates of Self-Reported and Direct Navigation Performance: The Effect of Real and Virtual Test Conditions Manipulation. *Front. Psychiatry* **2016**, *6*, 125. [CrossRef] [PubMed]

44. Nasreddine, Z.S.; Phillips, N.A.; Bedirian, V.; Charbonneau, S.; Whitehead, V.; Collin, I.; Cummings, J.L.; Chertkow, H.; Bédirian, V. The Montreal Cognitive Assessment, MoCA: A Brief Screening Tool for Mild Cognitive Impairment. *J. Am. Geriatr. Soc.* **2005**, *53*, 695–699. [CrossRef] [PubMed]
45. Buttaro, M. *Hooper Visual Organization Test*; Springer Nature: Basingstoke, UK, 2017; Volume 28, pp. 1–3.
46. Lopez, M.N.; Lazar, M.D.; Oh, S. Psychometric Properties of the Hooper Visual Organization Test. *Assessment* **2003**, *10*, 66–70. [CrossRef] [PubMed]
47. Hegarty, M. Development of a self-report measure of environmental spatial ability. *Intelligence* **2002**, *30*, 425–447. [CrossRef]
48. Brown, J. Some tests of the decay theory of immediate memory. *Q. J. Exp. Psychol.* **1958**, *10*, 12–21. [CrossRef]
49. Moffat, S.D.; Hampson, E.; Hatzipantelis, M. Navigation in a "Virtual" Maze: Sex Differences and Correlation with Psychometric Measures of Spatial Ability in Humans. *Evol. Hum. Behav.* **1998**, *19*, 73–87. [CrossRef]
50. Miceli, A.; Salkind, N. Teoria Statistica Delle Classi e Calcolo Delle Probabilità. In *Encyclopedia of Research Design*; SAGE Publications: Thousand Oaks, CA, USA, 2012.
51. Benjamini, Y.; Hochberg, Y. Controlling the False Discovery Rate: A Practical and Powerful Approach to Multiple Testing. *J. R. Stat. Soc. Ser. B* **1995**, *57*, 289–300. [CrossRef]
52. Ciaramelli, E. The role of ventromedial prefrontal cortex in navigation: A case of impaired wayfinding and rehabilitation. *Neuropsychologia* **2008**, *46*, 2099–2105. [CrossRef] [PubMed]
53. Moffat, S.D.; Kennedy, K.M.; Rodrigue, K.M.; Raz, N. Extrahippocampal Contributions to Age Differences in Human Spatial Navigation. *Cereb. Cortex* **2006**, *17*, 1274–1282. [CrossRef] [PubMed]
54. McCoy, S.L.; Tun, P.A.; Cox, L.C.; Colangelo, M.; Stewart, R.A.; Wingfield, A. Hearing loss and perceptual effort: downstream effects on older adults' memory for speech. *Q. J. Exp. Psychol. Sec. A* **2005**, *58*, 22–33. [CrossRef] [PubMed]
55. Gazova, I.; Laczo, J.; Rubinova, E.; Mokrisova, I.; Hyncicova, E.; Andel, R.; Vyhnalek, M.; Sheardova, K.; Coulson, E.J.; Hort, J. Spatial navigation in young versus older adults. *Front. Neuroinform.* **2013**, *5*, 94. [CrossRef] [PubMed]
56. Serino, S.; Cipresso, P.; Morganti, F.; Riva, G. The role of egocentric and allocentric abilities in Alzheimer's disease: A systematic review. *Ageing Res. Rev.* **2014**, *16*, 32–44. [CrossRef] [PubMed]
57. Siegel, A.W.; White, S.H. The Development of Spatial Representations of Large-Scale Environments. *Adv. Child Dev. Behav.* **1975**, *10*, 9–55. [PubMed]
58. Guderian, S.; Dzieciol, A.M.; Gadian, D.G.; Jentschke, S.; Doeller, C.F.; Burgess, N.; Mishkin, M.; Vargha-Khadem, F. Hippocampal Volume Reduction in Humans Predicts Impaired Allocentric Spatial Memory in Virtual-Reality Navigation. *J. Neurosci.* **2015**, *35*, 14123–14131. [CrossRef] [PubMed]
59. Fidalgo, C.; Martin, C.B. The Hippocampus Contributes to Allocentric Spatial Memory through Coherent Scene Representations. *J. Neurosci.* **2016**, *36*, 2555–2557. [CrossRef] [PubMed]
60. Graham, K.S.; Barense, M.D.; Lee, A.C. Going beyond LTM in the MTL: A synthesis of neuropsychological and neuroimaging findings on the role of the medial temporal lobe in memory and perception. *Neuropsychologia* **2010**, *48*, 831–853. [CrossRef] [PubMed]
61. Schacter, D.L.; Addis, D.R.; Hassabis, D.; Martin, V.C.; Spreng, R.N.; Szpunar, K.K. The Future of Memory: Remembering, Imagining, and the Brain. *Neuron* **2012**, *76*, 677–694. [CrossRef] [PubMed]
62. Maguire, E.A.; Mullally, S.L. The hippocampus: A manifesto for change. *J. Exp. Psychol. Gen.* **2013**, *142*, 1180–1189. [CrossRef] [PubMed]
63. Rendell, P.G.; Bailey, P.E.; Henry, J.D.; Phillips, L.H.; Gaskin, S.; Kliegel, M. Older adults have greater difficulty imagining future rather than atemporal experiences. *Psychol. Aging* **2012**, *27*, 1089–1098. [CrossRef] [PubMed]

8

A Homeostatic Model of Subjective Cognitive Decline

Akiko Mizuno [1,*], Maria Ly [1,2] and Howard J. Aizenstein [1,3]

1 Department of Psychiatry, University of Pittsburgh, Pittsburgh, PA 15213, USA; Ly.Maria@medstudent.pitt.edu (M.L.); aizen@pitt.edu (H.J.A.)
2 Department of Neuroscience, University of Pittsburgh, Pittsburgh, PA 15213, USA
3 Department of Bioengineering, University of Pittsburgh, Pittsburgh, PA 15213, USA
* Correspondence: akm82@pitt.edu

Abstract: Subjective Cognitive Decline (SCD) is possibly one of the earliest detectable signs of dementia, but we do not know which mental processes lead to elevated concern. In this narrative review, we will summarize the previous literature on the biomarkers and functional neuroanatomy of SCD. In order to extend upon the prevailing theory of SCD, compensatory hyperactivation, we will introduce a new model: the breakdown of homeostasis in the prediction error minimization system. A cognitive prediction error is a discrepancy between an implicit cognitive prediction and the corresponding outcome. Experiencing frequent prediction errors may be a primary source of elevated subjective concern. Our homeostasis breakdown model provides an explanation for the progression from both normal cognition to SCD and from SCD to advanced dementia stages.

Keywords: subjective cognitive decline; preclinical dementia; fMRI; compensation

---

1. Introduction

Subjective Cognitive Decline (SCD) refers to an individual's perception that their cognitive performance has declined, despite having no significant objective cognitive impairment. SCD may reflect one of the earliest signs of dementia, as it is a risk factor for developing mild cognitive impairment (MCI) and Alzheimer's disease (AD) [1,2]. However, SCD is quite understudied—which mental processes lead to SCD and the neural basis of SCD are yet to be understood. Here, we will provide a narrative review of the current literature for biomarkers, and the functional neuroanatomy associated with SCD. Then, we will propose a new model that integrates existing findings in SCD into a new neural system dysfunction model, which involves heightened prediction of error-signaling and homeostatic breakdown.

2. AD Biomarkers (Neurodegenerative Factors) and SCD

In order to investigate whether SCD represents a pre-clinical state of AD, the relationships between AD biomarkers in individuals with SCD were examined. In the traditional AD biomarker cascade, amyloid (Aβ) accumulation occurs prior to neurodegeneration and cognitive decline [3]. The most promising evidence that SCD precedes MCI and AD is that Aβ deposition is associated with SCD symptom severity, but not with objective memory performance [4–6]. Vogel and colleagues [7] found that amyloid status predicted future cognitive decline (on average, four years) among individuals with SCD. However, a larger longitudinal study [8] concluded that the Aβ-status by itself does not predict the progression of AD over a relatively brief time span of 2.5 years. More longitudinal studies are necessary to better understand the relationship between Aβ and objective cognitive decline in SCD. In addition to the accumulation of amyloid plaques, AD is also associated with neurofibrillary tangles composed of tau protein. Tau accumulation is believed to be more closely related to neurodegeneration and cognitive decline in AD, as compared with amyloid [9]. Tau has been shown to be more associated with SCD than with non-amnestic MCI [10]. Thus, like Aβ, the tau markers support the role SCD as an AD risk group.

Brain atrophy and white matter hyperintensities have been also reported in SCD, as seen in the early pre-clinical stages of AD progression. Several studies consistently reported cortical volume loss and thinning in the medial temporal regions in those with SCD [11–15], indicating the decreased structural integrity of the memory system. Longitudinal observations also reported the association between atrophy and future cognitive decline in SCD [16,17]. Whole-brain analysis by Verfaillie and colleagues [17] suggested that a steeper decline in cognition was not only associated with a thinner cortex of the temporal region but also the frontal and occipital cortices in SCD. Increased amounts of white matter hyperintensities in widespread regions have also been reported in SCD [18,19]. These studies provide support for the idea that SCD may be an early transitional stage prior to the onset of dementia (i.e., MCI and AD), especially as seen with the perturbations in the memory systems.

3. Functional Neuroanatomy and Compensation Theory in SCD

The neural basis of elevated subjective concern for cognitive decline among older individuals with normal cognition is the least investigated, but it represents a growing area of research (Table 1). Four functional magnetic resonance imaging (fMRI) studies investigated brain activation during memory-related tasks [20–23]. Most of these studies did not find group differences between participants with and without SCD in the behavioral performance of the task, but observed different functional brain activation patterns. The first study by Rodda and colleagues [23] measured brain activity while participants were encoding a list of semantically related words, which were later tested through a recognition paradigm. Whole-brain analysis demonstrated increased activation in the lateral part of the prefrontal cortex (PFC) in those with SCD. The level of the PFC activation was positively correlated with task performance. The authors interpreted that increased PFC activation served as neural compensation for the decreasing function of the primary hippocampal memory system, as indicated in previous structural imaging studies (summarized in the previous section). To test this compensation hypothesis, Erk et al. (2011) [20] investigated activation in the hippocampus and the PFC during memory encoding of faces and associated occupations, through a region-of-interest approach. Their results demonstrated decreased activation in the hippocampus, and increased activation in the dorsolateral PFC (dlPFC). Task performance was positively correlated with dlPFC activation only in the SCD group, which provided support for the compensation hypothesis in SCD.

Table 1. Summary of fMRI studies in SCD. Most of these studies demonstrate a pattern of regional hypoactivation, associated with hyperactivation elsewhere. This hyperactivation has been interpreted by authors as a compensatory response to the hypoactivation. Abbreviations: SCD: subjective cognitive decline, PFC: prefrontal cortex, BA: Brodmann area, DLPFC: dorsolateral prefrontal cortex, ROI: region-of-interest, SPL: superior parietal lobe, PCC: posterior cingulate cortex, DMN: default mode network, VMPFC: ventromedial prefrontal cortex, ACC: anterior cingulate cortex, MFG: middle frontal gyrus, WM: working memory.

Reference	fMRI Task	Participants	Hyperactivation (SCD > Control) or Positive Correlation with SCD Symptoms	Hypoactivation (Control > SCD) or Negative Correlation with SCD Symptoms	Behavioral Performance
Rodda et al. (2009) [23]	Memory encoding	10 memory clinic SCD vs. 10 controls (age: 64.2 vs. 68.0)	L PFC (BA6/9/44/46)		(1) No group differences in behavioral performance (2) Positive correlation between PFC activation and recognition performance in both groups.
Erk et al. (2011) [20]	Memory (encoding, recall, recognition) and working memory (n-back)	19 memory clinic SCD vs. 20 controls (age: 68.4 vs. 66.8)	R DLPFC during recall (ROI analysis)	Hippocampus during recall (ROI analysis)	(1) No group differences in behavioral performance (2) Positive correlation between DLPFC activation and recognition performance in SCD. (3) Positive correlation between hippocampal activation and recognition performance in controls
Rodda et al. (2011) [24]	Divided attention	11 memory clinic SCD vs. 10 controls (age: 64.6 vs. 68.0)	L medial temporal, bilateral thalamus, PCC, caudate		(1) No group differences in behavioral performance
Dumas et al. (2013) [25]	Working memory (n-back)	Postmenopausal women: 12 cognitive complainers vs. 11 controls (age = 56.8 vs. 57.1)	MFG (BA10/9), ACC (BA24/32), insula (BA 13), precuneus (increased activation as WM demand increased)	Caudate	(1) No group differences in behavioral performance
Hu et al. (2017) [22]	Future-oriented decision making	20 memory clinic SCD vs. 24 controls (age: 68.3 vs. 66.49)		Medial frontal polar cortex, ACC, insula	(2) SCD showed reduced future-oriented choices (3) Positive correlation between hippocampal activation (ROI analysis) and future-oriented choice in only the control.
Hayes et al. (2017) [21]	Memory: successful vs. unsuccessful encoding	23 SCD vs. 41 controls (age: 68.6 vs 67.5) 21 out of 23 were memory clinic SCD	(1) Negative subsequent memory effect in the occipital lobe, SPL, PCC (2) More complaints, more negative subsequence memory effects in DMN (PCC, precuneus, VMPFC)		(1) No group differences in behavioral performance

Hu et al. (2017) [22] utilized a task that emulated memory processes that were relevant to activities in daily life (future-oriented choice tasks). Brain activation was measured, while participants were required to select an immediate or delayed reward regarding a personally relevant episodic future event. Successful selection of the future-oriented choice (i.e., delayed reward) over the immediate reward requires the crucial involvement of episodic memory and valuation systems [26]. Unlike other studies, their study is the only one which observed group differences in task performance. The SCD group showed reduced preference for future-oriented choice, which was previously demonstrated in those with MCI [27]. A priori region-of-interest analysis showed that only participants in the control group showed an association between greater hippocampal activation and more future-oriented choices. The whole-brain analyses found reduced activation in medial frontal regions (medial frontal pole and anterior cingulate cortex (ACC)) and the insula in the SCD group, suggesting diminished valuation functioning. The authors suggested that reduced involvement in the episodic memory and valuation system in SCD during the decision-making process may reflect the attenuating attention and subjective evaluation system.

To address the possibility that increased PFC activation reflects a general cognitive processes rather than only memory encoding, Hayes et al. (2017) [21] used an event-related design to compare brain activation for high-confidence successful recall versus failed recall. The SCD group showed an increased activation for failed recall (i.e., negative subsequent memory) in the posterior areas (occipital, superior parietal, and precuneus). They also regressed activation on a continuous SCD symptom severity to identify the neural correlates of SCD, by combining participants in both groups. Participants with more severe SCD symptoms showed increased activation for failed recall in both the frontal and posterior nodes of the default mode network, which normally suppress its activity during cognitive tasks. They concluded that individuals with SCD rely on the altered neural system for successful memory encoding to maintain normal cognitive function.

Cognitive concerns in SCD mainly reflect the perceived decline of memory function, but the other domains of cognitive function may also contribute to elevated concerns [28]. There are two fMRI studies with non-episodic memory tasks. Dumas and colleagues [25] measured brain activation in SCD by using the n-back working memory task. Although this study was limited to females (i.e., a comparison between those with and without cognitive concerns among postmenopausal women without hormone therapy), their study is the first to report that activation increased with increasing cognitive load/effort among those with SCD. These effects were found in the extended working memory system, including middle frontal (BA 9/10), anterior cingulate cortex (BA 24/32), and the precuneus (BA 13). Both groups showed the same levels of behavioral performance. Another study by Rodda et al. (2011) [24] investigated brain activation during a divided attention task, where participants with SCD were required to respond to target stimuli while processing sequences of both visual and auditory information. Behavioral performance did not show group differences, but the SCD group demonstrated increased activation in two medial posterior regions: one in the cerebellum, and another in the thalamus, extending to the posterior cingulate cortex and the medial temporal lobe (hippocampus and parahippocampus). These two studies are consistent with the idea that early functional changes (i.e., increased activation) in executive function may manifest in SCD, despite the lack of impairment in behavioral performance or in the neuropsychological tests.

In summary, previous fMRI studies, along with the structural imaging studies (summarized in the previous section) have suggested three neural phenomena in SCD: (1) loss of integration of the memory system, (2) compensatory hyperactivation in the prefrontal cortex or the use of other alternative neural resources to maintain normal performance, and (3) decreased prefrontal activation for subtle yet declining higher-order cognitive functions. In other words, the direction of neural activation (increased or decreased) observed in SCD depends on whether the expected level of performance can be maintained. However, it is important to note that the sample sizes and statistical power in these studies were relatively low; likewise, inconsistencies between studies may have been partially due to sampling error. To extend our understanding of the functional neuroanatomy of SCD, more mechanistic and cohesive frameworks that can provide explanations for dysfunctional processes are necessary, regardless the level of task performance or cognitive domain. Furthermore, it is not yet understood which specific cognitive processes rely upon compensation, and how these processes are directly associated with SCD symptoms.

4. Current Theories of the Neural Basis of SCD

Compensatory hyperactivation of the prefrontal region is currently the most popular theory of the neural basis of SCD. Another theory is brain reserve [29], which proposes a structural basis for functional compensatory capacity. Alternatively, the dedifferentiation [30], a loss of specialization of neural function resulting in diffuse brain activations, is a theory which may explain hyperactivation in the prefrontal cortex. All of these versions of compensatory hyperactivation describe only the temporal transition from the pre-SCD state to the SCD state, and do not describe the dynamics of post-SCD neurodegeneration. Further, they do not describe how hyperactivation may contribute to post-SCD decline via harmful biological effects on the neural system, such as neurotoxicity or excitotoxicity. Here, we introduce homeostasis breakdown, a new mechanistic framework for comprehensive temporal dynamics in SCD and progression to AD.

5. Background of the Prediction Error Theory

Our brain functions as a statistical optimization engine that constantly makes implicit predictions of sensory inputs [31,32]. That is, rather than passively receiving sensory information, it is actively making inferences. These inferences are propagated as predicted expectations to heteromodal association areas and the PFC. These expectations are compared with the current environment, and a behavior is chosen. Moreover, the difference between predicted and observed behavior is used as learning signal to adapt for better performance in the future. This constant process of comparing internally generated predictions with external reality is called "predictive coding" [33]. This is why we think of the brain as learning and adapting across all behaviors.

Prediction errors refer to the mismatch between the internally generated prediction and the external reality. The most prominent brain region that responds to such errors is the dorsal anterior cingulate cortex (dACC). Both animal and human studies have demonstrated the increased activity in dACC to response to prediction errors [34,35]. Similar terms for prediction errors are conflict [34,36] and free-energy [37]. Although there is a general consensus that dACC mediates error-related signals; neuroscientists have different opinions about the specific processes in the dACC and the primary goal of the function [38]. Nonetheless (regardless of the diverse terminology and theories of dACC function), the minimization of prediction error is a core organizing principal for computational function at the local neural circuit. This error minimization optimizes our internal predictions, which facilitates successful goal-directed behaviors and survival.

6. Prediction Error and SCD Symptoms

Suppose a man who is very experienced with a computer notices that he is making more typing errors. If he experiences subtle yet frequent errors between his prediction ("I thought I typed out 'experience'") and actual outcome ("I accidentally typed 'exprience'"), his level of SCD symptoms may rise. This type of error signal raises the activation in the dACC, resulting in varying levels of awareness. We believe that an uncharacteristic accumulation of implicit errors may gradually lead to more effort being required to maintain cognitive performance, and then to having more explicit levels of error awareness. Another example that may highlight the relationship between error monitoring and the experience of cognitive tasks being more effortful in SCD would be the following: an individual may be accustomed to finishing the "New York Times" crossword puzzle in 20 minutes (their prediction). However, if that individual finds that they are now needing 30 minutes or more to complete the puzzle, this reflects both a prediction error and the experience of increased effort. Such awareness of errors could occur not only in memory, but rather across multiple cognitive domains, including attention, task switching, language, and mathematical operations.

Awareness of one's internal cognitive system is called metacognition. According to Nelson (1990) [39], metacognition has two primary operations: monitoring and control. Monitoring refers to the introspection of incoming sensory information and one's own performance, whereas control refers to an allocation of an action (i.e., self-regulation). These two operations are independent, but reciprocally interacted. Both the prediction error [31,32] and conflict monitoring [34,36] frameworks provide mechanistic models for the monitoring of errors or conflicts. These models, however, differ in the level of information processing that they are meant to explain. Prediction error refers to the process that can occur throughout the cortical network. Prediction errors provide a signal that our internal model need to be updated, and the signal is generated by distributed processes of our incoming sensory information [40]. These local prediction errors influence the local Hebbian learning model [41]. In this way, correct predictions are strengthened, and incorrect predictions are weakened [42]. On the other hand, conflict-monitoring framework refers to how the more extended controlled yet implicit cognitive process integrates generated error signals, such as prepotent response suppression. Unlike prediction error, which is a general network learning signal, conflict monitoring refers to the specific monitoring and control functions in the dACC. The prediction error [31,32] process may specifically infer to the earlier operation of monitoring, whereas conflict-monitoring [34,36] may associate with both monitoring and control operations, suggested in Nelson's framework [39].

In the framework of metacognition, SCD can be interpreted as the impairment of both monitoring and the early stages of control. The accumulated subjective experience of prediction errors and perceived increase in an effort to complete tasks may eventually lead to the elevated self-awareness of cognitive decline, as reflected in SCD. As these individuals develop frank cognitive decline, conflict-monitoring processes may then decrease, leading to an opposite pattern of decreased self-awareness of cognitive functioning. Experimental tasks that are sensitive to the suppression of the inappropriate responses to implicit prediction error may be able to capture an earlier objective process of decline in SCD. Furthermore, neuroimaging studies with these tasks will provide detailed neural mechanisms of dysfunctional metacognition in SCD.

7. Prediction Error and SCD Characteristics

Previous studies suggest that the cognitive implications of SCD symptoms depend on the level of education achievement [28]. Since higher level of education is considered to be a marker of cognitive reserve, Stern [43,44] postulated that cognitive reserve provides resilience to neurodegeneration. Levels of cognitive reserve may represent the sensitivity to prediction errors, and the utility of the error signals. Individuals with high cognitive reserve may be highly sensitive to prediction errors, and interpret them as important learning signals to update the internal model. These individuals constitute a lifestyle of using these learning signals more frequently and effectively to make higher achievements, resulting in having a high cognitive reserve.

Individuals with SCD are often highly anxious, and characterized by their tendency to worry [1], usually expressed as high neuroticism in the Big Five personality trait model [45]. It has been demonstrated that individuals with high neuroticism are highly sensitive to prediction errors [46]. In the course of progression of neurodegeneration, these individuals may start noticing prediction errors earlier than those with low neuroticism. The frequent experience of errors may not only raise an awareness, but may also elicit concern. Individual with high neuroticism may then interpret the perceived errors as important learning signals, resulting in symptoms of SCD.

The high prevalence of depressive symptoms is another characteristic that has been reported consistently in SCD [1]. Neuroticism is also highly associated with depression; however, the symptoms associated with neuroticism and depression may relate to different aspects of SCD. Neuroticism may serve as a predictor of how an individual may interpret prediction errors, whereas depressive symptoms may reflect the affective response to an individual's interpretation of their prediction errors.

Depressive symptoms in SCD, therefore, may be translated as a negative affective response (i.e., sad feeling) to frequently experiencing errors (i.e., the "monitoring" component of metacognition), leading to the persistence of depressive moods over time [47]. Depressive symptoms may also be a form of adjustment disorder, where an individual may have an emotional reaction to their new experience of difficulty in both internal prediction and performance (i.e., the "control" component of metacognition).

8. Homeostasis Breakdown

Homeostasis—or homeostatic regulation—is the ability to maintain stability and equilibrium of the system. As a classical example, the stability of our body temperature is a consequence of homeostatic processes that coordinate the activity of muscles, blood vessels, and sweat glands. When a cold environment decreases body temperature, the hypothalamus releases a signal to the skeletal muscles, promoting shivering as a mechanism of thermogenesis and a signal to the blood vessels to increase resistance of blood flow (i.e., vasoconstriction). Both of these responses minimize heat loss, helping to maintain body temperature.

Prior work by Li et al. has suggested that homeostatic dysregulation in multiple systems occur in aging, and may also serve as a key contributor to the biological mechanisms of aging [48]. While the authors have provided evidence in the systems of lipids, immune function, oxygen transport, liver functioning, vitamin levels, and electrolyte levels, they suggest that homeostatic dysregulation is not limited to these systems, and may occur in other systems in aging.

Thus, we propose that compensatory hyperactivation may represent a homeostatic process that serves to maintain the stability of cognition in a changing neurobiological environment. Homeostasis in the context of cognition serves to maintain cognitive functioning, despite the presence of neurodegeneration. Neurodegeneration may lead to prediction errors and corresponding SCD symptoms, much like the body temperature falling just enough to cause a sensation of coldness. Finally, the compensatory hyperactivation is one of the main homeostatic processes that we are currently aware of in cognition, and this is analogous to the onset of vasoconstriction of blood vessels to prevent hypothermia.

However, homeostatic processes can have negative side effects. For example, extreme vasoconstriction for an extended period of time can lead to vascular cell loss. Similarly, compensatory hyperactivation may lead to glutaminergic excitotoxicity, which may lead to neuronal death [49] or the production of Aβ [50]. Thus, although homeostasis can slow the onset of cognitive decline, this may come at the cost of negative side effects that weaken the core cognitive infrastructure. This may explain why individuals with SCD tend to experience a relatively rapid decline into AD [51].

This homeostatic model of SCD represents an extension of the prevailing compensatory hyperactivation model, as it may provide a mechanistic explanation for differing levels of neural activity. The compensation model is unclear as to what entity "drives" the change in activation levels, whereas the homeostatic model provides a dynamic control system that maintains cognitive functioning that is dependent on prediction error and conflict monitoring.

9. Future Directions

Clinicians do not yet have a standard intervention protocol for individuals with SCD. If the neural basis for SCD were better understood, an effective intervention may be developed. A recent meta-analysis of experimental interventions for SCD suggested that cognitive restructuring therapies may improve metacognition (i.e., alleviate self-perceived cognitive challenges) [52], indicating that SCD could be a modifiable risk factor of dementia. Alleviating SCD symptoms, along with associated psychological distress may slow neurodegeneration, such as atrophy and Aβ accumulation, by reducing hyperactivation.

More studies investigating the markers of neurotoxicity in SCD are necessary to provide basic evidence for psychotherapeutic interventions in the earliest stages of dementia. In this narrative review, we have proposed a homeostatic prediction error model for understanding how the progression of neural system dysfunction can manifest as SCD. fMRI studies can help in validating that increases in error prediction, and conflict monitoring is central to the subjective perception of cognitive impairment. Further research is also necessary to identify the working elements (neural control system, sensors, set point, etc.) of the homeostatic prediction error model. Moreover, fMRI studies coupled with behavioral interventions can be used as an outcome measure. This would help in the development and adaptation of behavioral interventions targeting SCD, and potentially mitigating the accelerated neurodegeneration that may be associated with hyperactivated stressed system that is out of homeostatic balance.

10. Conclusions

In common scientific practice, the term *subjective* may generally be disfavored, because it connotes a lack of objectivity, as the self-assessments that are used to diagnose SCD, presumably include individual biases. However, the presence of SCD symptoms appears to contain valuable information regarding cognitive decline over time and underlying neurophysiological pathologies. More studies and theoretical frameworks that can comprehensively explain temporal dynamics, including the positive and negative by-products of compensatory hyperactivation, are necessary. In this review, we proposed that prediction error, a metacognitive process, potentially leads to SCD symptoms. We also introduced homeostatic breakdown as a new framework that incorporates and integrates the current findings with the new prediction error perspective, to describe the cascading effect of neurodegeneration and cognitive decline in SCD. This framework has the potential to motivate new standard therapies for SCD that focus on alleviating not only the subjective symptoms, but also slow the progression of dementia, due to neurotoxicity from compensatory hyperactivation.

Acknowledgments: We thank the administrative staff of the Geriatric Psychiatry Neuroimaging lab for assistance with various logistics in the preparation of this manuscript.

References

1. Jessen, F.; Amariglio, R.E.; van Boxtel, M.; Breteler, M.; Ceccaldi, M.; Chetelat, G.; Dubois, B.; Dufouil, C.; Ellis, K.A.; van der Flier, W.M.; et al. A conceptual framework for research on subjective cognitive decline in preclinical Alzheimer's disease. *Alzheimers Dement.* **2014**, *10*, 844–852. [CrossRef] [PubMed]
2. Mitchell, A.J.; Beaumont, H.; Ferguson, D.; Yadegarfar, M.; Stubbs, B. Risk of dementia and mild cognitive impairment in older people with subjective memory complaints: Meta-analysis. *Acta Psychiatr. Scand.* **2014**, *130*, 439–451. [CrossRef] [PubMed]
3. Jack, C.R., Jr.; Knopman, D.S.; Jagust, W.J.; Shaw, L.M.; Aisen, P.S.; Weiner, M.W.; Petersen, R.C.; Trojanowski, J.Q. Hypothetical model of dynamic biomarkers of the Alzheimer's pathological cascade. *Lancet Neurol.* **2010**, *9*, 119–128. [CrossRef]
4. Amariglio, R.E.; Becker, J.A.; Carmasin, J.; Wadsworth, L.P.; Lorius, N.; Sullivan, C.; Maye, J.E.; Gidicsin, C.; Pepin, L.C.; Sperling, R.A.; et al. Subjective cognitive complaints and amyloid burden in cognitively normal older individuals. *Neuropsychologia* **2012**, *50*, 2880–2886. [CrossRef] [PubMed]
5. Perrotin, A.; Mormino, E.C.; Madison, C.M.; Hayenga, A.O.; Jagust, W.J. Subjective cognition and amyloid deposition imaging: A Pittsburgh Compound B positron emission tomography study in normal elderly individuals. *Arch. Neurol.* **2012**, *69*, 223–229. [CrossRef] [PubMed]
6. Snitz, B.E.; Weissfeld, L.A.; Cohen, A.D.; Lopez, O.L.; Nebes, R.D.; Aizenstein, H.J.; McDade, E.; Price, J.C.; Mathis, C.A.; Klunk, W.E. Subjective Cognitive Complaints, Personality and Brain Amyloid-beta in Cognitively Normal Older Adults. *Am. J. Geriatr. Psychiatry* **2015**, *23*, 985–993. [CrossRef] [PubMed]
7. Vogel, J.W.; Varga Dolezalova, M.; La Joie, R.; Marks, S.M.; Schwimmer, H.D.; Landau, S.M.; Jagust, W.J. Subjective cognitive decline and beta-amyloid burden predict cognitive change in healthy elderly. *Neurology* **2017**, *89*, 2002–2009. [CrossRef]
8. Dubois, B.; Epelbaum, S.; Nyasse, F.; Bakardjian, H.; Gagliardi, G.; Uspenskaya, O.; Houot, M.; Lista, S.; Cacciamani, F.; Potier, M.C.; et al. Cognitive and neuroimaging features and brain beta-amyloidosis in individuals at risk of Alzheimer's disease (INSIGHT-preAD): A longitudinal observational study. *Lancet Neurol.* **2018**, *17*, 335–346. [CrossRef]

9. Bejanin, A.; Schonhaut, D.R.; La Joie, R.; Kramer, J.H.; Baker, S.L.; Sosa, N.; Ayakta, N.; Cantwell, A.; Janabi, M.; Lauriola, M.; et al. Tau pathology and neurodegeneration contribute to cognitive impairment in Alzheimer's disease. *Brain* **2017**, *140*, 3286–3300. [CrossRef]
10. Eliassen, C.F.; Reinvang, I.; Selnes, P.; Grambaite, R.; Fladby, T.; Hessen, E. Biomarkers in subtypes of mild cognitive impairment and subjective cognitive decline. *Brain Behav.* **2017**, *7*, e00776. [CrossRef]
11. Hu, X.; Teunissen, C.; Spottke, A.; Heneka, M.T.; Duzel, E.; Peters, O.; Li, S.; Priller, J.; Burger, K.; Teipel, S.; et al. Smaller medial temporal lobe volumes in individuals with subjective cognitive decline and biomarker evidence of Alzheimer's disease-Data from three memory clinic studies. *Alzheimers Dement.* 2018.
12. Jessen, F.; Feyen, L.; Freymann, K.; Tepest, R.; Maier, W.; Heun, R.; Schild, H.H.; Scheef, L. Volume reduction of the entorhinal cortex in subjective memory impairment. *Neurobiol. Aging* **2006**, *27*, 1751–1756. [CrossRef] [PubMed]
13. Saykin, A.J.; Wishart, H.A.; Rabin, L.A.; Santulli, R.B.; Flashman, L.A.; West, J.D.; McHugh, T.L.; Mamourian, A.C. Older adults with cognitive complaints show brain atrophy similar to that of amnestic MCI. *Neurology* **2006**, *67*, 834–842. [CrossRef] [PubMed]
14. Striepens, N.; Scheef, L.; Wind, A.; Popp, J.; Spottke, A.; Cooper-Mahkorn, D.; Suliman, H.; Wagner, M.; Schild, H.H.; Jessen, F. Volume loss of the medial temporal lobe structures in subjective memory impairment. *Dement. Geriatr. Cognit. Disord.* **2010**, *29*, 75–81. [CrossRef] [PubMed]
15. van der Flier, W.M.; van Buchem, M.A.; Weverling-Rijnsburger, A.W.; Mutsaers, E.R.; Bollen, E.L.; Admiraal-Behloul, F.; Westendorp, R.G.; Middelkoop, H.A. Memory complaints in patients with normal cognition are associated with smaller hippocampal volumes. *J. Neurol.* **2004**, *251*, 671–675. [CrossRef] [PubMed]
16. Stewart, R.; Godin, O.; Crivello, F.; Maillard, P.; Mazoyer, B.; Tzourio, C.; Dufouil, C. Longitudinal neuroimaging correlates of subjective memory impairment: 4-year prospective community study. *Br. J. Psychiatry* **2011**, *198*, 199–205. [CrossRef] [PubMed]
17. Verfaillie, S.C.J.; Slot, R.E.; Tijms, B.M.; Bouwman, F.; Benedictus, M.R.; Overbeek, J.M.; Koene, T.; Vrenken, H.; Scheltens, P.; Barkhof, F.; et al. Thinner cortex in patients with subjective cognitive decline is associated with steeper decline of memory. *Neurobiol. Aging* **2018**, *61*, 238–244. [CrossRef] [PubMed]
18. Li, X.Y.; Tang, Z.C.; Sun, Y.; Tian, J.; Liu, Z.Y.; Han, Y. White matter degeneration in subjective cognitive decline: A diffusion tensor imaging study. *Oncotarget* **2016**, *7*, 54405–54414. [CrossRef]
19. Selnes, P.; Fjell, A.M.; Gjerstad, L.; Bjornerud, A.; Wallin, A.; Due-Tonnessen, P.; Grambaite, R.; Stenset, V.; Fladby, T. White matter imaging changes in subjective and mild cognitive impairment. *Alzheimers Dement.* **2012**, *8*, S112–S121. [CrossRef]
20. Erk, S.; Spottke, A.; Meisen, A.; Wagner, M.; Walter, H.; Jessen, F. Evidence of neuronal compensation during episodic memory in subjective memory impairment. *Arch. Gen. Psychiatry* **2011**, *68*, 845–852. [CrossRef]
21. Hayes, J.M.; Tang, L.; Viviano, R.P.; van Rooden, S.; Ofen, N.; Damoiseaux, J.S. Subjective memory complaints are associated with brain activation supporting successful memory encoding. *Neurobiol. Aging* **2017**, *60*, 71–80. [CrossRef]
22. Hu, X.; Uhle, F.; Fliessbach, K.; Wagner, M.; Han, Y.; Weber, B.; Jessen, F. Reduced future-oriented decision making in individuals with subjective cognitive decline: A functional MRI study. *Alzheimers Dement.* **2017**, *6*, 222–231. [CrossRef] [PubMed]
23. Rodda, J.E.; Dannhauser, T.M.; Cutinha, D.J.; Shergill, S.S.; Walker, Z. Subjective cognitive impairment: Increased prefrontal cortex activation compared to controls during an encoding task. *Int. J. Geriatr. Psychiatry* **2009**, *24*, 865–874. [CrossRef]
24. Rodda, J.; Dannhauser, T.; Cutinha, D.J.; Shergill, S.S.; Walker, Z. Subjective cognitive impairment: Functional MRI during a divided attention task. *Eur. Psychiatry* **2011**, *26*, 457–462. [CrossRef] [PubMed]
25. Dumas, J.A.; Kutz, A.M.; McDonald, B.C.; Naylor, M.R.; Pfaff, A.C.; Saykin, A.J.; Newhouse, P.A. Increased working memory-related brain activity in middle-aged women with cognitive complaints. *Neurobiol. Aging* **2013**, *34*, 1145–1147. [CrossRef] [PubMed]
26. Peters, J.; Buchel, C. Episodic future thinking reduces reward delay discounting through an enhancement of prefrontal-mediotemporal interactions. *Neuron* **2010**, *66*, 138–148. [CrossRef] [PubMed]
27. Lindbergh, C.A.; Puente, A.N.; Gray, J.C.; Mackillop, J.; Miller, L.S. Delay and probability discounting as candidate markers for dementia: An initial investigation. *Arch. Clin. Neuropsychol.* **2014**, *29*, 651–662. [CrossRef] [PubMed]

28. Rabin, L.A.; Smart, C.M.; Crane, P.K.; Amariglio, R.E.; Berman, L.M.; Boada, M.; Buckley, R.F.; Chetelat, G.; Dubois, B.; Ellis, K.A.; et al. Subjective Cognitive Decline in Older Adults: An Overview of Self-Report Measures Used Across 19 International Research Studies. *J. Alzheimers Dis.* **2015**, *48* (Suppl. 1), S63–S86. [CrossRef] [PubMed]
29. Katzman, R. Education and the prevalence of dementia and Alzheimer's disease. *Neurology* **1993**, *43*, 13–20. [CrossRef] [PubMed]
30. Cabeza, R. Hemispheric asymmetry reduction in older adults: The HAROLD model. *Psychol. Aging* **2002**, *17*, 85–100. [CrossRef] [PubMed]
31. Hohwy, J. Attention and conscious perception in the hypothesis testing brain. *Front. Psychol.* **2012**, *3*, 96. [CrossRef] [PubMed]
32. Hohwy, J. Priors in perception: Top-down modulation, Bayesian perceptual learning rate, and prediction error minimization. *Conscious. Cognit.* **2017**, *47*, 75–85. [CrossRef] [PubMed]
33. Rao, R.P.; Ballard, D.H. Predictive coding in the visual cortex: A functional interpretation of some extra-classical receptive-field effects. *Nat. Neurosci.* **1999**, *2*, 79–87. [CrossRef] [PubMed]
34. Botvinick, M.; Nystrom, L.E.; Fissell, K.; Carter, C.S.; Cohen, J.D. Conflict monitoring versus selection-for-action in anterior cingulate cortex. *Nature* **1999**, *402*, 179–181. [CrossRef] [PubMed]
35. Niki, H.; Watanabe, M. Prefrontal and cingulate unit activity during timing behavior in the monkey. *Brain Res.* **1979**, *171*, 213–224. [CrossRef]
36. Botvinick, M.M.; Cohen, J.D.; Carter, C.S. Conflict monitoring and anterior cingulate cortex: An update. *Trends Cognit. Sci.* **2004**, *8*, 539–546. [CrossRef] [PubMed]
37. Friston, K. The free-energy principle: A unified brain theory? *Nat. Rev. Neurosci.* **2010**, *11*, 127–138. [CrossRef] [PubMed]
38. Ebitz, R.B.; Hayden, B.Y. Dorsal anterior cingulate: A Rorschach test for cognitive neuroscience. *Nat. Neurosci.* **2016**, *19*, 1278–1279. [CrossRef] [PubMed]
39. Nelson, T.O. Metamemory: A theoretical framework and new findings. *Psychol. Learn. Motiv.* **1990**, *26*, 125–173.
40. McClelland, J.L.; Rumelhart, D.E. *Explorations in Parallel Distributed Processing: A Handbook of Models, Programs, and Exercises*; MIT Press: Cambridge, MA, USA, 1989.
41. Hebb, D.O. *The Organizations of Behavior: A Neuropsychological Theory*; Lawrence Erlbaum: New York, NY, USA, 1964.
42. Keysers, C.; Gazzola, V. Hebbian learning and predictive mirror neurons for actions, sensations and emotions. *Philos. Trans R. Soc. Lond. B Biol. Sci.* **2014**, *369*, 20130175. [CrossRef]
43. Stern, Y. Cognitive reserve. *Neuropsychologia* **2009**, *47*, 2015–2028. [CrossRef]
44. Stern, Y. Cognitive reserve in ageing and Alzheimer's disease. *Lancet Neurol.* **2012**, *11*, 1006–1012. [CrossRef]
45. McCrae, R.R.; Costa Jr, P.T. Brief versions of the NEO-PI-3. *J. Individ. Differ.* **2007**, *28*, 116–128. [CrossRef]
46. Pailing, P.E.; Segalowitz, S.J. The error-related negativity as a state and trait measure: Motivation, personality, and ERPs in response to errors. *Psychophysiology* **2004**, *41*, 84–95. [CrossRef] [PubMed]
47. Owens, H.; Maxmen, J.S. Mood and affect: A semantic confusion. *Am. J. Psychiatry* **1979**. [CrossRef]
48. Li, Q.; Wang, S.; Milot, E.; Bergeron, P.; Ferrucci, L.; Fried, L.P.; Cohen, A.A. Homeostatic dysregulation proceeds in parallel in multiple physiological systems. *Aging Cell* **2015**, *14*, 1103–1112. [CrossRef] [PubMed]
49. Dodd, P.R.; Scott, H.L.; Westphalen, R.I. Excitotoxic mechanisms in the pathogenesis of dementia. *Neurochem. Int.* **1994**, *25*, 203–219. [CrossRef]
50. Palop, J.J.; Chin, J.; Roberson, E.D.; Wang, J.; Thwin, M.T.; Bien-Ly, N.; Yoo, J.; Ho, K.O.; Yu, G.Q.; Kreitzer, A.; et al. Aberrant excitatory neuronal activity and compensatory remodeling of inhibitory hippocampal circuits in mouse models of Alzheimer's disease. *Neuron* **2007**, *55*, 697–711. [CrossRef]
51. Reisberg, B.; Shulman, M.B.; Torossian, C.; Leng, L.; Zhu, W. Outcome over seven years of healthy adults with and without subjective cognitive impairment. *Alzheimers Dement.* **2010**, *6*, 11–24. [CrossRef]
52. Bhome, R.; Berry, A.J.; Huntley, J.D.; Howard, R.J. Interventions for subjective cognitive decline: Systematic review and meta-analysis. *BMJ Open* **2018**, *8*, e021610. [CrossRef]

9

Changes in Nutritional Status and Musculoskeletal Health in a Geriatric Post-Fall Care Plan Setting

Romy Conzade [1,2,3], Steven Phu [1,2], Sara Vogrin [1,2], Ebrahim Bani Hassan [1,2], Walter Sepúlveda-Loyola [1,2,4], Barbara Thorand [3] and Gustavo Duque [1,2,*]

1. Australian Institute for Musculoskeletal Science (AIMSS), The University of Melbourne and Western Health, St. Albans, Victoria 3021, Australia
2. Department of Medicine—Western Health, Melbourne Medical School, The University of Melbourne, St. Albans, Victoria 3021, Australia
3. Institute of Epidemiology, Helmholtz Zentrum München, German Research Center for Environmental Health (GmbH), 85764 Neuherberg, Germany
4. Department of Physiotherapy, Londrina State University (UEL) and University North of Paraná (UNOPAR), Londrina, Paraná 86041-120, Brazil

* Correspondence: gustavo.duque@unimelb.edu.au

Abstract: Understanding how changes in nutritional status influence musculoskeletal recovery after falling remains unclear. We explored associations between changes in nutritional status and musculoskeletal health in 106 community-dwelling older adults aged ≥65 years, who attended the Falls and Fractures Clinic at Sunshine Hospital in St Albans, Australia after falling. At baseline and after 6 months, individuals were assessed for Mini Nutritional Assessment (MNA®), grip strength, gait speed, Timed Up and Go (TUG) test, Short Physical Performance Battery (SPPB), and bone turnover marker levels. Associations were examined using multiple linear regression, adjusted for baseline covariates and post-fall care plans. Over 6 months, the prevalence of malnutrition or risk thereof decreased from 29% to 15% using MNA <24/30. Specifically, 20 individuals (19%) improved, 7 (7%) deteriorated, and 73 (69%) maintained nutritional status, including 65 (61%) who remained well-nourished and 8 (8%) who remained malnourished/at risk. A 1-point increase in MNA score over 6 months was associated with an increase of 0.20 points (95% confidence interval 0.10, 0.31, $p < 0.001$) in SPPB score. Improvement in nutritional status was associated with improvement in physical performance, providing a basis for interventional studies to ascertain causality and evaluate nutritional models of care for post-fall functional recovery in older adults.

Keywords: malnutrition; MNA; nutrition; physical performance; bone turnover; sarcopenia; osteosarcopenia; falls; elderly; prospective

---

1. Introduction

About a third of community-dwelling older adults aged ≥65 years in Western countries fall each year and the frequency of falls and fall-related injuries (fractures or head trauma) increase with age [1]. Falls increase the risk of hospitalization and nursing home admission, as well as morbidity and mortality [2]. Investigating modifiable risk factors of falls is a key priority area for healthcare systems, which strive to identify conditions that prevent falls.

Poor nutritional status has been considered an important modifiable risk factor for falls [3]. Compared to well-nourished older adults, risk of experiencing falls has been shown in a meta-analysis of prospective studies to be 45% higher in malnourished individuals or those at risk of malnutrition (n = 9510) [4], based on the validated Mini Nutritional Assessment (MNA®) tool [5]. In an interventional study by Swanenburg et al., the combination of a three-month calcium/vitamin D supplementation plus protein/exercise was associated with a 89% reduction in the rate of falls over 12 months compared to only calcium/vitamin D supplementation in older women aged ≥65 years with low mineral density (n = 20) [6]. Altogether, these findings suggest that nutritional status should be properly considered when assessing the risk of falls in community-dwelling older adults; yet it is currently not included in most fall risk screening tools [7].

Poor nutritional status can be a consequence of underlying comorbid conditions [8], which may increase the risk of falls due to clinical and adverse effects on cognitive, functional, and physical performance [9]. Poor nutritional status due to inadequate nutritional intake, especially of proteins, can also be detrimental for maintaining the integrity and function of skeletal muscle and bone [10–12], possibly increasing the risk for sarcopenia, osteoporosis or both [13–16]. Sarcopenia-associated risk of falling and increased bone vulnerability have a synergistic impact on falls and fractures occurrence [17,18]. The impact of nutritional status on the risk of falls can thus be explored through the pathway of musculoskeletal health as an important contributor to falls risk [19,20].

Evidence suggests that malnutrition based on MNA is able to predict musculoskeletal decline in various healthcare settings [21–23], but the relationship between nutritional changes and musculoskeletal outcomes remains under-researched [24], in particular among those who fall. Improving knowledge about how nutritional changes may influence relevant musculoskeletal outcomes might be important to effective targeting of multidisciplinary post-fall interventions for older adults living in the community. This study aimed to investigate changes in nutritional status in older adults with a history of falling using the validated MNA®, and to determine associations between changes in nutritional status and relevant musculoskeletal outcomes. We hypothesized that improvement in nutritional status is associated with greater musculoskeletal recovery.

2. Materials and Methods

2.1. Study Design and Individuals

This retrospective observational study examined associations between changes in nutritional status and musculoskeletal outcomes among community-dwelling older adults who attended the Falls and Fractures Clinic at the Australian Institute for Musculoskeletal Science (Western Health-Sunshine Hospital) in St Albans, VIC, Australia. A multidisciplinary team at the clinic, including a geriatrician, a fracture liaison nurse, an accredited exercise physiologist, and a bone densitometrist, provides comprehensive care for older adults with a history of more than two falls in the previous year, or a single fall with established gait and/or balance problem, and/or clinical or radiological risk of falls and/or fractures. We analyzed information from baseline attendance between October 2016 and December 2018 and from follow-up attendance after a median time of 6 months (interquartile range (Q1–Q3) 6–8 months). All measurements obtained were part of standard care practices at this health service. The Western Health Low Risk Ethics Panel approved the registration of the Falls and Fractures Clinic Databank (DB2017.13, date of approval 23 October 2018) and the research protocol of the present study (QA2018.90_48118, date of approval 5 December 2018). Participant consent was waived due to use of de-identified data collected as part of standard care at the clinic and due to the low risk nature of the study beyond the initial consent to attend the clinic.

2.2. Demographic and Clinical Measures

Demographic data was obtained from the patient medical record including age, gender, and residential location. Comprehensive clinical assessment was performed by the geriatrician and the nurse as part of routine care practices on clinic attendance including comorbidities, family history, fracture history, osteoporosis risk assessment (e.g., hormone replacement therapy, menopause age, smoking, alcohol), falls risk (e.g., hearing and visual deficit, altered elimination, impaired mobility), assessment for postural drop, and list of current medications. For the purpose of this study, a Charlson age-comorbidity index (CACI) was generated, with an index of ≥5 being suggestive of severe comorbidity [25]. The CACI calculation is explained in Supplementary Table S1. Polypharmacy was defined as use of ≥5 prescribed or regularly taken medications, including drugs and dietary supplements. Depression was screened using the Short Form Geriatric Depression Scale (GDS), with a score of ≥6/15 points considered as "suggestive of depression" [26].

2.3. Nutritional Status

Nutritional status was evaluated by the nurse using the Mini Nutritional Assessment (MNA®), which is a validated screening and assessment tool for older adults in community and hospital settings. The full MNA consists of 18 items (6 questions in the screening part, also called the MNA Short-Form (MNA-SF), and 12 questions in the assessment part) capturing anthropometric measures, dietary intake, appetite, general health, and mobility [5]. The screening part first identifies older adults as "well-nourished" (MNA-SF ≥ 12/14) or "at nutritional risk" (MNA-SF < 12/14), so that the full MNA is performed only if an individual is "at nutritional risk". The full categorized MNA then classifies individuals into "malnourished" (MNA < 17/30), "at risk of malnutrition" (17/30 ≤ MNA < 24/30) or "well nourished" (MNA ≥ 24/30) [5]. To calculate a full continuous MNA score, individuals with MNA-SF ≥ 12/14 in the screening part were adjusted into a full MNA score (MNA-SF + 16 points) to obtain a full score ranging 0–30 points. Weight and height were measured using standardized scales to the nearest 0.1 kg and 0.01 m, respectively.

2.4. Biochemical Measures

Fasting venous blood was collected for the measurement of serum albumin, 25-hydroxyvitamin D (25OHD), parathyroid hormone (PTH), hemoglobin, and C-terminal telopeptide of type 1 collagen (CTx). Serum albumin, and hemoglobin levels were determined using automated standard laboratory methods. Serum 25OHD levels were measured by chemiluminescence immunoassay on a LIAISON® XL analyzer (DiaSorin S.p.A., Saluggia, Italy). Circulating intact PTH was measured by immunochemoluminometric assay performed on ADVIA Centaur® (Siemens Healthcare Diagnostics, Deerfield, MA, USA). Serum CTx levels were measured by electrochemiluminescence immunoassay on a Cobas® 6000 analyzer (Roche Diagnostics International Ltd, Rotkreuz Switzerland). Cut-off values for subnormal levels were 25OHD < 75 nmol/L [27], PTH > 6.9 pmol/L, and hemoglobin <130 g/L (men), <120 g/L (women). Estimated-glomerular filtration rate (eGFR) was calculated from serum creatinine as an indicator of renal function (MDRD formula [28]), with subnormal cut-off values of <60 mL/min/1.73 m^2. All measurements were performed at the pathology networks affiliated with the Western Health-Sunshine Hospital in St. Albans, Australia.

2.5. Post-Fall Care Plan

After review of the results of the complete assessment of the individuals' risk of falls and fractures by the multi-disciplinary team, individuals were provided with individualized care plans that included pharmacological (e.g., osteoporosis treatment, vitamin D supplements, protein supplements), and non-pharmacological recommendations (e.g., nutrition advice, physical exercise), with a focus on preventing new or recurrent episodes of falls and/or osteoporotic fractures. The care plan was patient-centered through consideration of the risk assessment, individual patient circumstances, and preferences. In consultation with their local general practitioners, individuals were involved in the management of their respective care plan. The current study looks into changes in nutritional status and musculoskeletal components over a period of 6 months.

2.6. Musculoskeletal Outcome Measures

Musculoskeletal outcome measures were evaluated by the exercise physiologist as part of standard patient assessment on attendance at baseline and 6-month follow-up. Grip strength (kg) was measured with a handheld JAMAR hydraulic dynamometer (Sammons Preston Inc., Bolingbrook, IL, USA). Individuals had to squeeze the device as hard as possible 3 times in each hand; the highest value was recorded. Gait speed (m/sec) was evaluated using a sensitive walkway (GAITRite system, 16′ model, CIR Systems Inc., Havertown, PA, USA), which recorded spatiotemporal gait speed over 4.8 m with individuals walking at usual speed. The best result of two trials was considered. The Timed Up and Go (TUG) test (sec) measured the time taken to stand up from a standard chair, walk a distance of 3 m, turn, walk back to the chair, and sit down again [29]. The Short Physical Performance Battery (SPPB) is a group of measures that combines the results of the gait speed, chair stand, and balance tests [30]. We included serum CTx levels (assessment described under biochemical measures) as a measure of bone turnover.

2.7. Osteopenia/Osteoporosis and Sarcopenia

Body composition and areal bone mineral density (BMD) at three sites (lumbar spine, total hip, and femoral neck) were assessed by the bone densitometrist using a Horizon dual energy X-ray absorptiometry (DXA) machine (Hologic Inc., Bedford, MA, USA). DXA scans were only performed at baseline, and osteopenia/osteoporosis was defined as a BMD T-score <-1.0 SD on at least one of the three regions. As recommended by the Australian and New Zealand Society for Sarcopenia and Frailty Research (ANZSSFR) [31], sarcopenia was defined according to the EWGSOP 2010 definition by fulfillment of low height-adjusted appendicular lean mass (ALM/height^2) combined with low grip strength or slow gait speed [32]. (ALM/height^2) was calculated automatically by the DXA machine. We applied the EWGSOP cut-offs for low ALM/height^2: $\leq$7.26 kg/m^2 (♂), $\leq$5.5 kg/m^2 (♀); for low grip strength: <30 kg (♂), <20 kg (♀) and for slow gait speed: $\leq$0.8 m/sec [32]. Osteosarcopenia was defined as the simultaneous presence of osteopenia/osteoporosis and sarcopenia.

2.8. Statistical Analysis

Statistical analysis was performed using SAS, version 9.4 (SAS Institute Inc., USA). Statistical significance was based on a two-sided p-value <0.05. Normality was assessed using the Shapiro-Wilk test. Mean (standard deviation (SD)) or median (25th percentile (Q1), and 75th percentile (Q3)) were reported for continuous data, and number (percentage (%)) for categorical data. Change (Δ) in continuous variables was calculated as the difference between follow-up and baseline, e.g., ΔMNA = [MNA score (follow-up)—MNA score (baseline)]. To compare baseline and follow-up results, differences were tested using paired t test or Wilcoxon signed-rank test for normally-distributed or not normally-distributed paired samples, respectively.

As proof of concept, multiple linear regression analyses were first performed to test the cross-sectional associations between baseline MNA score and baseline musculoskeletal outcomes. Analyses were adjusted for baseline variables (age, sex, GDS, CACI, and number of medications—all continuous except sex).

For main analysis, individuals were divided into four subgroups based on change in MNA category from baseline to follow-up: (1) Improved nutritional status from baseline to follow-up; (2) Deteriorated; (3) Maintained but remained malnourished or at risk of malnutrition; (4) Maintained and remained well-nourished (reference group). Comparison of clinical, biochemical and musculoskeletal outcome measures between the subgroups vs. the reference group was analyzed using t-test or Wilcoxon rank-sum test for normally-distributed or not normally-distributed variables, respectively.

To explore the longitudinal associations between changes in nutritional status and musculoskeletal outcomes, multiple linear regression analyses were performed for each of the musculoskeletal outcome. Change in nutritional status was considered as both continuous (ΔMNA) and categorized exposure. Analyses were adjusted for the baseline outcome, baseline variables (age, sex, GDS, CACI, and number of medications—all continuous except sex), and care plan variables (osteoporosis treatment, vitamin D supplements use, protein supplements use, and physical activity—all categorical). When change in nutritional status was used as continuous exposure (ΔMNA), analyses were additionally adjusted for baseline MNA score. To avoid deletion of information-rich participants, missing values for four binary variables were coded as a separate category. Scatter and residual plots were examined to determine if ΔMNA was related to musculoskeletal changes in a linear manner and if the errors components were independent, homogenous with respect to the variance, and had a mean of zero. If these assumptions were violated, the outcome and/or independent variables were log-transformed to ensure good model fit.

To control for multiple testing, we ranked our hypotheses. Our primary hypothesis is that improvement in nutritional status is associated with greater musculoskeletal recovery. Our secondary hypotheses are that individuals who deteriorated and remained malnourished or at risk of malnutrition are associated with poorer musculoskeletal recovery. As such, p-values from multiple linear regression analyses were interpreted in the view of multiple comparisons. If the p-value was fairly large ($0.01 \leq p < 0.05$), we did not interpret them as definitely true, but considered that they may be likely false positive, while very small p-values ($p < 0.01$ and $p < 0.001$) were interpreted as likely real findings.

3. Results

3.1. Descriptive Characteristics, Including Change in Nutritional Status

Out of 254 patients screened at the Falls and Fractures Clinic between October 2016 and December 2018, 106 (76% female) consecutive individuals with median age of 79 (Q1, Q3 72, 82) years were re-assessed at 6-month follow-up. Table 1 presents descriptive characteristics of this study sample. On attendance at baseline, polypharmacy and severe comorbidity were quite prevalent (67% taking ≥5 medications and 45% with a CACI ≥5). The median number of reported falls in the past year was 2 falls. Most individuals (92%) were osteopenic/osteoporotic, and 22% were sarcopenic. On attendance at follow-up, the median number of reported falls in the past 6 months decreased to 0 falls. Moreover, 91 (86%) individuals reported using vitamin D supplements and 5 (5%) protein supplements, 70 (66%) reported having an osteoporosis treatment, and 51 (48%) reported being physically active, as part of the post-fall care plans recommended.

Table 1. Descriptive characteristics of the study sample, including change in nutritional status.

Characteristic	Descriptive Statistics	All (n = 106)
Baseline		
Age, year	Median (Q1, Q3)	79 (72, 82)
Female	n (%)	80 (75.5)
BMI at baseline, kg/m^2	Median (Q1, Q3)	27.8 (23.8, 31.9)
Weight at baseline, kg	Median (Q1, Q3)	69.6 (58.5, 85.0)
Height, m	Mean (SD)	1.59 (0.09)
Current smoker [g]	n (%)	11 (10.4)
Number of falls (past 12 months)	Median (Q1, Q3)	2 (1, 2)
Number of fractures (past 5 years)	Median (Q1, Q3)	1 (1, 1)
Severe comorbidity (CACI ≥5)	n (%)	48 (45.3)
Polypharmacy (≥5 medications)	n (%)	71 (67.0)
Suggestive of depression [a] (GDS ≥6/15)	n (%)	26 (24.5)
Osteopenia/osteoporosis [c]	n (%)	97 (91.5)
Sarcopenia [b]	n (%)	22 (20.8)
Osteosarcopenia [b]	n (%)	22 (20.8)
Nutritional status		
MNA at baseline, score	Median (Q1, Q3)	29 (23, 30)
Malnourished or at risk at baseline (MNA <24/30)	n (%)	31 (29.3)

Table 1. *Cont.*

Characteristic	Descriptive Statistics	All (n = 106)
Follow-up		
ΔBMI [h], kg/m^2	Median (Q1, Q3)	0.6 (−0.2, 1.5) *
Δweight [f], kg	Median (Q1, Q3)	0.6 (−1.0, 3.0) *
Number of falls [d] (past 6 months)	Median (Q1, Q3)	0 (0, 1)
Number of fractures [d] (past 6 months)	Median (Q1, Q3)	0 (0, 0)
Osteoporosis treatment [e]	n (%)	70 (66.0)
Vitamin D supplement use [e]	n (%)	91 (85.9)
Protein supplement use [e]	n (%)	5 (4.7)
Physically active [j]	n (%)	51 (48.1)
Nutritional status		
ΔMNA [d], score	Median (Q1, Q3)	0 (0, 3.3) *
Malnourished or at risk at follow-up [d] (MNA <24/30)	n (%)	16 (15.1)

Q1, Q3 = 25th, 75th percentile; CACI = Charlson age-comorbidity index; GDS = Geriatric Depression Scale; MNA= Mini Nutritional Assessment; BMI = body mass index; number of missing values: [a] 1, [b] 3, [c] 5, [d] 6, [e] 10, [f] 14 [g] 15, [h] 16, [j] 27; *: $p < 0.05$ for paired t-test or Wilcoxon signed-rank test for the difference between baseline and follow-up values.

The prevalence of malnutrition or risk of malnutrition based on an MNA score <24/30 was 29% at baseline and 15% at 6-month follow-up. Most individuals maintained or improved nutritional status with at least 75% not having a decrease in MNA score (median change of 0.0 (0.0, 3.3) points, p = 0.001) (Table 1). Specifically, 73 individuals (69%) maintained nutritional status, including 65 (61%) who remained well-nourished and 8 (8%) who remained malnourished or at risk of malnutrition. Moreover, 20 individuals (19%) improved and 6 individuals (7%) deteriorated nutritional status, as illustrated in Figure 1.

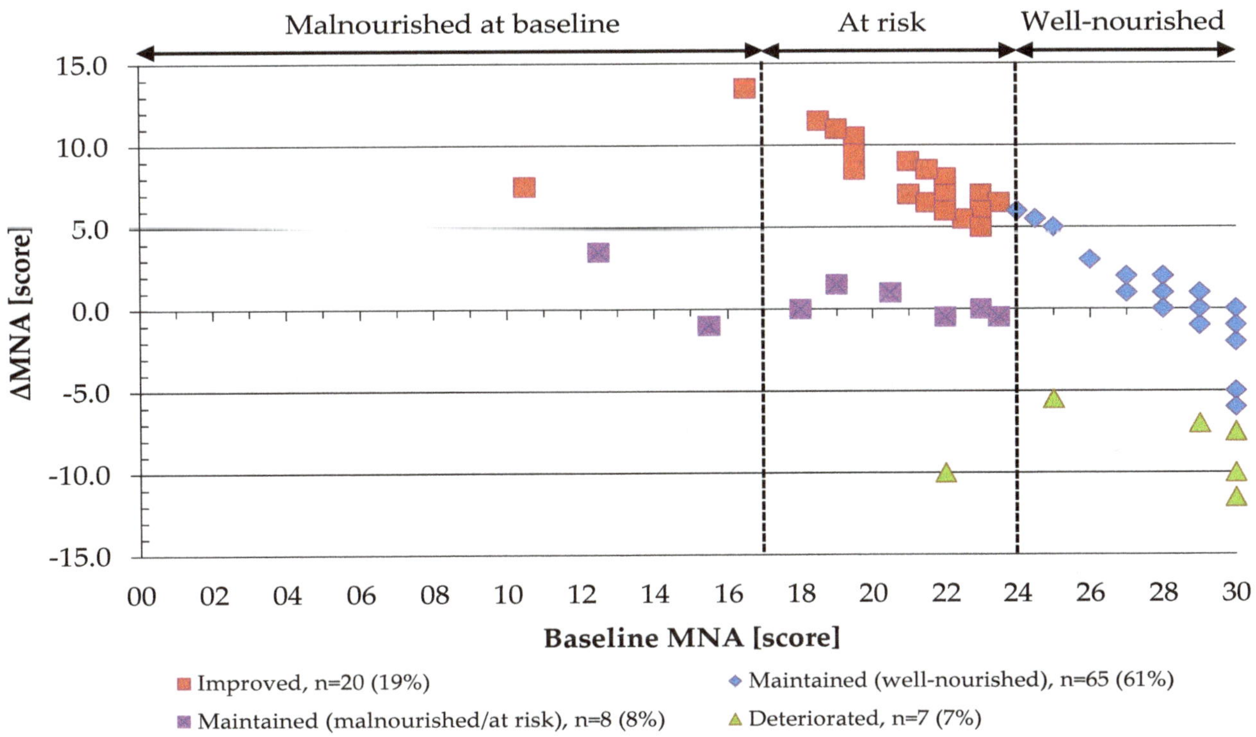

Figure 1. Change in MNA score (ΔMNA) by baseline MNA score across subgroups of nutritional status change. One dot represents one individual. Six participants could not be represented due to missing value in MNA score at follow-up.

3.2. *Nutritional Status and Musculoskeletal Health at Baseline*

In age-sex adjusted analyses, a 1-point increase in baseline MNA score was associated with an increase of 0.02 m/sec (95% CI 0.00, 0.03, $p = 0.022$) in gait speed and of 0.14 points (95% CI 0.05, 0.23, $p = 0.003$) in SPPB score. Additional adjustment for baseline variables weakened the associations, which became non-significant (Supplementary Table S2).

3.3. *Changes in Nutritional Status and Musculoskeletal Health*

Table 2 compares clinical, biochemical and musculoskeletal measures between subgroups of nutritional status change using the maintained (well-nourished) nutritional status group as reference group. The reference group was associated with significant increase in BMI ($p = 0.002$), weight ($p = 0.031$), 25OHD levels ($p = 0.013$), gait speed ($p < 0.001$), SPPB score ($p = 0.008$) and decrease in CTx levels ($p < 0.001$). Individuals who improved nutritional status were associated with greater increase in BMI ($p = 0.002$) and weight ($p = 0.006$) compared to the reference group, and similar increase in SPPB score ($p = 0.177$). They were not associated with significant improvement in gait speed ($p = 0.193$), but their TUG time significantly decreased ($p = 0.001$). Those who maintained (malnourished/at risk) or deteriorated nutritional status were not linked to significant improvement in any of the variables.

In multiple linear regression analyses (Table 3), change in nutritional status over 6 months showed the strongest associations with SPPB. After adjusting for baseline and care plan covariates, a 1-point increase in MNA score over 6 months was associated with an increase of 0.20 points (95% CI 0.10, 0.31, $p < 0.001$) in SPPB score. In subgroup analyses, individuals who improved nutritional status had for 3.30 sec (95% CI −6.34, −0.26, $p = 0.033$) a larger decrease in time for the TUG test compared to the reference group. Conversely, those who deteriorated in nutritional status had a larger decrease in SPPB score by 1.74 points (95% CI −3.29, −0.20, $p = 0.028$).

Table 2. Comparison of clinical, biochemical and musculoskeletal measures, stratified by subgroup of nutritional status change.

Characteristic	Descriptive Statistics	Maintained (Well-Nourished) n = 65 (*ref*)	Improved n = 20	Maintained (Malnourished/at Risk) n = 8	Deteriorated n = 7
Clinical and biochemical					
Age, year	Median (Q1, Q3)	77 (71, 81)	79 (73, 83)	80 (72, 84)	81 (79, 82)
BMI at baseline, kg/m^2	Median (Q1, Q3)	29.4 (24.8, 34.2)	25.6 (20.8, 29.6) †	23.8 (18.9, 29.8) †	24.1 (21.4, 27.9) †
ΔBMI [l], kg/m^2	Median (Q1, Q3)	0.4 (−0.3, 1.3) *	1.2 (0.7, 2.5) *,†	−0.8 (−2.5, 0.6)	0.0 (−0.3, 1.5)
Weight at baseline, kg	Median (Q1, Q3)	74.0 (64.0, 87.7)	64.1 (51.0, 76.6) †	64.8 (42.3, 70.4) †	64.7 (50.4, 74.0)
Δweight [k], kg	Median (Q1, Q3)	0.5 (−0.9, 2.4) *	3.0 (1.0, 5.9) *,†	−2.0 (−9.3, 0.0) †	−2.1 (−4.0, 2.8)
Number of falls at follow-up [f]	Median (Q1, Q3)	0 (0, 0)	0 (0, 1)	1 (0, 2)	2 (0, 2) †
Albumin at baseline, g/L	Median (Q1, Q3)	38.0 (36.0, 40.0)	38.0 (36.5, 40.0)	34.0 (29.5, 39.5)	38.0 (34.0, 41.0)
Δalbumin [c], g/L	Median (Q1, Q3)	0.0 (−2.0, 2.0)	0.0 (−2.0, 2.0)	0.5 (−1.5, 4.5)	1.0 (−2.0, 2.0)
25OHD at baseline, nmol/L	Mean (SD)	65.5 (22.5)	74.7 (20.2)	66.0 (23.7)	77.1 (28.3)
Δ25OHD [a], nmol/L	Median (Q1, Q3)	4.0 (−7.0, 25.0) *	9.5 (−11.0, 17.5)	8.5 (−5.0, 24.5)	12.0 (−1, 23.0)
PTH at baseline [f], pmol/L	Median (Q1, Q3)	6.9 (5.3, 10.3)	7.5 (5.8, 11.2)	6.0 (4.7, 10.5)	5.5 (3.9, 5.7) †
ΔPTH [g], pmol/L	Median (Q1, Q3)	−0.1 (−2.0, 2.3)	0.8 (−1.4, 3.8)	1.4 (1.1, 4.9) †	−0.1 (−1.4, 2.6)
Calcium, mmol/L	Mean (SD)	2.4 (0.1)	2.4 (0.1)	2.5 (0.1)	2.5 (0.1)
Phosphate, mmol/L	Mean (SD)	1.2 (0.2)	1.2 (0.2)	1.2 (0.2)	1.2 (0.1)
Hemoglobin at baseline [a], g/L	Mean (SD)	130.1 (13.7)	131.5 (13.2)	135.4 (18.9)	130.6 (13.5)
Δhemoglobin [c], g/L	Median (Q1, Q3)	1.0 (−4.0, 5.0)	1.0 (−5.0, 5.0)	1.5 (−6.5, 10.0)	5.0 (−11.0, 15.0)
eGFR at baseline, mL/min/1.73 m^2	Median (Q1, Q3)	75.0 (59.0, 86.0)	67.0 (52.5, 84.5)	85.0 (79.5, 87.5)	59.0 (55.0, 68.0)
ΔeGFR [d], mL/min/1.73 m^2	Median (Q1, Q3)	0.0 (−4.0, 4.0)	−3.0 (−8.0, 1.0)	−3.0 (−13.0, 0.0)	8.0 (0.0, 14.0) †
Musculoskeletal					
ALM/height^2 at baseline, kg/m^2	Median (Q1, Q3)	6.8 (6.0, 8.1)	6.0 (5.2, 6.8) †	6.2 (5.5, 6.3) †	5.7 (5.3, 6.6) †
Grip strength at baseline [a], kg	Median (Q1, Q3)	22.0 (17.0, 28.0)	20.5 (18.0, 26.0)	19.0 (15.0, 24.5)	16.0 (10.0, 24.0)
Δgrip strength [d], kg	Median (Q1, Q3)	0.0 (−3.0, 2.0)	0.0 (−2.0, 0.5)	0.5 (−1.5, 1.5)	−3.0 (−4.0, 2.0)
Gait speed at baseline [e], m/sec	Median (Q1, Q3)	0.7 (0.5, 1.0)	0.6 (0.5, 0.7)	0.7 (0.5, 0.9)	0.8 (0.6, 0.9)
Δgait speed [h], m/sec	Median (Q1, Q3)	0.1 (−0.1, 0.2) *	0.1 (−0.1, 0.2)	−0.0 (−0.1, −0.0) †	−0.1 (−0.2, 0) †
TUG at baseline [f], sec	Median (Q1, Q3)	15.2 (10.2, 21.3)	19.4 (16.5, 24.0) †	15.5 (10.9, 19.9)	18.3 (12.6, 22.0)
ΔTUG [k], sec	Median (Q1, Q3)	−0.5 (−2.2, 1.3)	−3.2 (−7.4, −0.6) *,†	−1.2 (−2.9, 3.4)	−2.6 (−2.9, 1.1)
SPPB at baseline [b], score (/12)	Median (Q1, Q3)	7.0 (5.0, 10.0)	6.0 (5.0, 7.0)	6.0 (4.0, 9.0)	7.0 (4.0, 8.0)
ΔSPPB [g], score	Median (Q1, Q3)	1.0 (0.0, 2.0) *	1.0 (0.0, 2.0) *	0.0 (−1.5, 1.0)	−1.5 (−2.0, 0.0) †
CTx at baseline [j], ng/L	Median (Q1, Q3)	330 (245, 447)	284 (204, 604)	278 (180, 361)	290 (162, 308)
ΔCTx [m], ng/L	Median (Q1, Q3)	−127 (−224, −15) *	−116 (−268, −9)	75.0 (−151.0, 102.0)	130 (8, 149) †

SD = standard deviation; Q1, Q3 = 25th, 75th percentile; ALM/height^2 = height-adjusted appendicular lean mass; BMI = body mass index; 25OHD = 25-hydroxyvitamin D; PTH = parathyroid hormone; EGFR = estimated glomerular filtration rate; TUG test = Timed Up and Go test; SPPB = Short Physical Performance Battery; CTX = C-terminal telopeptide of type 1 collagen; number of missing values: [a] 1, [b] 2, [c] 3, [d] 4, [e] 5, [f] 6, [g] 9, [h] 11, [j] 12, [k] 14, [l] 16, [m] 19; *: $p < 0.05$ for t-test or Wilcoxon signed-rank test for the difference between baseline and follow-up values within each group; †: $p < 0.05$ for t-test or Wilcoxon rank-sum test for the difference between the improved, maintained (malnourished/at risk) or deteriorated group vs. the maintained (well-nourished) nutritional status group (*ref*), respectively.

Table 3. Results of multiple linear regression analyses testing the association between changes in nutritional status and musculoskeletal outcomes.

Change in Musculoskeletal Outcome	Change in Nutritional Status		*n*	Age-Sex Adjusted β (95% CI)	Multivariable Adjusted β (95% CI)
Δgrip strength, kg	Categorized [a]	Improved vs. *ref*	20	−0.17 (−1.98, 1.63)	0.34 (−1.70, 2.73)
		Maintained (malnourished/at risk) vs. *ref*	8	−1.13 (−3.78, 1.52)	−1.22 (−4.07, 1.63)
		Deteriorated vs. *ref*	7	−2.12 (5.00, 0.75)	−1.48 (−4.41, 1.44)
	Continuous [b]	1-point higher in ΔMNA	96	0.10 (−0.10, 0.30)	0.09 (−0.11, 0.30)
Δgait speed, m/sec	Categorized [a]	Improved vs. *ref*	16	−0.03 (−0.12, 0.07)	0.04 (−0.07, 0.15)
		Maintained (malnourished/at risk) vs. *ref*	8	−0.14 (−0.27, −0.01) [i]	−0.07 (−0.21, 0.07)
		Deteriorated vs. *ref*	4	−0.15 (−0.33, 0.02)	−0.14 (−0.31, 0.04)
	Continuous [b]	1-point higher in ΔMNA	89	0.01 (0.00, 0.03) [i]	0.01 (0.00, 0.02) [i]
ΔTUG, sec	Categorized [a]	Improved vs. *ref*	17	−3.41 (−5.82, −0.99) [ii]	−3.30 (−6.34, −0.27) [i]
		Maintained (malnourished/at risk) vs. *ref*	8	0.04 (-3.25, 3.33)	−0.28 (−4.13, 3.56)
		Deteriorated vs. *ref*	3	−1.87 (−7.09, 3.34)	−1.74 (−7.35, 3.87)
	Continuous [b]	1-point higher in ΔMNA	86	−0.18 (−0.46, 0.10)	−0.13 (−0.41, 0.15)
ΔSPPB, score	Categorized [a]	Improved vs. *ref*	18	0.40 (−0.54, 1.33)	1.05 (−0.06, 2.15)
		Maintained (malnourished/at risk) vs. *ref*	8	−1.18 (−2.47, 0.11)	−0.72 (−2.13, 0.69)
		Deteriorated vs. *ref*	6	−2.21 (−3.69, −0.72) [ii]	−1.74 (−3.29, −0.20) [i]
	Continuous [b]	1-point higher in ΔMNA	91	0.21 (0.11, 0.31) [iii]	0.20 (0.10, 0.31) [iii]
Δlog (CTx), ng/L	Categorized [a]	Improved vs. *ref*	15	0.17 (−0.32, 0.66)	0.00 (−0.56, 0.56)
		Maintained (malnourished/at risk) vs. *ref*	5	0.10 (−0.69, 0.89)	0.10 (−0.79, 1.00)
		Deteriorated vs. *ref*	5	0.60 (−0.19, 1.40)	0.69 (−0.09, 1.48)
	Continuous [b]	1-point higher in ΔMNA	81	−0.02 (−0.08, 0.04)	−0.04 (−0.09, 0.02)

MNA = Mini Nutritional Assessment; TUG test = Timed Up and Go test; SPPB = Short Physical Performance Battery; CTX = C-terminal telopeptide of type 1 collagen; [iii] $p < 0.001$, [ii] $p < 0.01$, [i] $p < 0.05$: *p*-value of multiple linear regression models testing the associations between changes in nutritional status and musculoskeletal outcomes with the maintained (well-nourished) nutritional status group as reference group (*ref*); [a] β coefficient is the change in musculoskeletal outcome associated with change in MNA category from baseline to follow-up. Age-sex model adjusted for the baseline outcome, sex, and age. Multivariable model adjusted for the baseline outcome, baseline variables (sex, age, GDS, CACI, number of medications—all continuous except sex), and care plan variables (osteoporosis treatment, vitamin D supplement use, protein supplement use, physical activity—all categorical); [b] β coefficient is the change in musculoskeletal outcome associated with a unit increase in nutritional status over 6 months (ΔMNA). Models also adjusted for baseline MNA score.

4. Discussion

Poor nutritional status is subject to intense discussion in geriatric research mainly due to its high prevalence in older adults with falls, associations with higher morbidity and mortality risk, and effects on increased healthcare spending [33]. We assessed change in nutritional status in older adults with a history of falling and how it is related to relevant musculoskeletal changes during post-fall recovery. We found that improvement in nutritional status, based on increase in the MNA score over 6 months, was associated with improvement in physical performance, based on increase in the SPPB score over time.

4.1. Changes in Nutritional Status

Approximately one-third (29%) of the studied 106 older adults were malnourished or at risk of malnutrition at baseline. This prevalence is comparable to other studies of community-dwelling older adults using the MNA® (6%–32%) [34]. The prevalence of malnutrition or risk thereof decreased to 15% at follow-up. Comparable observational studies in community-dwelling older adults are lacking, but studies within inpatient settings reported a similar reduction in malnutrition prevalence (10%–13%) based on MNA category change between admission and discharge. However, older adults receiving inpatient services differ significantly in nutritional status and health recovery goals post-discharge to the community, so that results cannot be compared to community-dwelling older adults with confidence [24,35,36].

Most individuals (89%) maintained or improved nutritional status. It is worth noting that 8% of them remained malnourished or at risk of malnutrition at follow-up. A smaller number (7%) deteriorated to an extent sufficient to downgrade MNA category. This implies that while improvement or stabilization of nutritional status is possible during post-fall recovery, a number of individuals may not reach a well-nourished state, despite provision of individualized care plans, which included education and prescription of protein supplements, when indicated. This may have long-term implications for musculoskeletal recovery and quality of life and highlights the need for adequate follow-up of nutritional assessment. Moreover, while it is possible that subtle improvement or deterioration occurred within the stable group, the degree of change may not have been sufficient to alter MNA category.

Our study further demonstrated that MNA change was consistent with significant anthropometric (weight and BMI) changes. This is an important finding, as it is valuable to have a validated nutrition assessment tool to monitor nutrition progress over time, rather than relying only on anthropometric or biochemistry measures such as albumin, which may be confounded by clinical factors such as inflammation [37,38].

4.2. Changes in Nutritional Status and Musculoskeletal Health

Over 6 months, there were significant improvements in physical performance (based on gait speed, SPPB score, and TUG test performance) and in CTx levels. For gait speed and SPPB score, improvements were within a range indicating clinically meaningful changes [39], supporting that performance measures may offer a powerful mechanism to act on healthcare needs of older adults at risk for falls.

The observational design of this study prevents us from attributing changes of nutritional status and musculoskeletal outcomes to specific post-fall recommendations or other causes. Care plans were individualized through consideration of patient circumstances and treatment preferences. Incorporation of patients' decisions about treatment choices and their active involvement in managing their own care plan forms an integrative part of patient-centered medicine [40].

Our research investigated whether changes in nutritional status were reflected by changes in relevant musculoskeletal outcomes post-fall recovery. Improvement in nutritional status, based on a 1-point increase in MNA score over 6 months, was strongly associated with improvement in physical performance, based on an increase of 0.20 points (95% CI 0.10, 0.31, $p < 0.001$) in SPPB score over time. In subgroup analyses, the improved group was significantly associated with decrease in time to perform the TUG test and the deteriorated group with decrease in the SPPB score over time, compared to the reference group. These tools are interrelated and provide valid and reliable measurements of physical performance in community-dwelling older adults, incorporating elements of mobility and balance, with the addition of strength in both the SPPB and TUG test [41]. Nevertheless, caution is warranted when interpreting findings from subgroup analyses, because p-values were fairly large ($0.01 \leq p < 0.05$).

The impact of change in nutritional status on physical performance may be explained by direct or indirect mechanisms. First, increased adequacy of nutritional intake (in terms of quantity and quality) may contribute to recovery of muscle mass and function [42]. This affects physical performance, leading to functional and mobility improvements [10,11]. Improved nutritional status may also be an indicator of decreased comorbidity, which has positive effects on cognitive, functional, and physical performance [8]. Detailed data on changes in disease-related and medical factors could not be considered in this study and may have influenced changes between nutritional status groups and the time taken to recover musculoskeletal health. Finally, there was no association between changes in nutritional status and CTx levels. Physical performance may be more likely than bone turnover to improve alongside nutritional status due to recovery of muscle mass and function.

Our findings support the hypothesis that adequate nutritional follow-up support might increase relevant functional abilities during recovery from a fall. Two recent intervention studies, involving over 200 older adults aged ≥65 years each, showed that nutrition interventions (including enriched diets and/or oral nutritional supplements, home visits and/or telephone follow-ups) yielded significant improvements in weight and functional status over 3 months [43]. Another randomized control study involving over 150 geriatric patients aged >65 years at nutritional risk demonstrated the positive effect of individualized dietician counseling at home after discharge from hospital [44]. Perhaps this study design [44] can be used to conduct larger randomized controlled trials evaluating the effectiveness of specific nutritional interventions and models of care to improve nutritional and musculoskeletal measures in older adults at risk for falls.

4.3. Strengths and Limitations

Strengths of the study include the use of validated nutritional and musculoskeletal assessment tools, and the repeated measurements at two time points. The follow-up period of 6 months makes the study appropriate for documenting changes in nutritional status and musculoskeletal outcomes. There are also a number of limitations. The MNA lacks sensitivity to detect subtle changes in nutritional status [36]. As a result, the four nutritional status change subgroups are not evenly represented and are dominated by those who maintained well-nourished nutritional status. Another limitation arises from the selection bias associated with the follow-up design of this study, whereby only those willing to attend a follow-up session were assessed.

A control group was not feasible as routine geriatric care needed to be provided, which included individualized care plans for all patients. This limits the ability to attribute changes observed in musculoskeletal outcomes to specific recommendations. Importantly, it remains unclear whether change in nutritional status has a causal role in change in physical performance, or whether it is a case of reverse causation. The possibility of the temporal association between nutritional status and physical performance being due to residual confounding by unmeasured genetic, lifestyle or environmental factors cannot be ruled out. Finally, our findings may not be generalized because of the heterogeneous and convenience nature of the database.

5. Conclusions

Approximately one third of community-dwelling older adults with a history of falling were malnourished or at risk of malnutrition at baseline, and nearly one fifth improved nutritional status at

6-month follow-up. Improvement in nutritional status, based on increase in the MNA score over 6 months, was associated with improvement in physical performance, based on increase in the SPPB score over time. Larger intervention studies are required to ascertain causality and to evaluate specific nutritional interventions and models of care to improve nutritional status and functional recovery in older adults at risk for falls.

Author Contributions: R.C. and G.D. conceived and designed the study; S.P., E.G., and G.D. were involved in data collection and quality control; R.C. and G.D. coordinated the ethics application, R.C. analyzed the data, under the supervision of S.V., and wrote the first draft of the paper; W.S.-L. and B.T. helped interpreting the data; all authors contributed to the critical revision of the paper and approved the submitted version.

Acknowledgments: We thank all patients attending the Falls and Fractures Clinic for their extraordinary commitment and good will. We also thank Liz Liberts for her guidance on the ethics application process, Solange Bernardo for her assistance with the assessments of the participants, and Florian Schederecker for sharing his expertise on longitudinal data analysis.

Abbreviations

25OHD	25-hydroxyvitamin D
ALM	Appendicular lean mass
ANZSSFR	Australian and New Zealand Society for Sarcopenia and Frailty Research
BMD	Bone mineral density
BMI	Body mass index
CACI	Charlson age-comorbidity index
CI	Confidence interval
CTx	C-terminal telopeptide of type 1 collagen
DXA	Dual energy X-ray absorptiometry
EWGSOP	European Working Group on Sarcopenia in Older People
eGFR	Estimated glomerular filtration rate
GDS	Geriatric Depression Scale
MNA	Mini Nutritional Assessment
PTH	Parathyroid hormone
Q1	25th percentile
Q3	75th percentile
SD	Standard deviation
SPPB	Short Physical Performance Battery
TUG test	Timed Up and Go test

References

1. Gillespie, L.D.; Robertson, M.C.; Gillespie, W.J.; Lamb, S.E.; Gates, S.; Cumming, R.G.; Rowe, B.H. Interventions for preventing falls in older people living in the community. *Cochrane Database Syst. Rev.* **2009**. [CrossRef]
2. WHO (World Health Organization). WHO Global Report on Falls Prevention in Older Age. Available online: https://www.who.int/ageing/publications/Falls_prevention7March.pdf (accessed on 10 May 2018).
3. Torres, M.J.; Feart, C.; Samieri, C.; Dorigny, B.; Luiking, Y.; Berr, C.; Barberger-Gateau, P.; Letenneur, L. Poor nutritional status is associated with a higher risk of falling and fracture in elderly people living at home in France: the Three-City cohort study. *Osteoporos. Int.* **2015**, *26*, 2157–2164. [CrossRef]
4. Trevisan, C.; Crippa, A.; Ek, S.; Welmer, A.K.; Sergi, G.; Maggi, S.; Manzato, E.; Bea, J.W.; Cauley, J.A.; Decullier, E.; et al. Nutritional Status, Body Mass Index, and the Risk of Falls in Community-Dwelling Older Adults: A Systematic Review and Meta-Analysis. *J. Am. Med. Dir. Assoc.* **2018**. [CrossRef]
5. Vellas, B.; Villars, H.; Abellan, G.; Soto, M.E.; Rolland, Y.; Guigoz, Y.; Morley, J.E.; Chumlea, W.; Salva, A.; Rubenstein, L.Z.; et al. Overview of the MNA—Its history and challenges. *J. Nutr. Health Aging* **2006**, *10*, 456–463.

6. Swanenburg, J.; de Bruin, E.D.; Stauffacher, M.; Mulder, T.; Uebelhart, D. Effects of exercise and nutrition on postural balance and risk of falling in elderly people with decreased bone mineral density: randomized controlled trial pilot study. *Clin. Rehabil.* **2007**, *21*, 523–534. [CrossRef]
7. Park, S.H. Tools for assessing fall risk in the elderly: a systematic review and meta-analysis. *Aging Clin. Exp. Res.* **2018**, *30*, 1–16. [CrossRef]
8. Vellas, B.J.; Hunt, W.C.; Romero, L.J.; Koehler, K.M.; Baumgartner, R.N.; Garry, P.J. Changes in nutritional status and patterns of morbidity among free-living elderly persons: A 10-year longitudinal study. *Nutrition* **1997**, *13*, 515–519. [CrossRef]
9. Afrin, N.; Honkanen, R.; Koivumaa-Honkanen, H.; Lukkala, P.; Rikkonen, T.; Sirola, J.; Williams, L.J.; Kroger, H. Multimorbidity predicts falls differentially according to the type of fall in postmenopausal women. *Maturitas* **2016**, *91*, 19–24. [CrossRef]
10. Mithal, A.; Bonjour, J.P.; Boonen, S.; Burckhardt, P.; Degens, H.; El Hajj Fuleihan, G.; Josse, R.; Lips, P.; Morales Torres, J.; Rizzoli, R.; et al. Impact of nutrition on muscle mass, strength, and performance in older adults. *Osteoporos. Int.* **2013**, *24*, 1555–1566. [CrossRef]
11. Misu, S.; Asai, T.; Doi, T.; Sawa, R.; Ueda, Y.; Saito, T.; Nakamura, R.; Murata, S.; Sugimoto, T.; Yamada, M.; et al. Association between gait abnormality and malnutrition in a community-dwelling elderly population. *Geriatr. Gerontol. Int.* **2017**, *17*, 1155–1160. [CrossRef]
12. Bonjour, J.P. Dietary protein: an essential nutrient for bone health. *J. Am. Coll. Nutr.* **2005**, *24*, 526S–536S. [CrossRef]
13. Sanchez-Rodriguez, D.; Marco, E.; Ronquillo-Moreno, N.; Miralles, R.; Vazquez-Ibar, O.; Escalada, F.; Muniesa, J.M. Prevalence of malnutrition and sarcopenia in a post-acute care geriatric unit: Applying the new ESPEN definition and EWGSOP criteria. *Clin. Nutr.* **2017**, *36*, 1339–1344. [CrossRef]
14. Salminen, H.; Saaf, M.; Johansson, S.E.; Ringertz, H.; Strender, L.E. Nutritional status, as determined by the Mini-Nutritional Assessment, and osteoporosis: a cross-sectional study of an elderly female population. *Eur. J. Clin. Nutr.* **2006**, *60*, 486–493. [CrossRef]
15. Huo, Y.R.; Suriyaarachchi, P.; Gomez, F.; Curcio, C.L.; Boersma, D.; Gunawardene, P.; Demontiero, O.; Duque, G. Comprehensive nutritional status in sarco-osteoporotic older fallers. *J. Nutr. Health Aging* **2015**, *19*, 474–480. [CrossRef]
16. Reiss, J.; Iglseder, B.; Alzner, R.; Mayr-Pirker, B.; Pirich, C.; Kassmann, H.; Kreutzer, M.; Dovjak, P.; Reiter, R. Sarcopenia and osteoporosis are interrelated in geriatric inpatients. *Z. Gerontol. Geriatr.* **2019**. [CrossRef]
17. Zhang, X.; Huang, P.; Dou, Q.; Wang, C.; Zhang, W.; Yang, Y.; Wang, J.; Xie, X.; Zhou, J.; Zeng, Y. Falls among older adults with sarcopenia dwelling in nursing home or community: A meta-analysis. *Clin. Nutr.* **2019**. [CrossRef]
18. Hirschfeld, H.P.; Kinsella, R.; Duque, G. Osteosarcopenia: where bone, muscle, and fat collide. *Osteoporos. Int.* **2017**, *28*, 2781–2790. [CrossRef]
19. Tinetti, M.E.; Kumar, C. The patient who falls: "It's always a trade-off". *Jama* **2010**, *303*, 258–266. [CrossRef]
20. Deandrea, S.; Lucenteforte, E.; Bravi, F.; Foschi, R.; La Vecchia, C.; Negri, E. Risk factors for falls in community-dwelling older people: a systematic review and meta-analysis. *Epidemiology* **2010**, *21*, 658–668. [CrossRef]
21. Nuotio, M.; Tuominen, P.; Luukkaala, T. Association of nutritional status as measured by the Mini-Nutritional Assessment Short Form with changes in mobility, institutionalization and death after hip fracture. *Eur. J. Clin. Nutr.* **2016**, *70*, 393–398. [CrossRef]
22. Inoue, T.; Misu, S.; Tanaka, T.; Kakehi, T.; Ono, R. Acute phase nutritional screening tool associated with functional outcomes of hip fracture patients: A longitudinal study to compare MNA-SF, MUST, NRS-2002 and GNRI. *Clin. Nutr.* **2019**, *38*, 220–226. [CrossRef]
23. Vivanti, A.; Ward, N.; Haines, T. Nutritional status and associations with falls, balance, mobility and functionality during hospital admission. *J. Nutr. Health Aging* **2011**, *15*, 388–391. [CrossRef]
24. Whitley, A.; Skliros, E.; Graven, C.; McIntosh, R.; Lasry, C.; Newsome, C.; Bowie, A. Changes in Nutritional and Functional Status in Longer Stay Patients Admitted to a Geriatric Evaluation and Management Unit. *J. Nutr. Health Aging* **2017**, *21*, 686–691. [CrossRef]
25. Charlson, M.E.; Pompei, P.; Ales, K.L.; MacKenzie, C.R. A new method of classifying prognostic comorbidity in longitudinal studies: Development and validation. *J. Chronic Dis.* **1987**, *40*, 373–383. [CrossRef]

26. Sheikh, J.I.; Yesavage, J.A. Geriatric Depression Scale (GDS): Recent evidence and development of a shorter version. *Clin. Gerontol. J. Aging Ment. Health* **1986**, *5*, 165–173.
27. Vitamin, D. Supplementation Guidelines-Osteoporosis Australia. Available online: https://www.osteoporosis.org.au/sites/default/files/files/oa_medical_vitd_2nd_ed.pdf (accessed on 4 July 2019).
28. Levey, A.S.; Bosch, J.P.; Lewis, J.B.; Greene, T.; Rogers, N.; Roth, D. A more accurate method to estimate glomerular filtration rate from serum creatinine: a new prediction equation. Modification of Diet in Renal Disease Study Group. *Ann. Intern. Med.* **1999**, *130*, 461–470. [CrossRef]
29. Podsiadlo, D.; Richardson, S. The timed "Up & Go": A test of basic functional mobility for frail elderly persons. *J. Am. Geriatr. Soc.* **1991**, *39*, 142–148.
30. Guralnik, J.M.; Simonsick, E.M.; Ferrucci, L.; Glynn, R.J.; Berkman, L.F.; Blazer, D.G.; Scherr, P.A.; Wallace, R.B. A short physical performance battery assessing lower extremity function: Association with self-reported disability and prediction of mortality and nursing home admission. *J. Gerontol.* **1994**, *49*, M85–M94. [CrossRef]
31. Zanker, J.; Scott, D.; Reijnierse, E.M.; Brennan-Olsen, S.L.; Daly, R.M.; Girgis, C.M.; Grossmann, M.; Hayes, A.; Henwood, T.; Hirani, V.; et al. Establishing an Operational Definition of Sarcopenia in Australia and New Zealand: Delphi Method Based Consensus Statement. *J. Nutr. Health Aging* **2019**, *23*, 105–110. [CrossRef]
32. Cruz-Jentoft, A.J.; Baeyens, J.P.; Bauer, J.M.; Boirie, Y.; Cederholm, T.; Landi, F.; Martin, F.C.; Michel, J.P.; Rolland, Y.; Schneider, S.M.; et al. Sarcopenia: European consensus on definition and diagnosis: Report of the European Working Group on Sarcopenia in Older People. *Age Ageing* **2010**, *39*, 412–423. [CrossRef]
33. Agarwal, E.; Miller, M.; Yaxley, A.; Isenring, E. Malnutrition in the elderly: A narrative review. *Maturitas* **2013**, *76*, 296–302. [CrossRef]
34. Kaiser, M.J.; Bauer, J.M.; Ramsch, C.; Uter, W.; Guigoz, Y.; Cederholm, T.; Thomas, D.R.; Anthony, P.S.; Charlton, K.E.; Maggio, M.; et al. Frequency of malnutrition in older adults: a multinational perspective using the mini nutritional assessment. *J. Am. Geriatr. Soc.* **2010**, *58*, 1734–1738. [CrossRef]
35. Collins, J.; Porter, J.; Truby, H.; Huggins, C.E. How does nutritional state change during a subacute admission? Findings and implications for practice. *Eur. J. Clin. Nutr.* **2016**, *70*, 607–612. [CrossRef]
36. McDougall, K.E.; Cooper, P.L.; Stewart, A.J.; Huggins, C.E. Can the Mini Nutritional Assessment (MNA) Be Used as a Nutrition Evaluation Tool for Subacute Inpatients over an Average Length of Stay? *J. Nutr. Health Aging* **2015**, *19*, 1032–1036. [CrossRef]
37. Kruizenga, H.M.; Wierdsma, N.J.; van Bokhorst-de van der Schueren, M.A.; Haollander, H.J.; Jonkers-Schuitema, C.F.; van der Heijden, E.; Melis, G.C.; van Staveren, W.A. Screening of nutritional status in The Netherlands. *Clin. Nutr.* **2003**, *22*, 147–152. [CrossRef]
38. Cabrerizo, S.; Cuadras, D.; Gomez-Busto, F.; Artaza-Artabe, I.; Marín-Ciancas, F.; Malafarina, V. Serum albumin and health in older people: Review and meta analysis. *Maturitas* **2015**, *81*, 17–27. [CrossRef]
39. Perera, S.; Mody, S.H.; Woodman, R.C.; Studenski, S.A. Meaningful change and responsiveness in common physical performance measures in older adults. *J. Am. Geriatr. Soc.* **2006**, *54*, 743–749. [CrossRef]
40. Morley, J.E.; Vellas, B. Patient-Centered (P4) Medicine and the Older Person. *J. Am. Med. Dir. Assoc.* **2017**, *18*, 455–459. [CrossRef]
41. Mijnarends, D.M.; Meijers, J.M.; Halfens, R.J.; ter Borg, S.; Luiking, Y.C.; Verlaan, S.; Schoberer, D.; Cruz Jentoft, A.J.; van Loon, L.J.; Schols, J.M. Validity and reliability of tools to measure muscle mass, strength, and physical performance in community-dwelling older people: A systematic review. *J. Am. Med. Dir. Assoc.* **2013**, *14*, 170–178. [CrossRef]
42. Robinson, S.M.; Reginster, J.Y.; Rizzoli, R.; Shaw, S.C.; Kanis, J.A.; Bautmans, I.; Bischoff-Ferrari, H.; Bruyere, O.; Cesari, M.; Dawson-Hughes, B.; et al. Does nutrition play a role in the prevention and management of sarcopenia? *Clin. Nutr.* **2018**, *37*, 1121–1132. [CrossRef]
43. Neelemaat, F.; Bosmans, J.E.; Thijs, A.; Seidell, J.C.; van Bokhorst-de van der Schueren, M.A. Post-discharge nutritional support in malnourished elderly individuals improves functional limitations. *J. Am. Med. Dir. Assoc.* **2011**, *12*, 295–301. [CrossRef] [PubMed]
44. Beck, A.M.; Kjaer, S.; Hansen, B.S.; Storm, R.L.; Thal-Jantzen, K.; Bitz, C. Follow-up home visits with registered dietitians have a positive effect on the functional and nutritional status of geriatric medical patients after discharge: A randomized controlled trial. *Clin. Rehabil.* **2013**, *27*, 483–493. [CrossRef] [PubMed]

10

Tele-Follow-Up of Older Adult Patients from the Geriatric Emergency Department Innovation (GEDI) Program

Lucy Morse [1], Linda Xiong [1], Vanessa Ramirez-Zohfeld [1], Scott Dresden [2] and Lee A. Lindquist [1,*]

[1] Division of General Internal Medicine & Geriatrics, Northwestern University Feinberg School of Medicine, Chicago, IL 60611, USA; Lucy.Morse@northwestern.edu (L.M.); Linda.Xiong@northwesten.edu (L.X.); Vanessa-Ramirez-0@northwesten.edu (V.R.-Z.)

[2] Department of Emergency Medicine, Northwestern University Feinberg School of Medicine, Chicago, IL 60611, USA; S-Dresden@northwestern.edu

* Correspondence: LAL425@NORTHWESTERN.EDU

Abstract: The objective of this study was to characterize the content and interventions performed during follow-up phone calls made to patients discharged from the Geriatrics Emergency Department Innovation (GEDI) Program and to demonstrate the benefit of these calls in the care of older adults discharged from the emergency department (ED). This study utilizes retrospective chart review with qualitative analysis. It was set in a large, urban, academic hospital emergency department utilizing the Geriatric Emergency Department Innovations (GEDI) Program. The subjects were adults aged 65 and over who visited the emergency department for acute care. Follow-up telephone calls were made by geriatric nurse liaisons (GNLs) at 24–72 h and 10–14 days post-discharge from the ED. The GNLs documented the content of the phone calls, and these notes were analyzed through a constant comparative method to identify emergent themes. The results showed that the most commonly arising themes in the patients' questions and nurses' responses across time-points included symptom management, medications, and care coordination (physician appointments, social services, therapy, and medical equipment). Early follow-up presented the opportunity for nurses to address needs in symptom management and care coordination that directly related to the ED admission; later follow-up presented a unique opportunity to resolve sub-acute issues that were not addressed by the initial discharge plan and to manage newly arising symptoms and patient needs. Thus, telephone follow-up after emergency department discharge presents an opportunity to better connect older adults with appropriate outpatient care and to address needs arising shortly after discharge that may not have otherwise been detected. By following up at two discrete time-points, this intervention identifies and addresses distinct patient needs.

Keywords: Emergency department; follow-up phone calls; older adults

---

1. Introduction

Providing affordable, quality health care to older adults in the emergency department (ED) is of paramount concern in the present and future medical landscapes. The number of adults ages 65 and over in the United States (US) is projected to more than double in the next 40 years, comprising nearly 25% of the total population by 2069 [1]. This older adult population is more likely to be admitted to the hospital following a visit to the emergency department relative to younger adults, and nearly half are readmitted within six months. Moreover, hospital admission is both costly and associated with a number of adverse outcomes for older patients, especially [2–4]. Several novel interventions have been designed to identify at-risk older adults interfacing with the emergency department in an effort to streamline impactful care and to reduce the financial and personnel burdens that accompany the hospital admission of older adults [5–7].

One such point of intervention is avoidable admission for reasons other than acute illness, including functional decline, polypharmacy, dementia, and an unstable living environment. Although these conditions may not be grounds for admission independently, in combination with acute illness and complex medical needs, they may lead to imminent risk to the patient if discharged [8,9].

1.1. The Geriatric Emergency Department Innovation (GEDI) Program

The GEDI program was developed to optimize the treatment of older adult patients entering the emergency department in order to shorten ED visits and reduce hospital admissions, while connecting patients with the social and outpatient medical services best suited to their needs [9]. At Northwestern Memorial Hospital (NMH), nurses specially trained in geriatrics—geriatric nurse liaisons (GNLs)—identify older adults through the Identify Seniors at Risk (ISAR) tool and perform further screens for common geriatric syndromes by assessing for cognition (Short Portable Mental Status Questionnaire), delirium (Confusion Assessment Method), functional status, (Katz Activities of Daily Living), fall risk (Timed Up and Go test), caregiver strain (Modified Caregiver Strain Index), and transition readiness (Care Transitions Measure-3) [9,10]. GNLs assess the patient and determine if the patient can receive optimal treatment at home with outpatient follow-up instead of being admitted to the hospital. Hospitalization is well-established to be detrimental for older adults with resulting decreased physical function, worsening cognition, medication issues, and a multitude of other adverse effects. Based on results from the GNL testing series, patients are referred to primary care and specialist services, physical therapy, occupational therapy, and social and home care services as appropriate. The GNL designs a care plan for discharge, and then, the patient is sent home from the ED. After discharge, the GNL makes follow-up phone calls at two time-points following the ED admission to assess the continuing needs in care and answer any medical or logistical questions that may have arisen since the ED discharge [9,10].

The results from NMH's GEDI program have shown that the intervention results in a significant decrease in the hospital admission of older adults presenting to the emergency department [9]. Individual components of the GEDI program's effectiveness and impact, however, remain to be analyzed. Specifically, the impact of the telephone follow-up care provided to patients discharged from the GEDI program and ED has yet to be examined.

1.2. Follow-Up in Emergency and Ambulatory Care Settings

Previous research on the impact of follow-up care in the medical setting strongly indicates its important role in high-value, low-cost care. Follow-up phone calls made by pharmacists 48 h after hospital discharge at an academic medical center resulted in greater patient satisfaction, medication resolution, and medical referral for a subset of patients and fewer ED readmissions 30 days post-discharge for patients receiving the phone calls [11]. Similar interventions in pediatric, geriatric, and adult populations have demonstrated that calls can present an opportunity to assist a significant proportion of patients with medical questions and issues arising post-discharge and can increase patient adherence to appointments and care instructions in post-discharge and traditional clinic settings [12–15]. While the value of follow-up phone calls in the setting of the GEDI program at NMH is strongly indicated, the outcomes of these calls remain unexamined. Furthermore, the value of these follow-up calls in addressing patient needs as it relates to timepoint post-discharge remains, to our knowledge, unstudied in the context of care for older adults.

The objective of this study was to characterize the content and interventions performed during follow-up phone calls made to discharged patients who presented at the GEDI program academic medical center and to demonstrate the benefit of these calls to the care of older adults discharged from the emergency department.

2. Materials and Methods

2.1. Participants

All the patients over the age of 65 presenting to the emergency room and meeting the ISAR criteria for further work-up through the GEDI program received the follow-up phone calls that were the subject of this analysis. The data were anonymized prior to qualitative analysis. This project was considered exempt by the Northwestern University Institutional Review Board.

2.2. Data Collection

GEDI follow-up phone calls were made at two time-points: 24–72 h and 10–14 days following the primary ED admission. The GNL responsible for the patient case performed the follow-up phone call and transcribed the conversation in an open-response format; notes from the patient charts were abstracted, and these notes were the subject of the data analysis, until saturation of themes was achieved.

2.3. Data Analysis

The transcripts were then de-identified and analyzed by 3 authors (LL, LM, and LX) using content and constant comparative techniques [16], through which the coders independently assessed the participant responses for focal themes. The authors then convened to compare and compile their findings to create a list of major themes, which were discussed through further meetings, such that a consensus was reached in all the cases of initial discrepancy. The coders independently organized the content into an overarching categorical system: Multiple coders were allowed to independently develop categorical systems in order to control for the subjective bias each coder brings to the analytic process [17]. From these overarching categories, the coders synthesized the relevant themes and compared them across time-points.

3. Results

3.1. Obtaining Thematic Saturation

The responses to telephone follow-up were consecutively abstracted and qualitatively analyzed, until thematic saturation was reached (e.g., consensus of the research team that no new information was emerging in the data collection) [18–20]. Hematic saturation was determined to be completed after 57 charts. Prior qualitative research has shown that as few as 8–12 interviews are needed to reach thematic saturation [21,22].

3.2. Subject Characteristics

For the 57 subjects, the mean age was 88.6 years (range 66–96 years). The subjects had a mean ISAR score of 4 (range 1–6). From a cognitive perspective, the subjects scored a mean 1.65 (range 0–7) on the Short Portable Mental Status Questionnaire (SPMSQ, normal is less than 2). From a functional perspective, of the six basic activities of daily living (ADLs: eating, bathing, getting dressed, toileting, transferring, and continence), the subjects were able to do a mean of 5.28 (range 0–6) independently without assistance. These data were self-reported. A total of 14 subjects used an assistive device (cane or walker) and scored a mean of 15.5 s (range 8–34 s) on the Timed Up and Go test.

3.3. Key Themes

Key themes in the patients' concerns and the nurses' responses emerged in both time-points. The emergent themes in the patient concerns included clinical symptoms, medication questions, medical equipment, therapy or home health services, and follow-up with specialists or primary care providers (Table 1). The emergent themes in the nurse responses included providing clinical information, medication counseling, care coordination relating to appointments, and communication with social workers to arrange other social services (Table 2). These themes were largely overlapping across time-points; however, certain themes were unique to the later time point, and notably, certain themes were much more frequently encountered in one time point or the other. Upon further investigation of frequency disparities in theme across the time-points, certain content specificities within the overarching categories were found to vary, leading to the demonstrated differences.

Table 1. Patient concerns at follow-up: Patient concerns arising 24–72 h and 10–14 days post-discharge.

Emergent Themes	Selected Quotes
Clinical/symptom management	"The patient discussed how long her eye might remain red...informed to follow-up with ophthalmologist or emergency department if increased discharge, draining, bleeding from the eye, pain, or visual disturbances."
Medication	"Taking acetaminophen only 2 times a day. Afraid of aggravating liver." "Did quiz him about the use of his insulin and he states that his blood sugars have been in the 130-150 range. States he is checking his sugars two times a day"
Therapy, home health, or medical equipment	"Patient concerned about being alone and having to take shower without having someone check on her" "Questions in regard to when home health care and physical therapy would come to evaluate the patient"
Physician follow-up	"Has appointment on the 23rd. Will be receiving home occupational therapy in addition to home physical therapy. Patient lost list of geriatric psychiatrists, asked to resend to home. Mailed today."
Transitions of care **	"Discharged home from skilled nursing facility on 4/18. Scheduled for blood draw and evaluation in the Coumadin Clinic today. Appointment with cardiologist scheduled for 4/29."

** Theme only present at the 10–14-day follow-up. Quotes edited for grammar and clarity.

Table 2. Nurse response at follow-up: nurses' responses to patient concerns identified at 24–72 h and 10–14 days post-discharge.

Emergent Themes	Selected Quotes
Symptom counseling	"Informed to elevate, apply ice or take Tylenol, as needed" "instructed on warm compresses and stretching"
Medication counseling	"Not discharged from emergency department observation unit with any pain medications. Encouraged acetaminophen 650 mg every 4 h as needed"
Physician care coordination	"Encouraged to follow-up with primary care physician (PCP) and Gastroenterologist as scheduled for increased pain" "... Physician referral services contacted and made appointment for patient for follow-up with primary care physician for Wednesday this week."
Therapy, home health, or medical equipment coordination	"Having difficulty obtaining walker, which was told was ordered two weeks ago, but home care agency said they are waiting on physician order. Will contact our social worker to help facilitate. 1445: Prescription obtained for walker from emergency department physician faxed by the Geriatric Emergency Department Innovation (GEDI) nurse liaison and will facilitate walker delivery to pt." "Patient required multiple calls to help facilitate outpatient physical therapy. Prescription faxed to rehabilitation center with diagnosis."
Social work/services coordination	"...To have endoscopy and colonoscopy at the end of May. Looking into Medical Alert Systems. Given several names from Social worker list."
Caregiver coordination **	"Patient states he is not aware of visits; caregiver daughter is in charge. Called daughter and left a message if she needs any assistance with appointment scheduling."

** Theme only present at 10–14-day follow-up. Quotes edited for grammar and clarity.

3.4. Comparison across Timepoints

3.4.1. Clinical Symptoms

Clinical symptoms made up a large portion of issues discussed at both the 24–72-h and 10–14-day time-points; however, the concerns differed in content within this theme. Clinical concerns raised shortly after discharge were typically found to relate to the concern for which the patient presented to the ED initially, as exemplified by this follow-up note: "*The patient discussed how long her eye might remain red...informed to follow-up with ophthalmologist or ED if increased discharge, draining, bleeding from the eye, pain, or visual disturbances.*" By contrast, symptom-related concerns at 10–14 days were sometimes unrelated to the cause for ED admission, as shown by this note: "*Has an appt. with primary care physician in another week. I asked her to speak with the doctor about her elevated blood pressure. Patient was concerned that it has not been controlled with her current medication but will seek guidance from primary care physician.*" A subset of clinical concerns presenting at the 10–14-day time-point was entirely unrelated to the chief concern at the ED admission: *"Complaining of productive cough and occasional wheezing. Using inhaler with some relief"*. By contrast, none of the clinical concerns identified at 24–72 h were entirely new or unrelated to the concern precipitating the ED visit. In short, while clinical/symptom-related concerns were a common feature of the follow-up calls at both time-points, the later time-point demonstrated use in identifying sub-acute or unrelated clinical concerns that had not been apparent at the earlier time-point.

3.4.2. Physician Follow-Up Appointment Scheduling

Although follow-up physician scheduling was managed at both time-points, concerns and new information were more frequently elicited at the later time-point; while instructions were given to follow up and appointments were scheduled by the GNLs at the earlier time-point, the later time-point allowed the nurses to follow up on planned/recommended appointments that had not successfully been made, as shown in this note: *"Spoke with patient to verify that she called the ophthalmology clinic for an appointment...notified her that I would call back tomorrow to be sure she was ok and had made her follow-up appt...addendum: scheduled follow-up ophthalmology appointment for 4/23/13 at 1500."*

3.4.3. Durable Medical Equipment (DME), Physical Therapy (PT), and Home Health Nursing (HN) Coordination

Nurse coordination of durable medical equipment (DME), physical therapy (PT), and home health nursing (HN) took place more frequently at the 24–72-h follow-up relative to the 10–14-day follow-up. Early communication is critical for quick access to DMEs and HN services, such as home safety evaluations: *"Having difficulty obtaining walker, which was told was ordered 2 weeks ago, but home health agency said they are waiting on physician order. Will contact our social worker to help facilitate. 1445: Prescription obtained for walker from emergency department physician, faxed by the Geriatric Emergency Department Innovation (GEDI) nurse liaison and will facilitate walker delivery to patient."*

However, calls at the second time-point added value in that they allowed nurses to connect patients with services that were identified as potentially beneficial upon the initial physician follow-up, as shown here: *"The patient states her primary care physician suggested physical therapy. Will call office to see about order for physical therapy."*

4. Discussion and Conclusions

This study set out to characterize the content and interventions performed during follow-up phone calls made to discharged patients who presented at the GEDI program academic medical center and to demonstrate the potential benefit of these calls to the care of older adults discharged from the emergency department. Qualitative analysis revealed key emergent themes in both the patient concerns expressed during the calls, as well as the nurse responses to the patient needs raised during in the follow-up. Concerns regarding clinical symptoms, medications, specialist and primary care physician follow-up, and durable medical equipment, physical therapy, and home health nursing services arose frequently across both time-points. The nurses responded to such concerns by providing clinical symptom and medication counseling, confirming or scheduling physician follow-up appointments and interfacing with case managers in order to navigate patient access to durable medical equipment, physical therapy, and home health nursing services; these actions were taken by nurses at both time-points. Some patient concerns and nurse responses were only encountered at the later time-point, including caregiver coordination and management of transitions of care.

4.1. Significance of Cross-Timepoint Comparisons

While there was a great amount of consistency across time-points where the emergent themes were concerned, a variation of content within themes, as well as differences in frequency of theme presence across time points, was identified. Clinical concerns and symptom management at the 24–48-h time-point was consistently related to the chief concern that precipitated the ED intake, while this theme at the 10–14-day follow-up included newly identified clinical concerns, as well as issues that were sub-acute or secondary at the time of the ED admission. This finding suggests the added value of the later follow-up, as it has the potential to support the increased identification of underlying or newly arising patient needs that may have gone unmet without a later follow-up. Later follow-up also presented a unique opportunity for improved transitions of care and care management relating to physician follow-up. The later time-point appears to facilitate scheduling of appointments that were recommended but had not yet been initiated, which was a pattern more commonly observed at this stage. The early follow-up proved critical for establishing initial connections to medical equipment, therapy, and home nursing services; however, later follow-up also added value where apparent 'missed connections' with services were concerned.

In examining the patient concerns and interventions directly from the telephone calls, our qualitative results show that there is a benefit to telephone follow-up after an emergency department visit. While Biese et al. found no benefit of a telephone call to older adults from the ED on readmission or death in primary outcomes, our results show that there are unmet needs after a hospital visit that benefit from phone follow-up and interventions [23]. The singular outcomes of readmission or death may not provide a complete picture as to the effects or benefits of a telephone follow-up after an ED visit. Hwang et al. encouraged expanding the scope of the outcomes assessed, beyond hospital admissions and ED revisits, as a necessary starting point for future work—including how ED interventions affect important outcomes such as perceived social support, use of home care services and physician referrals, and functional decline [24]. Our results show that during telephone follow-up after an ED visit, issues relating to older adult patients that can be eased by essential interventions, such as home services, medical equipment, social support, and physician referrals, can be initiated to improve quality of care.

4.2. Strengths and Limitations

The qualitative design of this study allowed for the identification of novel patterns and themes that elucidate the value of two distinct time-points for follow-ups with patients admitted to the emergency department. The comparison of themes between two time-points illustrated the distinct benefits of each stage of follow-up. The study is limited, however, in that the nature of these data and methods do not permit for parametric statistical analysis; therefore, the frequencies with which these themes arose in early and late follow-up, while informative descriptively, cannot be applied to establish the significance of the observed differences.

4.3. Recommendations and Future Directions

Follow-up phone calls following an emergency department visit, occurring at two time-points, identified the questions and unmet needs of older adult patients after emergency department discharge. The geriatrics nurse liaisons (GNLs) were able to remedy these concerns and needs, thus establishing the value of follow-up phone calls within the context of the GEDI program. These findings suggest that both short-term and longer-term follow-up telephone calls are critical, as they each promote the management of distinct problems by allowing the GNLs to identify needs that arise at different stages post-discharge.

A future focus for the investigation of GEDI follow-up will be establishing the impact of these telephone calls on quantitative, outcomes-based metrics, such as 30-day readmission. The readmission of older adults following emergency room discharge is a pressing issue for patients and hospitals, with rates of 30-day readmission estimated to reach between 12 and 20% [18,19]. Based on our findings, GEDI follow-up calls provide an opportunity to connect older adults with the care that they need and demonstrate concrete incidences of direct intervention taken by GNLs to promote patient access to medical care, as well as non-medical services. Important next steps in this line of research include demonstrating the downstream impacts of reaching patients in this way on outcome measures and using the newly identified themes to direct the improvement of discharge interventions, such as the GEDI program.

Author Contributions: All the authors made substantial contributions to the conception/design of the work. L.M.: Data analysis, preparation of the draft manuscript, and finalization of the manuscript. L.X.: Data analysis and preparation and finalization of the manuscript. S.D.: Concept, study design, and preparation and finalization of the manuscript. V.R.-Z.: Study design and preparation and finalization of the manuscript. L.A.L.: Concept, study design, data analysis, and preparation and finalization of the manuscript.

Impact Statement: We certify that this work is novel or confirmatory of recent novel clinical research. The potential impact of this research on clinical care or health policy includes the following: (1) Providing data supporting the use of follow-up phone calls in emergency department protocols for the care of older adults. (2) Identifying key care needs of older adults discharged from the emergency department that may be addressed through follow-up phone calls.

References

1. U.S. Census Bureau. The Population 65 Years and Older in the United States. Available online: https://www.census.gov/library/publications/2018/acs/acs-38.html (accessed on 5 December 2018).
2. Rui, P.; Kang, K. National Hospital Ambulatory Medical Care Survey: 2014 Emergency Department Summary Tables. HHS 2014. United States Department of Health and Human Services (Online). Available online: https://www.cdc.gov/nchs/data/nhamcs/web_tables/2014_ed_web_tables.pdf (accessed on 2 January 2018).
3. McCusker, J.; Cardin, S.; Bellavance, F.; Belzile, E. Return to the emergency department among elders: Patterns and predictors. *Acad. Emerg. Med.* **2000**, *7*, 249–259. [CrossRef] [PubMed]
4. Pines, J.M.; Mullins, P.M.; Cooper, J.K.; Feng, L.B.; Roth, K.E. National trends in emergency department use, care patterns, and quality of care of older adults in the United States. *J. Am. Geriatr. Soc.* **2013**, *61*, 12–17. [CrossRef] [PubMed]
5. Creditor, M.C. Hazards of hospitalization of the elderly. *Ann. Intern. Med.* **1993**, *118*, 219–223. [CrossRef] [PubMed]
6. Carpenter, C.R.; Bromley, M.; Caterino, J.M.; Chun, A.; Gerson, L.W.; Greenspan, J.; Hwang, U.; John, D.P.; Lyons, W.L.; Platts-Mills, T.F.; et al. Optimal older adult emergency care: Introducing multidisciplinary geriatric emergency department guidelines from the American College of Emergency Physicians, American Geriatrics Society, Emergency Nurses Association, and Society for Academic Emergency Medicine. *J. Am. Geriatr. Soc.* **2014**, *62*, 1360–1363. [PubMed]
7. McCusker, J.; Bellavance, F.; Cardin, S.; Trepanier, S.; Verdon, J.; Ardman, O. Detection of older people at increased risk of adverse health outcomes after an emergency visit: The ISAR screening tool. *J. Am. Geriatr. Soc.* **1999**, *47*, 1229–1237. [CrossRef] [PubMed]
8. Mion, L.C.; Palmer, R.M.; Anetzberger, G.J.; Meldon, S.W. Establishing a case-finding and referral system for at-risk older individuals in the emergency department setting: The SIGNET model. *J. Am. Geriatr. Soc.* **2001**, *49*, 1379–1386. [CrossRef] [PubMed]
9. Aldeen, A.Z.; Courtney, D.M.; Lindquist, L.A.; Dresden, S.M.; Gravenor, S.J.; GEDI-WISE Investigators. Geriatric emergency department innovations: Preliminary data for the geriatric nurse liaison model. *J. Am. Geriatr. Soc.* **2014**, *62*, 1781–1785. [CrossRef] [PubMed]
10. Hwang, U.; Rosenberg, M.S.; Dresden, S.M. Geriatrics Emergency Department—The GEDI WISE Program. In *Geriatrics Models of Care*; Springer: Berlin/Heidelberg, Germany, 2015; pp. 201–209.
11. Dudas, V.; Bookwalter, T.; Kerr, K.M.; Pagentilat, S.Z. The impact of follow-up telephone calls to patients after hospitalization. *Am. J. Med.* **2001**, *111*, 26–30. [CrossRef]
12. Harrison, J.D.; Auerbach, A.D.; Quinn, K.; Kynoch, E.; Mourad, M. Assessing the impact of nurse post-discharge telephone calls on 30-day hospital readmission rates. *J. Gen. Intern. Med.* **2014**, *29*, 1519–1525. [CrossRef] [PubMed]
13. Chande, V.T.; Exum, V. Follow-up phone calls after an emergency department visit. *Pediatrics* **1994**, *93*, 513–514. [PubMed]
14. Dockery, F.; Rajkumar, C.; Chapman, C.; Bulpitt, C.; Nicholl, C. The effect of reminder calls in reducing non-attendance rates at care of the elderly clinics. *Postgrad. Med. J.* **2001**, *77*, 37–39. [CrossRef] [PubMed]

15. Karam, G.; Radden, Z.; Berall, L.E.; Cheng, C.; Gruneir, A. Efficacy of emergency department-based interventions designed to reduce repeat visits and other adverse outcomes for older patients after discharge: A systematic review. *Geriatr. Gerontol. Int.* **2015**, *15*, 1107–1117. [CrossRef] [PubMed]
16. Nasreddine, Z.S.; Phillips, N.A.; Bédirian, V.; Charbonneau, S.; Whitehead, V.; Collin, I.; Cummings, J.L.; Chertkow, H. The Montreal Cognitive Assessment, MoCA: A brief screening tool for mild cognitive impairment. *J. Am. Geriatr. Soc.* **2005**, *53*, 695–699. [CrossRef] [PubMed]
17. Guba, E.G.; Lincoln, Y.S. Competing paradigms in qualitative research. *Handb. Qual. Res.* **1994**, *2*, 105.
18. Charmaz, K. Qualitative interviewing and grounded theory analysis. In *Handbook of Interview Research: Context and Method*; Gubrium, J.F., Holstein, J.A., Eds.; Sage: Thousand Oaks, CA, USA, 2011; pp. 675–694.
19. Morse, J.M. The significance of saturation. *Qual. Health Res.* **1995**, *5*, 147–149. [CrossRef]
20. Morse, J.M. Determining sample size. *Qual. Health Res.* **2000**, *10*, 3–5. [CrossRef]
21. Guest, G.; Bunce, A.; Johnson, L. How many interviews are enough? An experiment with data saturation and variability. *Field Methods* **2006**, *18*, 59–82. [CrossRef]
22. Crouch, M.; McKenzie, H. The logic of small samples in interview based qualitative research. *Soc. Sci. Inf.* **2006**, *45*, 483–499. [CrossRef]
23. Biese, K.; Busby-Whitehead, J.; Cai, J.; Stearns, S.C.; Roberts, E.; Mihas, P.; Emmett, D.; Zhou, Q.; Farmer, F.; Kizer, J.S. Telephone follow-up for older adults discharged to home from the emergency department: A pragmatic randomized controlled trial. *J. Am. Geriatr. Soc.* **2018**, *66*, 452–458. [CrossRef] [PubMed]
24. Ula Hwang, S. Nicole Hastings and Katherine Ramos, Improving Emergency Department Discharge Care with Telephone Follow-Up. Does It Connect? *J. Am. Geriatr. Soc.* **2017**, *66*, 436–438. [CrossRef] [PubMed]

11

High Prevalence of Hypovitaminosis D in Institutionalized Elderly Individuals is Associated with Summer in a Region with High Ultraviolet Radiation Levels

Sara Estéfani S. Sousa [1], Márcia Cristina Sales [2], José Rodolfo T. Araújo [3], Karine C.M. Sena-Evangelista [1,4], Kenio C. Lima [3,5] and Lucia F.C. Pedrosa [1,3,4,*]

1 Postgraduate Program in Nutrition, Federal University of Rio Grande do Norte, Av. Senador Salgado Filho, 3000, Lagoa Nova, 59078970 Natal, RN, Brazil

2 School of Medicine, State University of Roraima, Rua Sete de Setembro, 231, Canarinho, 69306530 Boa Vista, RR, Brazil

3 Postgraduate Program of Health Sciences, Federal University of Rio Grande do Norte, Rua General Gustavo Cordeiro de Farias, Petrópolis, 59010180 Natal, RN, Brazil

4 Department of Nutrition, Federal University of Rio Grande do Norte, Av. Senador Salgado Filho, 3000, Lagoa Nova, 59078970 Natal, Brazil

5 Department of Dentistry, Federal University of Rio Grande do Norte, Av. Senador Salgado Filho, 1787, Lagoa Nova, 59056000 Natal, RN, Brazil

* Correspondence: lfcpedrosa@gmail.com

Abstract: Vitamin D may play a significant role in regulating the rate of aging. The objective of the study was to assess vitamin D status and its associated factors in institutionalized elderly individuals. A total of 153 elderly individuals living in Nursing Homes (NH) were recruited into the study. Serum 25-hydroxyvitamin D [25(OH)D] concentration was used as the biomarker of vitamin D status, and it was considered as the dependent variable in the model. The independent variables were the type of NH, age-adjusted time of institutionalization, age, sex, skin color, body mass index, waist and calf circumference, physical activity practice, mobility, dietary intake of vitamin D and calcium, vitamin D supplementation, use of antiepileptics, and season of the year. Serum 25(OH)D concentrations less than or equal to 29 ng/mL were classified as insufficient vitamin D status. The prevalences of inadequate dietary intake of vitamin D and calcium were 95.4% and 79.7%, respectively. The prevalence of hypovitaminosis D was 71.2%, and the mean serum concentration of 25(OH)D was 23.9 ng/mL (95% confidence interval [CI]: 22.8–26.1). Serum 25(OH)D concentration was associated with the season of summer ($p = 0.046$). There were no associations with other independent variables (all $p > 0.05$). The present results showed that a high prevalence of hypovitaminosis D was significantly associated with summer in institutionalized elderly individuals.

Keywords: vitamin D; elderly individuals; nursing homes

---

1. Introduction

The population aged 60 or over is growing at a faster rate than the total population in almost all regions worldwide. Most notably, the current challenge in demographics is the rapidly increasing population of older adults. In 2012, people aged 60 or over represented almost 11.5 per cent of our total global population of 7 billion. By 2050, the proportion is projected to nearly double to 22 per cent [1].

The number of elderly individuals in Brazil was estimated to be more than 30.2 million in 2017. Thus, they represented approximately 7 per cent of the Brazilian population of 209.3 million inhabitants in this period. In the Northeast of Brazil, the proportion of elderly individuals increased from 5.8% in 2000 to 7.2% in 2010 [2].

A widespread health problem experienced among elderly individuals is multiple micronutrient inadequacy, including vitamin D, which may lead mainly to frailty, sarcopenia, and cognitive decline [3,4].

Vitamin D regulates aging by controlling the activity of autophagy, which slows down aging processes by removing dysfunctional mitochondria. Vitamin D also reduces mitochondrial dysfunction, oxidative stress, inflammation, calcium signaling, epigenetic changes and DNA disorders, including telomere shortening, which act upon aging processes [5].

The diagnosis of vitamin D deficiency is a controversial issue. Serum levels of 25-hydroxyvitamin D [25(OH)D] above 30 ng/mL are associated with increased efficacy of intestinal calcium absorption and stabilization of serum parathyroid hormone (PTH) values, which are suggested as being the threshold for fracture prevention [6]. The Endocrine Society suggests that the 25(OH)D concentrations that are considered deficient, insufficient, and sufficient are ≤20, ≥21 and ≤29, and ≥30 ng/mL, respectively [7]. However, the Brazilian Society of Clinical Pathology/Laboratory Medicine and the Brazilian Society of Endocrinology and Metabolism recently proposed concentrations of 25(OH)D above 20 ng/mL as being adequate for the health of the population up to 60 years old, while values between 30 and 60 ng/mL are adopted for groups at risk of vitamin D deficiency, including elderly individuals [8].

Vitamin D deficiency among elderly individuals can result in cardiovascular risk, mortality, low quality-of-life scores, decreased physical functionality, secondary hyperparathyroidism, and increased risk of fractures [3,9–11]. Age-related changes in body composition, such as decreased muscle mass and increased adipose tissue, can lead to a decrease in serum vitamin D concentrations. Furthermore, the muscular weakness presented by the elderly population can be potentiated by the deficiency of vitamin D [12]. Moreover, Pilz et al. (2012) observed a significantly increased mortality risk in the female Nursing Home (NH) residents with the lowest 25(OH)D levels [13].

Several factors are involved in changes in vitamin D status in aging, such as the seasonality, which is currently observed as being an important predictor because it has an impact on the behavior and lifestyle of individuals [6,14,15]. Even under favorable environmental conditions, vitamin D bioavailability in elderly individuals can be negatively affected by the reduced capacity of its cutaneous synthesis. Furthermore, this population can be vulnerable to vitamin D deficiency as a result of low exposure to sunlight, their particular type of skin pigmentation, adiposity, use of antiepileptic medications, reduced kidney function, and low dietary vitamin D intake [9,15–17].

In light of these considerations, hypovitaminosis D has been frequently found among institutionalized elderly individuals living in countries with low ultraviolet radiation (UV) indexes, where elderly people spend more time indoors [13,18], as well as in high-latitude regions where there is a high UV index [16,19,20].

Although several studies carried out on elderly people have revealed a poorer vitamin D status during the winter seasons because of the lower sunlight exposure [19–22], contradictory findings have been found in the literature. One study developed with elderly people from a Mediterranean area suggested significant differences in serum 25(OH)D concentrations between seasons, with the lowest concentrations occurring in the summer and the highest during the autumn, although their vitamin D intake was significantly lower in the autumn and winter [23].

Based on these findings, our study was developed to answer the question about the status of vitamin D in institutionalized elderly individuals living in a region with high levels of UV radiation, while considering various particularities of aging. For this reason, we have drawn up a theoretical model that encompasses diverse variables and contemplates these conditions.

In addition to this, institutionalization impacts the interactions of elderly individuals with the environment as well as their nutritional status, which, in turn, are influenced by their social status, psychological disorders, and general health conditions [24,25]. In this scenario, the objective of the present study is to assess serum 25(OH)D concentrations and associated factors in institutionalized elderly individuals living in a region of northeastern Brazil with high ultraviolet radiation levels.

2. Materials and Methods

2.1. Study Population

The study was carried out with 304 elderly individuals living in nine Nursing Homes (NH) in the city of Natal (Rio Grande do Norte state), which is in the northeast of Brazil. All the individuals included in the study were at least 60 years old and living in these NHs. In Brazil, the Statute of the Elderly [26] considers elderly individuals to be aged 60 years or older. Elderly individuals who had marked physical and mental impairments, as well as difficult venous access, were excluded from the study. After exclusion, the initial sample of 304 elderly individuals was narrowed down to 153 participants (Figure 1).

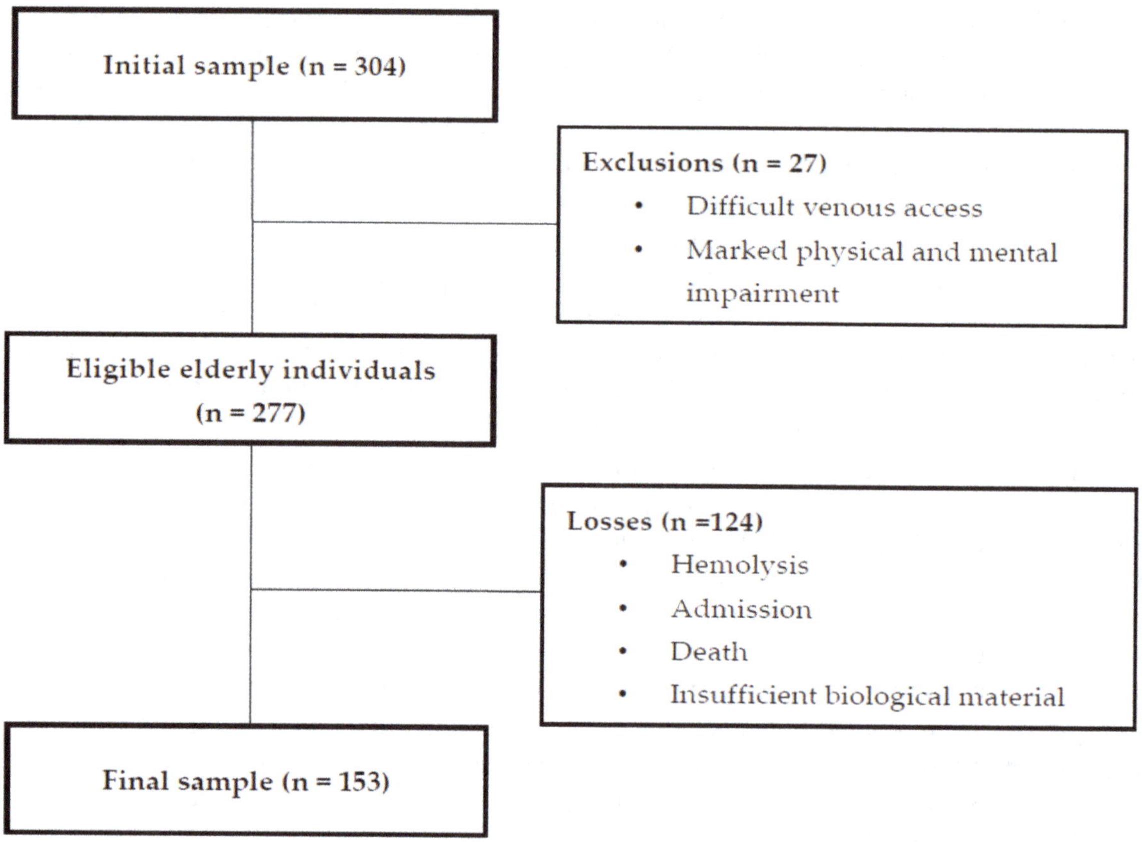

Figure 1. Flowchart of the study participants.

The study was conducted in accordance with the Declaration of Helsinki, and the protocol was approved by the Research Ethics Committee of the Federal University of Rio Grande do Norte (#263/11; CAAE 0290.0.051.000-11). All participants or their guardians provided written informed consent before they participated in the study.

The sample size calculation for the cross-sectional studies was defined on the basis of the mean and standard deviation of the concentration of 24.0 (7.6) ng/mL of 25(OH)D, corresponding to 10 random subjects in the sample of this study, and to the power of the test of 95%, resulting in 154 elderly individuals. Thus, this study obtained a response rate of 99.3%. For association studies, the sample size would be 156 elderly individuals, considering the population size of 304 elderly individuals, a hypothetical frequency of vitamin D deficiency of 71.2% [19], a confidence limit of 5%, and a design effect equal to 1 [27].

2.2. Theoretical Model of the Study

The theoretical model of this study was developed according to determinant factors of vitamin D status. Serum 25(OH)D concentration was defined as the dependent variable, and the independent variables were those likely to influence vitamin D status: Age, sex, skin color, body mass index (BMI), physical activity practice, mobility, diet, use of vitamin D supplements, and use of antiepileptic medications. The sociodemographic, nutritional, lifestyle, and biological variables were included in the "proximal" layers. Type of NH, age-adjusted time of institutionalization, and level of education were components of the "distal" layer. The season of the year was considered as a cross-sectional influence because it has a direct relationship with 25(OH)D concentrations (Figure 2). This study also addressed the relationship between the dependent variable and possible clinical implications in cases of vitamin D-deficient elderly individuals—multimorbidity, falls, sarcopenia, depression, cognition, and functional status.

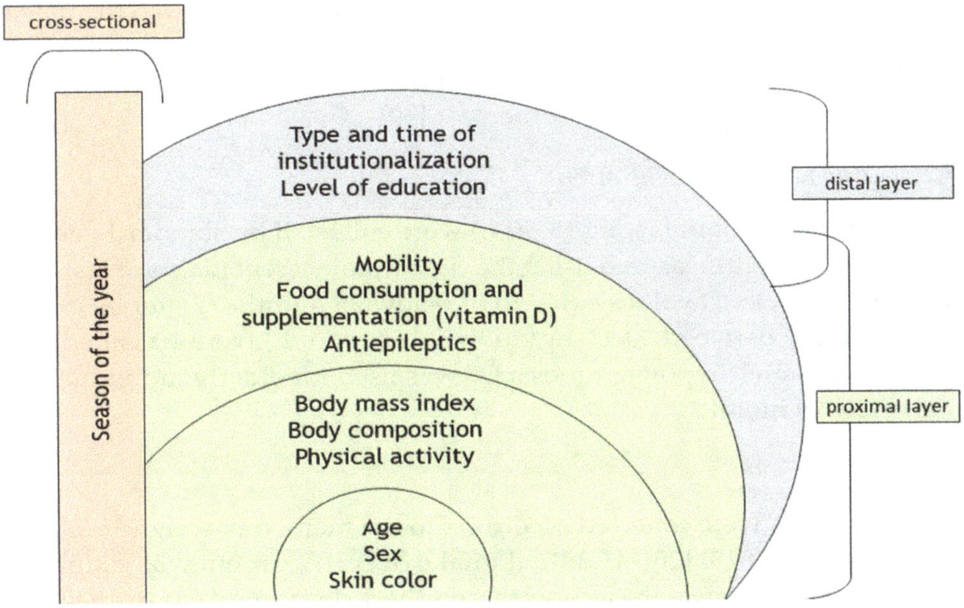

Figure 2. Theoretical model of the determinants of vitamin D status in institutionalized elderly individuals.

Age-adjusted time of institutionalization was calculated to determine how much time after the advanced age period (as a percentage, defined as the time after turning 60 years of age) elderly individuals remained institutionalized, according to a previous study [28].

Weight, height, and waist and calf circumference were measured to determine the anthropometric variables. Skin color was obtained by self-classification among the five categories adopted by the Brazilian Institute of Geography and Statistics (IBGE): Black, mixed race ("pardo" in official Portuguese), Caucasian, Asian, and indigenous (Native Brazilian) [29]. Body weight was assessed with a Balmak® electronic scale (Santa Barbara do Oeste, Brazil) with a capacity of 300 kg and an accuracy of 50 g. In elderly individuals with disabilities or permanent mobility restrictions, weight was measured with a Seca® 985 bed scale (Bolton, England). Height was defined using the average of the two measurements and a portable Caumaq® stadiometer (Cachoeira do Sul, Brazil). For physically impaired elderly individuals, height was estimated using the equation of Chumlea et al. (1987) [30]. BMI was classified while considering the cutoff points proposed by Lipschitz [31].

Calf perimeter values less than 31 cm were indicative of loss of muscle mass in elderly individuals. Results for waist perimeter greater than 102 cm in males and 88 cm in females were considered to indicate a higher risk of diseases [32].

Physical activity practice was determined through information provided by caregivers, categorized into "yes" or "no" answers. Information on diseases, multimorbidity, polypharmacy, use of antiepileptic drugs, and vitamin D supplementation was collected from the medical records of the NHs. Multimorbidity was considered as the presence of two or more diseases with clinical diagnoses included in medical records. Polypharmacy was characterized for those individuals who took five or more medications daily [33].

Data on the mobility variable were collected from the caregivers of the elderly individuals using a Barthel scale [34]. Sarcopenia was measured according to previously defined criteria [35], based on discrimination of reduced muscle mass concentrations (calf circumference assessment) associated with a reduction in strength (grip test) and/or functional status. Functional status was assessed according to the scale set by Katz [36]. Cognitive function was assessed according to Pfeiffer's Short Portable Mental Status Questionnaire, which evaluates short- and long-term memory, orientation, information on everyday facts, and mathematical reasoning. Individuals were classified into four categories: intact mental function (0–2 errors), mild cognitive impairment (3–4 errors), moderate (5–7 errors), and severe (8–10 errors) [37,38].

The elderly subjects were categorized by seasons. The season used was the date corresponding to 30 days prior to blood collection. This was to take into account the half-life of 25(OH)D [39]. The Laboratory of Environmental and Tropical Variables of the Federal University of Rio Grande do Norte provided UV values for each season of the year [39].

2.3. *Analysis of 25(OH)D Serum Concentration*

Blood samples after overnight fasting (8–12 h) were collected by standard venipuncture. Serum concentrations of 25(OH)D were measured using the chemiluminescent Liaison® test from kit DiaSorin® (Saluggia, Italy). Serum 25(OH)D values equal to or below 29 ng/mL (72 nmol/L) were considered as "insufficient", while values between 30–60 ng/mL (75–150 nmol/L) were classified as "sufficient" [8]. In the present study, the name "hypovitaminosis D" was used for elderly individuals with a 25(OH)D value equal to or below 29 ng/mL.

2.4. *Dietary Intake*

Food consumption data were collected according to the method of weighed food records (WFRs), as described by Sales et al. (2018) [28]. Habitual intake of each nutrient was estimated by removing the effect of intrapersonal variance, based on the method developed by Nusser et al. (1996) [40]. Subsequently, the results were adjusted for energy intake [41]. The prevalences of inadequate intake of calcium and vitamin D were estimated by using the Estimated Average Requirement (EAR) as the cut-off point [42].

2.5. *Statistical Analysis*

The data were analyzed using the statistical software IBM SPSS Statistics 21 (IBM Corp, Armonk, NY, USA). Initially, a descriptive analysis was performed with variables at the individual level, which allowed the sample to be characterized for socioeconomic, health, anthropometric, nutritional, and vitamin D statuses. Data on serum levels of 25(OH)D and dietary intake were checked for missing data and outliers that could hinder a multivariate analysis. In addition, variables were excluded from further analysis when they had more than 25% of missing data and outliers, identified under a multivariate perspective through measurement of the Mahalanobis distance (D^2)—distance greater than 3.0. There was no record of sample losses and multivariate outliers after adjustment of intrapersonal variability, interpersonal variability, and energy from dietary intake. The normality was checked by using the Kolmogorov–Smirnov test. Subsequently, the variables color, body mass index, cognition, functional status, and seasons of the year were dichotomized according to the predominance of elderly individuals in groups and/or clinical characteristics. Subsequently, to check for statistical associations, Pearson's chi-square test was run, considering the outcome variable (25(OH)D) and other variables relative to the theoretical model. The magnitude of the association was assessed using prevalence ratios (PR) with the corresponding confidence intervals (CIs). The significance level α was set at $p < 0.05$ (two-tailed test).

3. Results

The power of the study was 99.7% (with continuity correction), considering a 95% confidence interval. The calculation was obtained from 109 exposed participants and 44 unexposed participants, resulting in a prevalence of vitamin D insufficiency of 71% and 28%, respectively. Thus, the prevalence ratio (PR) was equal to 2.5, with a difference of 43% among the prevalences.

The mean age of the elderly individuals was 81.7 (9.2) years, ranging from 60–103. Thus, they were a long-living population, and there were more females (78.4%) than males. It was found that 64.5% of them had some level of education, 70.6% lived in nonprofit institutions, and that the average age-adjusted time of institutionalization was 29.4%. The BMI values indicated that 46.4% of the elderly individuals were thin.

It was found that 60.3% showed signs of loss of muscle mass, according to calf circumference. Most of the elderly individuals did not practice physical activity, had moderate-to-severe cognitive impairment, and showed multimorbidity (Table 1).

Table 1. General, anthropometric, lifestyle, and health characteristics of institutionalized elderly individuals (n = 153).

Variables	n (%)	95% CI
Sex		
Male	33 (21.6)	3.30–15.00
Female	120 (78.4)	3.30–71.90
Skin color [a]		
White	70 (54.7)	46.10–54.10
Black	25 (19.5)	12.50–26.60
Brown	27 (21.1)	14.10–28.90
Other	6 (4.7)	1.60–8.60
Marital status [b]		
Single	66 (52.0)	42.50–60.60
Widowed	32 (25.2)	18.10–33.10
Married	17 (13.4)	7.90–19.70
Separated/Divorced	12 (9.4)	3.70–17.30
Level of education [c]		
Illiterate	43 (35.5)	27.30–43.80
Literate	32 (26.4)	18.20–34.70
Elementary I (years 1–5)	16 (13.2)	6.60–19.00
Elementary II (years 6–9)	6 (5.0)	1.70–9.10
High School	18 (14.9)	8.30–21.50
Higher Education	6 (5.0)	1.70–9.10
Type of institution		
Profit	45 (29.4)	22.20–37.20
Nonprofit	108 (70.6)	62.80–77.80
Time of institutionalization (mean) [d]	29.38%	24.72–34.04
BMI (kg/m^2) [e]		
Thin	55 (46.4)	39.10–54.00
Normal weight	37 (31.1)	23.90–39.50
Excess weight	27 (22.7)	15.10–29.40
Abdominal circumference [f]		
Obese	51 (40.5)	31.80–50.00
Non-obese	75 (59.5)	50.00–68.20
Calf circumference [g]		
Sign of lean mass loss	88 (60.3)	51.10–68.50
No sign of lean mass loss	58 (39.7)	31.50–47.90

Table 1. *Cont.*

Variables	*n* (%)	95% CI
Physical activity [h]		
Inactive	87 (70.2)	67.80–81.50
Active	37 (29.8)	18.50–32.20
Mobility		
Without mobility	20 (13.1)	7.80–19.00
With mobility	133 (86.9)	81.00–92.20
Sarcopenia [g]	66 (45.2)	46.60–63.00
Cognition [i]		
Preserved mental function	13 (9.0)	4.90–13.90
Mild cognitive impairment	9 (6.3)	2.80–10.40
Moderate cognitive impairment	26 (18.1)	11.80–25.00
Severe cognitive impairment	96 (66.7)	58.40–74.30
Multimorbidity [b]	84 (66.1)	57.50–74.00
Polypharmacy [j]	59 (38.6)	34.80–50.70
Use of antiepileptic medications	27 (18.8)	12.50–25.70

[a] n = 128; [b] n = 127; [c] n = 121; [d] n = 133; [e] n = 151; [f] n = 126; [g] n = 146; [h] n = 124; [i] n = 144; [j] n = 139.

Concerning functional status, 31.8% of the elderly individuals were classified as "A" (independent for eating, continence, locomotion, toilet use, dressing, and bathing), followed by 16.2% in the item "G" (dependent on performing the above six functions). Dietary intake of vitamin D was 2.8 (3.2) µg/day, resulting in a high prevalence of inadequacy (95.4%), in addition to low frequency in the use of vitamin D supplementation (5.9%). The prevalence of hypovitaminosis D in the study population was 71.2%, with a mean value of 23.9 (16.6) ng/mL for 25(OH)D/mL. No participant was categorized in the winter season according to the criteria applied to the distribution of elderly individuals by seasons (Table 2).

Table 2. Dietary and environmental characteristics of institutionalized elderly individuals (n = 153).

Variables	Mean (SD)	95% CI
Vitamin D intake (µg/day)	2.8 (3.2)	2.32–3.33
Calcium intake (mg/day)	997.9 (291.8)	921.18–1074.64
Serum 25(OH)D (ng/mL) [a]	23.9 (16.6–31.0)	-
Local UV Index		
Summer	6.6 (0.5)	6.45–6.66
Spring	6.6 (0.5)	6.51–6.80
Fall	6.3 (0.4)	6.48–6.99
Vitamin D intake		
Possibly inadequate	146 (95.4)	92.20–98.70
Possibly adequate	7 (4.6)	1.30–7.80
Calcium intake		
Possibly inadequate	122 (79.7)	73.20–85.60
Possibly adequate	31 (20.3)	14.40–26.80
Vitamin D status [b]		
Insufficient	109 (71.2)	64.70–78.40
Sufficient	44 (28.8)	21.60–35.30
Distribution by seasons		
Summer	92 (60.1)	51.60–68.00
Spring	46 (30.1)	22.90–37.90
Fall	15 (9.8)	5.20–15.00

[a] median (inter-quartile range between 25 and 75, respectively); [b] according to the diagnosis of vitamin D status.

There was an association between 25(OH)D and summer (p = 0.046), and there were no associations with any other independent variables (all p > 0.05) (Table 3).

Table 3. Association between serum 25(OH)D concentration and variables of the theoretical model.

	Serum 25(OH)D (ng/mL)					
	Hypovitaminosis D (≤29)		**Sufficient (30–60)**			
	n	%	*n*	%	**PR [a] (95% CI)**	*p*
Sex						
Male	25	75.8	8	24.2	1.08 (0.86–1.36)	0.518
Female	84	70.0	36	30.0		
Age						
75 years or older	84	73.0	31	27.0	1.11 (0.86–1.43)	0.392
60–74 years	25	65.8	13	34.2		
Skin color						
Non-white	36	62.1	22	37.9	0.80 (0.63–1.02)	0.063
White	54	77.1	16	22.9		
Type of institution						
Nonprofit	72	66.7	36	33.3	0.43 (0.18–1.03)	0.053
Profit	37	82.2	8	17.8		
Body Mass Index						
Non-normal weight	83	72.3	31	27.2	0.63 (0.25–1.57)	0.314
Normal weight	30	81.1	7	18.9		
Abdominal circumference						
With abdominal fat	39	76.5	12	23.5	0.85 (0.68–1.06)	0.181
Without abdominal fat	49	65.3	26	34.7		
Calf circumference						
Sign of muscle mass loss	62	70.5	26	29.5	1.05 (0.86–1.29)	0.628
No sign of muscle mass loss	43	74.1	15	25.9		
Physical activity						
Inactive	75	68.8	34	31.2	0.43 (0.16–1.12)	0.078
Active	31	83.8	6	16.2		
Mobility						
Yes	17	85.0	3	15.0	1.23 (0.99–1.53)	0.145
No	92	69.2	41	30.8		
Multimorbidity						
Yes	59	70.2	25	29.8	0.91 (0.77–1.23)	0.828
No	31	72.1	12	27.9		
Falls						
Yes	4	80.0	1	20.0	1.12 (0.72–1.76)	0.669
None	99	71.2	40	28.8		
Sarcopenia						
Yes	57	71.3	23	28.8	1.00 (0.81–1.23)	0.996
No	47	71.2	19	28.8		
Cognition						
Moderate to severe impairment	89	73.0	33	27.0	1.33 (0.90–1.99)	0.083
Preserved to mild impairment	12	54.5	10	45.5		
Depression						
Depressed	6	54.5	5	45.5	0.75 (0.13–1.30)	0.198
Non-depressed	86	72.9	32	27.1		
Functional status						
Reduced independence	68	67.3	33	32.7	0.88 (0.71–1.08)	0.251
Independent	36	76.6	11	23.4		
Seasons of the year						
Other seasons	38	62.3	23	37.7	0.49 (0.24–1.00)	0.046
Summer	71	77.2	21	22.8		

Table 3. *Cont.*

	Serum 25(OH)D (ng/mL)					
	Hypovitaminosis D (≤29)		Sufficient (30–60)			
	n	%	*n*	%	PR [a] (95% CI)	*p*
Vitamin D intake						
Possibly inadequate	104	71.2	42	28.8	1.00 (0.62–1.61)	0.991
Possibly adequate	5	71.4	2	28.6		
Dietary Calcium						
Possibly inadequate	117	95.9	5	4.1	1.02 (0.93–1.13)	0.576
Possibly adequate	29	93.5	2	6.5		
Vitamin D supplementation						
Yes	87	70.2	37	29.8	1.05 (0.65–1.69)	0.825
No	6	66.7	3	33.3		
Antiepileptic medications						
Yes	19	70.4	8	29.6	0.98 (0.75–1.28)	0.882
No	84	71.8	33	28.2		

[a] Prevalence Ratio.

4. Discussion

The high prevalence of hypovitaminosis D found in the institutionalized elderly individuals of the present study was only significantly associated with the summer season, and this was found in the theoretical model involving several proximal and distal factors that determine vitamin D status. Moreover, the seasons of the year were considered as cross-sectional variables. The evaluation of the seasons of the year together with the assessment of the dietary intake of vitamin D (whether it was adequate or inadequate) was a relevant point of the present study, in that it was necessary to consider the two external sources of vitamin D obtained by the population.

Vitamin D is the only nutrient acquired from external sources, e.g., natural sunlight. It is estimated that an individual's highest daily vitamin D intake can be obtained by exposure to sunlight. However, in elderly individuals, the capacity of the cutaneous synthesis of vitamin D is undermined by the gradual loss of this physiological mechanism [9,17].

In epidemiological studies on vitamin D status, physical activity is often used as a proxy for time spent outdoors and, indirectly, for exposure to sunlight. Consequently, the elderly individuals who spend their lives at home indoors and those who spend less time doing outdoor physical activities have decreased levels of 25(OH)D [43].

Many of the elderly individuals were distributed by the summer season (60.1%), but although the region where the study was conducted has an annual average of UV indexes ranging from high to very high [44], it can be inferred that the studied population did not benefit from this environmental factor, as shown by the contradictory significant association between hypovitaminosis D and summer. We know that in tropical regions, the summer heat is extremely uncomfortable, causing most elderly individuals to avoid sunlight exposure. Similar reasons for this paradoxical finding were previously discussed, emphasizing different weather conditions between areas or countries [23]. In addition, their failure to benefit from the summer season can also be explained because activities in the NHs follow a pattern—they start early in the day with personal hygiene and provision of food and medicines, and end with little or no sunlight exposure, because the times are inappropriate. Furthermore, factors such as health problems, logistics of the NH, and indoor leisure activities affect the access of the elderly individuals to sunlight exposure more often when compared to their non-institutionalized peers [19,45].

Other findings from our study, such as the high inadequacies of dietary vitamin D and calcium, physical inactivity, and multimorbidities may additionally have nullified the response to environmental conditions that would otherwise be favorable for vitamin D status. In regard to elderly Brazilian subjects, even in the summer, Caucasian males in the youngest group of individuals presented a significant increase in 25(OH)D levels, demonstrating that a seasonal variation in 25(OH)D concentrations was influenced by factors such as gender, ethnicity, and age [20].

Okan et al. noted that 25(OH)D levels and the UV index of elderly people living in NHs were significantly lower than those living in their own homes, though there was a positive correlation between UV index and 25(OH)D observed in both groups [46].

These data reinforce the need to discuss vitamin D status in the context of the institutionalization of elderly individuals, and demands a model that encompasses diversified variables, such as those used in our study.

Although aging has been reported as a factor that interferes with vitamin D metabolism [9,17], the 25(OH)D concentrations in elderly Brazilian individuals with regular sunlight exposure and physical activity practice were similar to the values found in young and healthy individuals. These results confirm that vitamin D metabolism is activated by sunlight exposure, despite the physiological limitations of elderly individuals [20]. Physical activity is considered to be one of the factors associated with higher 25(OH)D levels [14]. In light of this evidence, some benefits can be achieved with changes in the lifestyles of elderly individuals.

Most of the elderly individuals lived in nonprofit institutions and had lived 29% of their life as an elderly individual in an institutional setting, which was considered a distal factor of the study model and was associated with an increased risk of vitamin D insufficiency and hypovitaminosis D when compared to elderly individuals living in the community [19]. In the same study, the prevalences of hypovitaminosis D in institutionalized elderly individuals and outpatients from a city in southeastern Brazil were 71.2% and 43.8%, respectively. This result is similar to that found in the present study. In this regard, confounding factors arising from disease burden in elderly individuals may also account for the high prevalence of vitamin D insufficiency. In a previous study, frail elderly individuals who had been recently institutionalized showed a 41% prevalence of vitamin D deficiency and a 45% prevalence of vitamin D insufficiency [47].

In our study, the population profiles and the infrastructures of the NHs were similar. Therefore, the studied elderly individuals did not show significant differences, whether they were in nonprofit public or for-profit private institutions. As shown in Table 3, the high prevalence of hypovitaminosis D in for-profit private institutions demonstrates that the institutionalization, by itself, can be addressed as a determinant of health problems in NHs. Furthermore, the study population lives in the Northeast of Brazil, a region with high social inequalities that may affect genetic distinctions in comparison to other areas of the country. A study developed in the same region found evidence that longevity in this region was characterized by the presence of longer telomeres in women associated with a low level of education [48].

All these factors may partly explain the findings reported in this study. However, the high prevalence of vitamin D insufficiency, per se, in the context of low dietary intake of vitamin D and calcium as well as physical inactivity, represents signs of deterioration in vitamin D status, thus affecting the health of institutionalized elderly individuals.

Other points should be addressed in the field of aging. This study focuses on this particular generation of long-living individuals, and according to the theoretical model proposed, age is a proximal factor of interference in 25(OH)D concentrations. In this regard, there is increasing evidence that aging can proceed at variable rates and be regulated by vitamin D. Normal concentrations of vitamin D are capable of maintaining these processes at their regular low rates, and this slows down the aging process and also helps to prevent the onset of some age-related diseases. When vitamin D is deficient, there is an increase in the activities of these aging processes, which not only accelerates the rate of aging, but also creates conditions that initiate the onset of age-related diseases [5].

The present study showed limitations regarding its temporal approach (cross-sectional), hindering the establishment of a causal relationship, and also due to lack of evaluation of sun exposure. Future studies should focus on reproducibility, involving a protocol with longitudinal observation and comparison among institutionalized and non-institutionalized elderly individuals. Furthermore, as shown by the benefits found in institutionalized elderly individuals in Finland [49] who received vitamin D food fortification, the literature reinforces the need for special attention in health care for elderly people, with a focus on modifiable risk factors.

5. Conclusions

A high prevalence of hypovitaminosis D was found in institutionalized elderly individuals living in a region with high ultraviolet radiation levels, and this was significantly associated with summer. These findings suggest the probability of the presence of interfering vitamin D factors mediated by aging. In this scenario, aging conditions which increase the risk of vitamin D deficiency have to be taken into consideration. Furthermore, the institutionalization of elderly individuals needs to be carefully handled to create alternatives that mitigate aging-related health problems.

Author Contributions: Conceptualization, S.E.S.S., K.C.L., and L.F.C.P.; data curation, S.E.S.S., M.C.S., and J.R.T.A.; formal analysis, S.E.S.S. and K.C.L.; funding acquisition, K.C.L. and L.F.C.P.; investigation, S.E.S.S. and L.F.C.P.; methodology, S.E.S.S., M.C.S., J.R.T.A., K.C.M.S.-E., K.C.L., and L.F.C.P.; project administration, K.C.L. and L.F.C.P.; supervision, K.C.M.S.-E., K.C.L., and L.F.C.P.; validation, S.E.S.S., M.C.S., J.R.T.A., K.C.L., and L.F.C.P.; visualization, S.E.S.S.; writing—original draft, S.E.S.S. and L.F.C.P.; writing—review & editing, S.E.S.S., M.C.S., J.R.T.A., K.C.M.S.-E., K.C.L., and L.F.C.P.

References

1. UNFPA. *Ageing in the Twenty-First Century: A Celebration and A Challenge*; UNFPA: New York, NY, USA, 2012; ISBN 9780897149815.
2. BRASIL Sinopse Do Censo Demográfico. Available online: http://www.ibge.gov.br/home/estatistica/populacao/censo2010/sinopse/default_sinopse.shtm (accessed on 22 August 2017).
3. Veldurthy, V.; Wei, R.; Oz, L.; Dhawan, P.; Jeon, Y.H.; Christakos, S. Vitamin D, calcium homeostasis and aging. *Bone Res.* **2016**, *4*, 16041. [CrossRef] [PubMed]
4. Ter Borg, S.; Verlaan, S.; Hemsworth, J.; Mijnarends, D.M.; Schols, J.M.G.A.; Luiking, Y.C.; De Groot, L.C. Micronutrient intakes and potential inadequacies of community-dwelling older adults: A systematic review. *Br. J. Nutr.* **2015**, *113*, 1195–1206. [CrossRef] [PubMed]
5. Berridge, M.J. Vitamin D deficiency accelerates ageing and age-related diseases: A novel hypothesis. *J. Physiol.* **2017**, *595*, 6825–6836. [CrossRef] [PubMed]
6. Holick, M.F. Vitamin D Deficiency. *N. Engl. J. Med.* **2007**, *357*, 266–281. [CrossRef] [PubMed]
7. Holick, M.F.; Binkley, N.C.; Bischoff-Ferrari, H.A.; Gordon, C.M.; Hanley, D.A.; Heaney, R.P.; Murad, M.H.; Weaver, C.M. Endocrine Society Evaluation, treatment, and prevention of vitamin D deficiency: An Endocrine Society clinical practice guideline. *J. Clin. Endocrinol. Metab.* **2011**, *96*, 1911–1930. [CrossRef] [PubMed]
8. Ferreira, C.E.S.; Maeda, S.S.; Batista, M.C.; Lazaretti-Castro, M.; Vasconcellos, L.S.; Madeira, M.; Soares, L.M.; Borba, V.Z.C.; Moreira, C.A. Posicionamento oficial da Sociedade Brasileira de Patologia Clínica/Medicina Laboratorial (SBPC/ML) e da Sociedade Brasileira de Endocrinologia e Metabologia (SBEM) sobre intervalos de referência da vitamina D [25(OH)D]. *J. Bras. Patol. Med. Lab.* **2017**, *53*, 377–381.
9. Flicker, L. Vitamin D and the endocrinology of ageing. *Curr. Opin. Endocr. Metab. Res.* **2019**, *5*, 7–10. [CrossRef]
10. Feng, X.; Guo, T.; Wang, Y.; Kang, D.; Che, X.; Zhang, H.; Cao, W.; Wang, P. The vitamin D status and its effects on life quality among the elderly in Jinan, China. *Arch. Gerontol. Geriatr.* **2016**, *62*, 26–29. [CrossRef]
11. Salminen, M.; Saaristo, P.; Salonoja, M.; Vaapio, S.; Vahlberg, T.; Lamberg-Allardt, C.; Aarnio, P.; Kivelä, S.-L. Vitamin D status and physical function in older Finnish people: A one-year follow-up study. *Arch. Gerontol. Geriatr.* **2015**, *61*, 419–424. [CrossRef]
12. Dawson-Hughes, B. Vitamin D and muscle function. *J. Steroid Biochem. Mol. Biol.* **2017**, *173*, 313–316. [CrossRef]
13. Pilz, S.; Dobnig, H.; Tomaschitz, A.; Kienreich, K.; Meinitzer, A.; Friedl, C.; Wagner, D.; Piswanger-Sölkner, C.; März, W.; Fahrleitner-Pammer, A. Low 25-hydroxyvitamin D is associated with increased mortality in female nursing home residents. *J. Clin. Endocrinol. Metab.* **2012**, *97*, 653–657. [CrossRef] [PubMed]

14. Skaaby, T.; Husemoen, L.L.N.; Thuesen, B.H.; Pisinger, C.; Hannemann, A.; Jørgensen, T.; Linneberg, A. Longitudinal associations between lifestyle and vitamin D: A general population study with repeated vitamin D measurements. *Endocrine* **2016**, *51*, 342–350. [CrossRef] [PubMed]
15. Liu, B.A.; Gordon, M.; Labranche, J.M.; Murray, T.M.; Vieth, R.; Shear, N.H. Seasonal prevalence of vitamin D deficiency in institutionalized older adults. *J. Am. Geriatr. Soc.* **1997**, *45*, 598–603. [CrossRef] [PubMed]
16. Mosekilde, L. Vitamin D and the elderly. *Clin. Endocrinol.* **2005**, *62*, 265–281. [CrossRef] [PubMed]
17. De Jongh, R.T.; Van Schoor, N.M.; Lips, P. Changes in vitamin D endocrinology during aging in adults. *Mol. Cell. Endocrinol.* **2017**, *453*, 144–150. [CrossRef] [PubMed]
18. Samefors, M.; Östgren, C.J.; Mölstad, S.; Lannering, C.; Midlöv, P.; Tengblad, A. Vitamin D deficiency in elderly people in Swedish nursing homes is associated with increased mortality. *Eur. J. Endocrinol.* **2014**, *170*, 667–675. [CrossRef]
19. Saraiva, G.L.; Cendoroglo, M.S.; Ramos, L.R.; Araújo, L.M.Q.; Vieira, J.G.H.; Maeda, S.S.; Borba, V.Z.C.; Kunii, I.; Hayashi, L.F.; Lazaretti-Castro, M. Prevalência da deficiência, insuficiência de vitamina D e hiperparatiroidismo secundário em idosos institucionalizados e moradores na comunidade da cidade de São Paulo, Brasil. *Arq. Bras. Endocrinol. Metabol.* **2007**, *51*, 437–442. [CrossRef]
20. Maeda, S.S.; Kunii, I.S.; Hayashi, L.F.; Lazaretti-Castro, M. Increases in summer serum 25-hydroxyvitamin D (25OHD) concentrations in elderly subjects in São Paulo, Brazil vary with age, gender and ethnicity. *BMC Endocr. Disord.* **2010**, *10*, 12. [CrossRef]
21. Andersen, R.; Mølgaard, C.; Skovgaard, L.T.; Brot, C.; Cashman, K.D.; Chabros, E.; Charzewska, J.; Flynn, A.; Jakobsen, J.; Karkkainen, M.; et al. Teenage girls and elderly women living in northern Europe have low winter vitamin D status. *Eur. J. Clin. Nutr.* **2005**, *59*, 533–541. [CrossRef]
22. Mowé, M.; Bohmer, T.; Haug, E. Serum calcidiol and calcitriol concentrations in elderly people: Variations with age, sex, season and disease. *Clin. Nutr.* **1996**, *15*, 201–206. [CrossRef]
23. Pérez-Llamas, F.; López-Contreras, M.J.; Blanco, M.J.; López-Azorín, F.; Zamora, S.; Moreiras, O. Seemingly paradoxical seasonal influences on vitamin D status in nursing-home elderly people from a Mediterranean area. *Nutrition* **2008**, *24*, 414–420. [CrossRef] [PubMed]
24. Pereira Machado, R.S.; Santa Cruz Coelho, M.A. Risk of malnutrition among Brazilian institutionalized elderly: A study with the Mini Nutritional Assessment (MNA) questionnaire. *J. Nutr. Health Aging* **2011**, *15*, 532–535. [CrossRef] [PubMed]
25. Hoffman, R. Micronutrient deficiencies in the elderly—Could ready meals be part of the solution? *J. Nutr. Sci.* **2017**, *6*, 4. [CrossRef]
26. Brazil. The Statute of the Elderly, Law 10741. 2003. Available online: http://www.planalto.gov.br/ccivil_03/leis/2003/l10.741.htm (accessed on 15 April 2017).
27. Open Source Epidemiologic Statistics for Public Health. Available online: https://www.openepi.com (accessed on 22 January 2018).
28. Sales, M.C.M.C.; de Oliveira, L.P.; de Araújo Cabral, N.L.; de Sousa, S.E.S.; das Graças Almeida, M.; Lemos, T.M.A.M.; de Oliveira Lyra, C.; de Lima, K.C.; Sena-Evangelista, K.C.M.; de Fatima Campos Pedrosa, L.; et al. Plasma zinc in institutionalized elderly individuals: Relation with immune and cardiometabolic biomarkers. *J. Trace Elem. Med. Biol.* **2018**, *50*, 615–621. [CrossRef] [PubMed]
29. Instituto Brasileiro de Geografia e Estatística (IBGE). *Características étnico-raciais da população: Classificações e identidades*, 2nd ed.; IBGE: Rio de Janeiro, Brazil, 2013; ISBN 978-85-240-4244-7.
30. Chumlea, W.A.; Roche, A.F.; Mukherjee, D. *Nutritional Assessment of the Elderly Through Anthropometry*; Ross Laboratories: Columbus, OH, USA, 1987.
31. Lipschitz, D.A. Screening for nutritional status in the elderly. *Prim. Care* **1994**, *21*, 55–67.
32. National Cholesterol Education Program (NCEP) Expert Panel on Detection, Evaluation; Treatment of High Blood Cholesterol in Adults (Adult Treatment Panel III). Third report of the National Cholesterol Education Program (NCEP) expert panel on detection, evaluation, and treatment of high blood cholesterol in adults (Adult Treatment Panel III) fin. *Circulation* **2002**, *106*, 3143–3421. [CrossRef]
33. Kennerfalk, A.; Ruigómez, A.; Wallander, M.-A.; Wilhelmsen, L.; Johansson, S. Geriatric Drug Therapy and Healthcare Utilization in the United Kingdom. *Ann. Pharmacother.* **2002**, *36*, 797–803. [CrossRef]

34. Cincura, C.; Pontes-Neto, O.M.; Neville, I.S.; Mendes, H.F.; Menezes, D.F.; Mariano, D.C.; Pereira, I.F.; Teixeira, L.A.; Jesus, P.A.P.; de Queiroz, D.C.L.; et al. Validation of the National Institutes of Health Stroke Scale, Modified Rankin Scale and Barthel Index in Brazil: The Role of Cultural Adaptation and Structured Interviewing. *Cerebrovasc. Dis.* **2009**, *27*, 119–122. [CrossRef]
35. De Oliveira Neto, L.; Agrícola, P.M.D.; de Andrade, F.L.J.P.; de Oliveira, L.P.; Lima, K.C.; de Oliveira Neto, L.; Agrícola, P.M.D.; de Andrade, F.L.J.P.; de Oliveira, L.P.; Lima, K.C. What is the impact of the European Consensus on the diagnosis and prevalence of sarcopenia among institutionalized elderly persons? *Rev. Bras. Geriatr. Gerontol.* **2017**, *20*, 754–761. [CrossRef]
36. Katz, S.; Ford, A.B.; Moskowitz, R.W.; Jackson, B.A.; Jaffe, M.W. Studies of illness in the aged. The index of adl: A standardized measure of biological and psychosocial function. *JAMA* **1963**, *185*, 914–919. [CrossRef]
37. Pfeiffer, E. A short portable mental status questionnaire for the assessment of organic brain deficit in elderly patients. *J. Am. Geriatr. Soc.* **1975**, *23*, 433–441. [CrossRef] [PubMed]
38. Martínez de la Iglesia, J.; Dueñas Herrero, R.; Onís Vilches, M.C.; Aguado Taberné, C.; Albert Colomer, C.; Luque Luque, R. Spanish language adaptation and validation of the Pfeiffer's questionnaire (SPMSQ) to detect cognitive deterioration in people over 65 years of age. *Med. Clin.* **2001**, *117*, 129–134.
39. LAVAT Laboratório de Váriaveis Ambientais e Tropicais. Available online: http://www.crn.inpe.br/lavat/ (accessed on 8 May 2019).
40. Nusser, S.M.; Carriquiry, A.L.; Dodd, K.W.; Fuller, W.A. A semiparametric transformation approach to estimating usual daily intake distributions. *J. Am. Stat. Assoc.* **1996**, *91*, 1440–1449. [CrossRef]
41. Willett, W.; Stampfer, M.J. Total energy intake: Implications for epidemiologic analyses. *Am. J. Epidemiol.* **1986**, *124*, 17–27. [CrossRef] [PubMed]
42. Institute of Medicine (US) Subcommittee on Interpretation and Uses of Dietary Reference Intakes; Institute of Medicine (US) Standing Committee on the Scientific Evaluation of Dietary Reference Intakes. *Standing Committee on the Scientific Evaluation of Dietary Reference Intakes. Dietary Reference Intakes: Applications in Dietary Assessment*; National Academies Press: Washington, DC, USA, 2000; ISBN 978-0-309-07183-3.
43. Van Dam, R.M.; Snijder, M.B.; Dekker, J.M.; Stehouwer, C.D.; Bouter, L.M.; Heine, R.J.; Lips, P. Potentially modifiable determinants of vitamin D status in an older population in the Netherlands: The Hoorn Study. *Am. J. Clin. Nutr.* **2007**, *85*, 755–761. [CrossRef] [PubMed]
44. World Health Organization (WHO). *Global Solar UV Index: A Practical Guide. A Joint Recommendation of World Health Organization, World Meteorological Organization, United Nations Environment Programme and the International Commission on Non-Ionizing Radiation Protection*; Library Cataloguing-in-Publication; WHO: Geneva, Switzerland, 2002; ISBN 92 4 159007 6.
45. Lin, T.-C.; Liao, Y.-C. The impact of sunlight exposure on the health of older adults. *J. Nurs.* **2016**, *63*, 116–122.
46. Okan, F.; Okan, S.; Zincir, H. Effect of Sunlight Exposure on Vitamin D Status of Individuals Living in a Nursing Home and Their Own Homes. *J. Clin. Densitom.* **2018**. In Press. [CrossRef]
47. Komar, L.; Nieves, J.; Cosman, F.; Rubin, A.; Shen, V.; Lindsay, R. Calcium Homeostasis of an Elderly Population upon Admission to a Nursing Home. *J. Am. Geriatr. Soc.* **1993**, *41*, 1057–1064. [CrossRef]
48. Oliveira, B.S.; Zunzunegui, M.V.; Quinlan, J.; Batistuzzo de Medeiros, S.R.; Thomasini, R.L.; Guerra, R.O. Lifecourse Adversity and Telomere Length in Older Women from Northeast Brazil. *Rejuvenation Res.* **2018**, *21*, 294–303. [CrossRef]
49. Jääskeläinen, T.; Itkonen, S.T.; Lundqvist, A.; Erkkola, M.; Koskela, T.; Lakkala, K.; Dowling, K.G.; Hull, G.L.; Kröger, H.; Karppinen, J.; et al. The positive impact of general vitamin D food fortification policy on vitamin D status in a representative adult Finnish population: Evidence from an 11-y follow-up based on standardized 25-hydroxyvitamin D data. *Am. J. Clin. Nutr.* **2017**, *105*, 1512–1520. [CrossRef]

12

Age-Related Deficits in Memory Encoding and Retrieval in Word List Free Recall

Dorina Cadar [1], Marius Usher [2] and Eddy J. Davelaar [3,*]

[1] Department of Behavioural Science and Health, University College London, London WC1E 7HB, UK; d.cadar@ucl.ac.uk
[2] Department of Psychology, Tel-Aviv University, Tel-Aviv 69978, Israel; marius@tauex.tau.ac.il
[3] Department of Psychological Sciences, Birkbeck, University of London, London WC1E 7HX, UK
* Correspondence: e.davelaar@bbk.ac.uk

Abstract: Although ageing is known to affect memory, the precise nature of its effect on retrieval and encoding processes is not well understood. Here, we examine the effect of ageing on the free recall of word lists, in which the semantic structure of word sequences was manipulated from unrelated words to pairs of associated words with various separations (between pair members) within the sequence. We find that ageing is associated with reduced total recall, especially for sequences with associated words. Furthermore, we find that the degree of semantic clustering (controlled for chance clustering) shows an age effect and that it interacts with the distance between the words within a pair. The results are consistent with the view that age effects in memory are mediated both by retrieval and by encoding processes associated with frontal control and working memory.

Keywords: ageing; memory encoding; memory retrieval; free recall; semantic clustering

---

1. Introduction

Episodic memory is known to decline with age, and this decline affects some tasks and processes more than others. For example, the largest age-related declines are found in tasks, such as free recall, which depend on retrieval strategies, while smaller deficits are found in recognition memory [1]. This conclusion is supported by studies of free recall [2], which reported that older adults have lower temporal contiguity effects (a reduction in the conditional probability of sequentially reporting items in proximal list positions). This is an effect which is associated with the use of retrieved context to guide subsequent retrieval [3]. Furthermore, an ageing retrieval deficit is suggested by verbal fluency studies, showing that older adults retrieve fewer words in a semantic fluency task, in which as many animal names as possible have to be generated within a fixed time period [4]. As no encoding is required in verbal fluency, this strongly supports an ageing effect on memory retrieval. While such studies suggest that age-related decline in episodic memory is due to a retrieval deficit, encoding deficits have also been demonstrated, as older participants are less likely to form rich, elaborative memory traces [5]. Furthermore, smaller age differences in memory are found when the initial encoding is equated [6].

The ageing deficit has been explained in terms of a reduction in frontal lobe functioning [7]. This hypothesis is supported by significant correlations between neuropsychological measures of frontal lobe functions and memory tests sensitive to ageing [8]. Morphological [9] and neuroimaging studies [10,11] give further support to this hypothesis by showing reduced activation in the left prefrontal cortex (PFC, associated with memory encoding and the processing of semantic information) during memory encoding and semantic processing. Further support for the "ageing as PFC reduction" perspective comes from the observation that like older adults, frontal patients show clear deficits in tests of free recall but not in memory recognition [12,13] and source memory (more than in item memory [14]).

Moscovitch [15] argued that both encoding and retrieval of consciously apprehended information are supported by the medial temporal lobes and hippocampus [16–18], and that these processes are under voluntary control. He noted that the frontal lobes operate on these structures and guide the encoding, retrieval, monitoring, and organisation of information: "By operating on the medial temporal and diencephalic system, the frontal lobes act as working-with-memory structures that control the more reflexive medial temporal and diencephalic system and confer a measure of intelligence and direction to it" ([15], p. 8, see also [19]).

Although evidence suggests that ageing affects both encoding and retrieval, a recurrent problem of interpretation is that different tasks and methods are used to provide support in favour of the encoding or retrieval interpretation. Here, we focus on the task of free recall (a single task from which metrics of encoding and retrieval can be extracted) in which the effect of age can be investigated.

Free recall of word list sequences can be used to quantify the contributions of encoding and retrieval processes in ageing. In a typical experimental paradigm, participants memorise a sequence of words consisting of exemplars from a small number of categories (e.g., four words from each of four categories). The words may be presented sequentially in a blocked-by-category fashion or randomized, and the recall is scored both in terms of the total number of correctly reported words and in terms of the degree of semantic clustering (see Section 2.4). One rationale for examining clustering performance is that it could provide a measure of retrieval strategies and memory organisation [20], uncontaminated by differences in total recall. Ageing studies have shown that semantic clustering scores are lowered for older adults and frontal patients compared with controls [20,21], but the evidence on the ageing effect remains mixed [22,23]. However, differences in semantic clustering scores in free recall may reflect both encoding and retrieval processes [24]. For example, memorising a word is easier when a semantically related word was just committed to memory. In that case, the semantics will help to encode the words in an episodic chunk, which during retrieval leads to a clustered output. In the absence of a semantically supported chunk, having just retrieved a word might prime the retrieval of a semantically related word. This would also produce a clustered output. Both processes are sensitive to ageing effects, but relative sensitivities are unclear.

The aim of our study is to estimate whether age deficits in a single task of word free recall are mediated by retrieval, by encoding processes, or by both. Based on previous studies [21,25], we expect to find age-related differences in both total recall and clustering. These studies, however, were able to assess only encoding or retrieval effects, but not both. To dissociate or isolate encoding and retrieval deficits within a single task, we employed a method that is sensitive to associative processes at encoding, while keeping the retrieval demands constant. This design is created by systematically varying the separation between semantic associates within a word list as part of a free recall paradigm, which is adapted from Glanzer [26] (see also [27]), who presented participants with lists made of pairs of weakly associated words (e.g., "stomach–liver").

The critical manipulation is the separation between associated pair members in the list. There are four conditions: Three related and one unrelated. The related ones are divided into three separation levels, i.e., the number of unrelated intervening words between a pair of associates. Thus, for the related conditions, each list contains one separation condition: separation-0 corresponds to a1, a2, b1, b2...; separation-1 to a1, b1, a2, b2 . . . ; and separation-5 to a1, b1, c1, d1, e1, f1, a2, b2 . . . . Using such a design, Glanzer [26] reported that memory recall was higher for lists with associated, compared with unrelated words, and was higher when the associates were separated by fewer unrelated words (small separation). As proposed by Glanzer, and demonstrated in simulation models [27,28], this separation effect can be explained as a result of semantic-associative processes during encoding in a capacity-limited working memory [27,29]. We have shown how encoding processes supported by the prefrontal cortex (PFC) operate on sequences that include an associative structure [24]. Specifically, when members of a pair reside in working memory simultaneously, the associative link between the words is increased (see also [30]), by recruiting category units that are linked with the list context and support subsequent retrieval. Thus, total recall, as well as semantic clustering, are predicted to be higher for word pairs whose members are separated by fewer unrelated words, as they are more likely to co-occupy working memory. Such a differential effect observed with a separation design is thus an encoding effect.

Using this paradigm, the separation-1 condition (i.e., one intervening item between pair members) is critical in demonstrating the age deficits that are in part due to declines in working memory assisted encoding. At separation-1, older participants may be more strongly affected in their recall of related words, because those words were less likely to have been maintained within their reduced working memory. Therefore, if ageing affects memory encoding, we predict an age-related reduction in semantic clustering at separation-1, which will differ from separation-5, as recall of word pairs separated by five intervening words is not assumed to be mediated by working memory. Thus, with this paradigm, we can demonstrate the additional influence of encoding processes on top of retrieval within a single task, based on the separation between associates.

To summarise, we expect age differences at encoding to result in an interaction between age and separation, either on total recall or on clustering, while age differences at retrieval to result in an interaction between age and relatedness with a long-separation (separation-5).

2. Materials and Methods

2.1. Participants

Forty native English speakers, who reported being in good health, took part in this study. The younger (n = 20, age range 19–35, mean 27) and older (n = 20, age range 55–65, mean 61) groups were balanced in educational background (young: 55% high-school; 45% university; older: 50% high-school, 50% university). Both groups were tested on a Test Of English as Foreign Language (TOEFL) as part of a standard test of general knowledge. The Quick test format used in the study was composed of 10 words, each followed by a four-alternative multiple choice question probing the word's meaning. The vocabulary test was administered after the free recall memory task. The mean score for young adults was 6.05 (SD = 2.19) and for the older adults it was 5.4 (SD = 2.52). No group differences were present ($t < 1$). Thus, any group differences in memory recall or clustering cannot be attributed to group differences in background vocabulary. The study was approved by the Birkbeck ethics committee.

2.2. Materials

For the memory task, we used a pool of 240 words consisting of common one- and two-syllable nouns with 90 pairs of weak associates (e.g., "stomach–liver", see [28]); weak associates were used in order to avoid guessing strategies. The words have a mean written word frequency of 66.9 per million, and the average associative strength was 0.15 (SD = 0.14; [31]). Each memory list consisted of 12 words and was constructed in accordance with one of four separation conditions. The five lists in the unrelated condition contained twelve words that did not have a semantic relation. We created three types of related lists by varying the number of intervening unrelated n items separating the members of a pair. We used separation-0, -1, and -5. With separation-0, the members of an associated pair, a1–a2, appeared in temporally adjacent list positions (e.g., a1, a2, b1, b2, c1, c2, d1, d2, e1, e2, f1, f2). In separation-1, the pair members were separated by one unrelated word, which was a member of a different pair (e.g., a1, b1, a2, b2, c1, d1, c2, d2, e1, f1, e2, f2), whereas in the separation-5 condition, five words separated the pair members (e.g., a1, b1, c1, d1, e1, f1, a2, b2, c2, d2, e2, f2). There were a total of 23 lists: three practice trials and 20 experimental trials.

2.3. Procedure

Participants were tested individually in noise-attenuated conditions and presented with the computerised memory task followed by the vocabulary test. Instructions were presented on the computer screen as well as verbally to ensure comprehension. Presentation of the memory test was visual. Participants were seated in front of the monitor, fixating the centre of the screen. Each trial started with a row of three question marks in the middle of the screen. These were replaced by words presented at a rate of one word per second. Participants were required to read each word silently and immediately after the final word to perform the arithmetic distractor task. This distractor task consisted of a mix of 12 additions and subtractions of the form A +/− B = C, where A, B and C were positive single digit numbers such as e.g., "1 + 2 = 3". The participant was instructed to quickly press the "k" (when correct) or "s" button on the keyboard to indicate the accuracy of the mathematical expression. A row of three question marks prompted the participants to recall aloud as many words from the list as possible, in any order. The experimenter wrote down the recalled items.

2.4. Semantic Clustering Scores

Semantic clustering was estimated using the pair frequency score, which is identical to the original clustering metric proposed by Bousfield and Bousfield [32]. This metric looks at the memory recall protocol and focuses on the number of within-category repetitions. To illustrate, consider a two-category word list, made of *cat, dog, rabbit, fork, knife, spoon*, with a recall output of *cat, dog, fork, knife, rabbit*. The pair frequency is the difference between the observed number of within-cluster transitions, which is 2 (cat → dog, fork → knife) and the expected number of within-cluster transitions, which is calculated using the following formula:

$$\sum_{i=1}^{N_c} \frac{n_i(n_i - 1)}{r} \tag{1}$$

where n_i is the number of correct words for category i, out of N_c recalled categories, and r is the total recall. In the example, $i = 2$, $n_1 = 3$ (cat, dog, rabbit), $n_2 = 2$ (fork, knife), and r is 5. This leads to an expected number of within-cluster transitions of $3 \times 2/5 + 2 \times 1/5 = 1.6$, and the overall clustering score of $2 - 1.6 = 0.4$.

In addition, we also estimated semantic clustering, using the California Verbal Learning Test (CVLT: [33]) measure. As the results are the same, we only report the pair-frequency measure here.

3. Results

Figure 1A,B show the average number of words recalled in the four conditions (three separations and one unrelated) and for the related (averaged across separation) and unrelated conditions, for young and older adults, respectively. Participants recalled more words in the related than in the unrelated condition. Younger adults reported more words than older adults, especially in the related condition. A 2 (age: young, older) × 2 (association: related, unrelated) mixed ANOVA revealed a main effect of age (F (1,38) = 15.83, MSe = 1.16, $p < 0.001$, $\eta^2 = 0.29$), a main effect of association (F (1,38) = 102.85, MSe = 0.31, $p < 0.001$, $\eta^2 = 0.73$), and an interaction (F (1,38) = 5.23, MSe = 0.31, $p < 0.05$, $\eta^2 = 0.12$). The interaction was due to a larger increase in total recall with related lists for younger than for older adults (t (38) = 2.29, $p < 0.05$). The same conclusions were obtained when the ANOVA was limited to unrelated versus separation-5.

Both groups showed equivalent decrease in recall performance with increasing separation between pair members. A 2 (age: young, older) × 3 (separation: 0, 1, 5) mixed ANOVA revealed a significant main effect of age (F (1,38) = 18.42, MSe = 2.52, $p < 0.001$, $\eta^2 = 0.33$) and a main effect of separation (F (2,76) = 12.25, MSe = 0.74, $p < 0.001$, $\eta^2 = 0.24$). The interaction between age and separation was not significant (F < 1).

We computed, for each separation, a semantic clustering score. Several metrics have been developed to measure semantic clustering [20,34]. Here, we use the pair frequency, which is identical to the original clustering metric proposed by Bousfield and Bousfield [32]. If, for example, a participant saw the words light_1 man_2 candle_1 father_2 hat_3 river_4 cap_3 lake_4 door_5 thief_6 wall_5 crook_6 (separation-1) and then reported lake_4 river_4 light_1 man_2 candle_1 (numbers are only added for illustration and were not present in the experiment), the clustering score would be 0.20 (OBS − EXP = 1 − (2 × 1/5 + 2 × 1/5 + 1 × 0/5) = 0.2). See Methods for details.

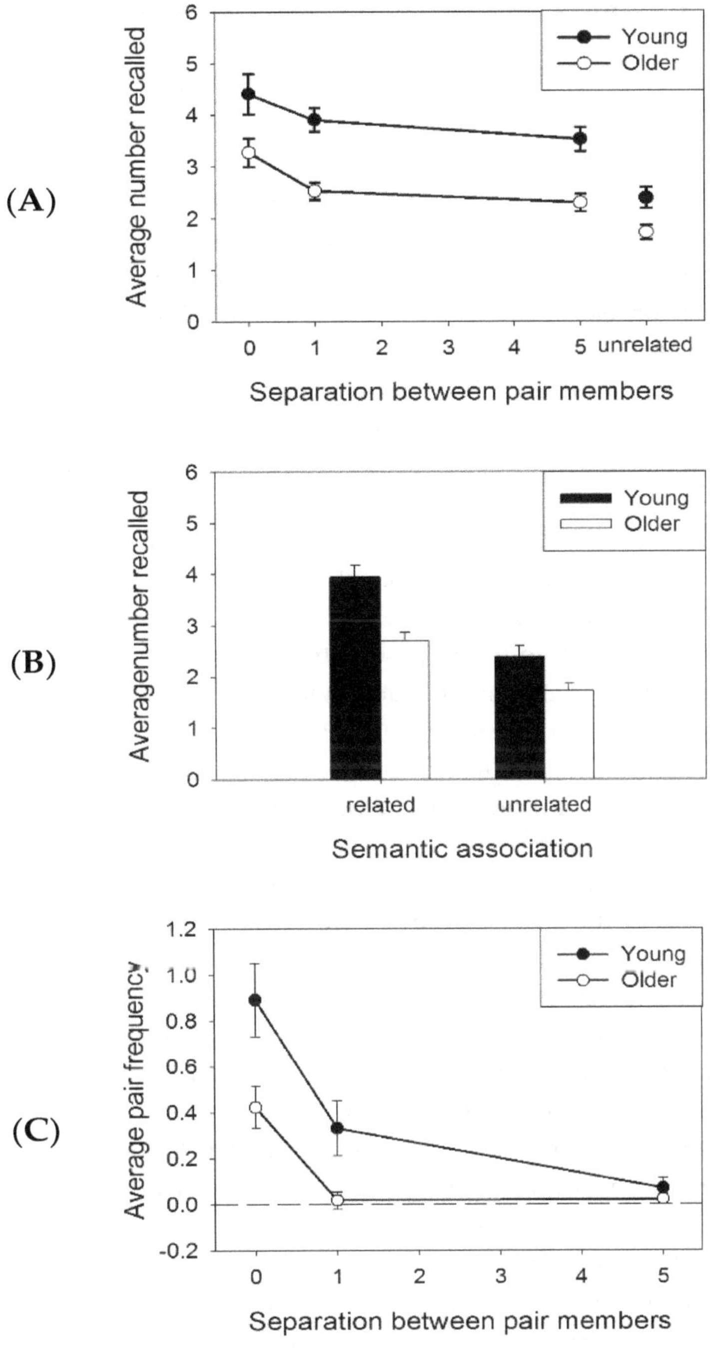

Figure 1. (**A**) Average number of words recalled as a function of the separation between the members of an associated pair and age. The separations in the related condition are presented. (**B**) The same as in panel A, but the related condition is averaged across separations. (**C**) Clustering scores in the related conditions as a function of the separation between pair members and age. The error bars represent standard error of the mean.

Figure 1C presents the clustering scores for each separation. Younger adults (filled circles) clustered the members of a pair more often than older adults (open circles). In addition, increasing the separation between pair members during encoding lowered the clustering effect for both age groups. A 2 (age: younger, older) × 3 (separation: 0, 1, 5) mixed ANOVA revealed a significant main effect of separation ($F(2,76) = 39.39$, $MSe = 0.11$, $p < 0.001$, $\eta^2 = 0.51$) and age ($F(2,76) = 7.34$, $MSe = 0.31$, $p < 0.01$, $\eta^2 = 0.16$) and an interaction between separation and age ($F(2,76) = 4.29$, $MSe = 0.11$, $p < 0.05$, $\eta^2 = 0.10$). This interaction was due to an absence of an age effect for separation 5 ($p > 0.34$). Also, older adults did not cluster the words when the pair members were separated by one or more unrelated words (all $ps > 0.10$).

4. Discussion

We tested for age-related differences in memory recall of word lists made of associated pairs, with various degrees of separation (number of unrelated intervening words) between the pair members. First, we found that lists containing associated pairs are recalled better than lists of un-associated words in both age groups and that this difference is larger for young adults. In particular, we found only small age differences for lists of unrelated words (0.67 words) and we found larger age differences for lists containing associated pairs (1.32 words). This interaction is also present when comparing the unrelated and separation-5 conditions. As word associates, which are separated by five intervening unrelated words, are not likely to co-occupy working memory, this interaction is likely to indicate a retrieval deficit: younger participants might be better in using the last word recalled, as a cue to memory search [2].

Second, we found that for both age groups, the association effect (better recall of associated than unrelated words) also depends on the separation of the pair members in the memory list, with better performance at short separation. This replicates the results by Glanzer [26], indicating that the encoding of the list is more effective when associated pairs co-occupy a capacity-limited working memory [27,29]. If older participants have reduced working memory capacity, one could expect that they will benefit less of associated pairs at separation-1; in both conditions, the pairs are unlikely to co-occupy working memory. Although the difference in total recall for separations 1 and 5 was numerically larger for young than for older participants, this difference was not statistically significant.

Third, we examined the clustering measures, of the two age groups, at each level of separation. Participants produced more clustered output, at short separations, consistent with an encoding mechanism (co-occupation of the associates in working memory, enhances their association). As we predicted, younger participants produced more clusters at separation-1 than at separation-5, consistent with an age-dependent working memory-assisted encoding. The clustering frequency for the old group at separation-1 was not different from that at separation-5, which was at chance level. Thus, older adults show reduced beneficial effect of closer temporal proximity, as expected from a reduced encoding of relations between words that co-occupy working memory. The absence of clustering at separation-1 critically supports the suggestion that older adults' working memory capacity is just too small to have both members of a pair active simultaneously after a single intervening unrelated item. This prevents the detection of the semantic similarity and the associative boost that is needed for these items to be recalled consecutively. While we report the pair frequency measure for semantic clustering, we also looked at other clustering measures such as the one used for the CVLT. Age-effects at separation-1 were present in these measures at separation-1, with older adults showing no clustering beyond what is expected by chance.

We suggest that the results indicate age effects in both the retrieval and encoding of a list of words, which are due to a reduced ability to encode relations between list-words (see also [35] for similar findings using a memory recognition paradigm). This is consistent with previous age studies of clustering, which used the CVLT [33], reporting marked age-related decline [25]. In a previous study, we have shown that ageing is associated with a significant deficit in a test that shares some features with the CVLT—The conceptual-span task [36]. Furthermore, our results parallel those obtained in memory studies in frontal patients, who do not show enhanced recall with related, compared with unrelated word lists [37], and who do not spontaneously utilise cues to enhance their memory encoding and retrieval, and show reduced semantic clustering [12]. These frontal memory deficits are well accounted for by neuropsychological models of memory, such as Hemispheric Encoding-Retrieval Asymmetry (HERA) [38], which postulate a role for the left PFC in semantic processing and memory encoding and by computational models that unpack the PFC mechanisms involved in memory encoding and retrieval [24,39]. For example, in the Categorization–Activation–Novelty (CAN; [24]) model, the PFC detects the semantic differences and similarities among list items that co-occupy WM. Semantic associates get an encoding boost, but only if their relatedness has been detected.

We believe that these similarities are explained best by the hypothesis that ageing deficits in memory are caused by a frontal mechanism [7,40]. As previously reviewed, this hypothesis is supported by neuropsychological, neurological, and neuroimaging evidence, showing changes in frontal lobe structures and functioning with advancing age. This interpretation is also consistent with the finding that older adults are less likely to form rich, elaborative memory traces [5]. The results presented here provide convergent evidence within a single paradigm suggesting that age-related declines in total recall are associated with a decrease in the use of associative information during both encoding and retrieval.

Author Contributions: Formal analysis, D.C., M.U., and E.J.D.; Investigation, D.C.; Methodology, D.C., M.U., E.J.D.; Writing—Original draft, D.C., M.U., and E.J.D.

References

1. Craik, F.I.M.; McDowd, J.M. Age differences in recall and recognition. *J. Exp. Psychol. Learn. Mem. Cogn.* **1987**, *13*, 474–479. [CrossRef]
2. Kahana, M.J.; Howard, M.W.; Zaromb, F.; Wingfield, A. Age dissociates recency and lag recency effects in free recall. *J. Exp. Psychol. Learn. Mem. Cogn.* **2002**, *3*, 530–540. [CrossRef]
3. Howard, M.W.; Kahana, M.J. A distributed representation of temporal context. *J. Math. Psychol.* **2002**, *46*, 269–299. [CrossRef]
4. Wingfield, A.; Lindfield, K.C.; Kahana, M.J. Adult age differences in the temporal characteristics of category free recall. *Psychol. Aging* **1998**, *13*, 256–266. [CrossRef]
5. Craik, F.I.M.; Jennings, J.M. Human memory. In *Handbook of Aging and Cognition*, 1st ed.; Craik, F.I.M., Salthouse, T.A., Eds.; Erlbaum: Hillsdale, NJ, USA, 1992; pp. 51–110.
6. Rybarczyk, B.D.; Hart, R.P.; Harkins, S.W. Age and forgetting rate with pictorial stimuli. *Psychol. Aging* **1987**, *2*, 404–406. [CrossRef] [PubMed]
7. West, R. An application of prefrontal cortex function theory to cognitive aging. *Psychol. Bull.* **1996**, *120*, 272–292. [CrossRef] [PubMed]
8. Parkin, A.J.; Walter, B.M. Recollective experience, normal aging, and frontal dysfunction. *Psychol. Aging* **1992**, *7*, 290–298. [CrossRef] [PubMed]
9. Haug, H.; Eggers, R. Morphometry of the human cortex cerebri and human striatum during aging. *Neurobiol. Aging* **1991**, *12*, 336–338. [CrossRef]
10. Cabeza, R.; Grady, C.L.; Nyberg, L.; McIntosh, A.R.; Tulving, E.; Kapur, S.; Jennings, J.M.; Houle, S.; Craik, F.I.M. Age-related differences in neural activity during memory encoding and retrieval: A positron emission tomography study. *J. Neurosci.* **1997**, *17*, 391–400. [CrossRef]
11. Stebbins, G.T.; Carrillo, M.C.; Dorman, J.; Dirksen, C.; Desond, J.E.; Turner, D.A.; Bennett, D.A.; Wilson, R.S.; Glover, G.; Gabrieli, J.D. Aging effects on memory encoding in the frontal lobes. *Psychol. Aging* **2002**, *17*, 44–55. [CrossRef]
12. Baldo, J.V.; Delis, D.; Kramer, J.; Shimamura, A.P. Memory performance on the California Verbal Learning Test II: Finding from patients with local frontal lesions. *J. Int. Neuropsychol. Soc.* **2002**, *8*, 539–546. [CrossRef] [PubMed]
13. Janowsky, J.S.; Shimamura, A.P.; Squire, L.R. Source memory impairment in patients with frontal lobe lesions. *Neuropsychologia* **1989**, *27*, 1043–1056. [CrossRef]

14. Simons, J.S.; Verfaellie, M.; Galton, C.J.; Miller, B.L.; Hodges, J.R.; Graham, K.S. Recollection-based memory in frontotemporal dementia: Implications for theories of long-term memory. *Brain* **2002**, *125*, 2523–2536. [CrossRef]
15. Moscovitch, M. Amnesia. In *The International Encyclopedia of Social and Behavioural Sciences*; Smesler, N.B., Baltes, O.B., Eds.; Pergamon/Elsevier Science: Oxford, UK, 2004; pp. 1–26.
16. Moscovitch, M.; Westmacott, R.; Gilboa, A.; Addis, D.R.; Rosenbaum, R.S.; Viskontas, I.; Priselac, S.; Svoboda, E.; Ziegler, M.; Black, S.; et al. Hippocampal complex contribution to retention and retrieval of recent and remote episodic and semantic memories: Evidence from behavioral and neuroimaging studies of healthy and brain-damaged people. In *Dynamic Cognitive Processes*; Ohta, N., MacLeod, C.M., Uttl, B., Eds.; Springer: Tokyo, Japan, 2005; pp. 333–380.
17. Nadel, L.; Moscovitch, M. Memory consolidation, retrograde amnesia and the hippocampal complex. *Curr. Opin. Neurobiol.* **1997**, *7*, 217–227. [CrossRef]
18. Nadel, L.; Samsonovich, A.; Ryan, L.; Moscovitch, M. Multiple trace theory of human memory: Computational, neuroimaging, and neuropsychological results. *Hippocampus* **2000**, *10*, 352–368. [CrossRef]
19. Simons, J.S.; Spiers, H.J. Prefrontal and medial temporal lobe interactions in long-term memory. *Nat. Rev. Neurosci.* **2003**, *4*, 637–648. [CrossRef] [PubMed]
20. Stricker, J.L.; Brown, G.G.; Wixted, J.T.; Baldo, J.V.; Delis, D. New semantic and serial clustering indices for the California Verbal Learning Test 2: Background, rationale, and formulae. *J. Int. Neuropsychol. Soc.* **2002**, *8*, 425–435. [CrossRef] [PubMed]
21. Taconnat, L.; Raz, N.; Tocze, C.; Bouazzaoui, B.; Sauzeon, H.; Fay, S.; Isingrini, M. Ageing and organisation strategies in free recall: the role of cognitive flexibility. *Eur. J. Cogn. Psychol.* **2009**, *21*, 347–365. [CrossRef]
22. Backman, L.; Larsson, M. Recall of organizable words and objects in adulthood: Influences of instructions, retention interval, and retrieval cues. *J. Gerontol.* **1992**, *47*, P273–P278. [CrossRef] [PubMed]
23. Verhaeghen, P.; Marcoen, A. More or less the same? A memorability analysis on episodic memory tasks in young and older adults. *J. Gerontol.* **1993**, *48*, P172–P178. [CrossRef] [PubMed]
24. Elhalal, A.; Davelaar, E.J.; Usher, M. The role of the frontal cortex in memory: An investigation of the Von Restorff effect. *Front. Hum. Neurosci.* **2014**, *8*, 410. [CrossRef] [PubMed]
25. Norman, M.A.; Evans, J.D.; Miller, S.W.; Heaton, R.K. Demographically corrected norms for the California Verbal Learning Test. *J. Clin. Exp. Neuropsychol.* **2000**, *22*, 80–94. [CrossRef]
26. Glanzer, M. Distance between related words in free recall: Trace of the STS. *J. Verbal Learn. Verbal Behav.* **1969**, *8*, 105–111. [CrossRef]
27. Davelaar, E.J.; Haarmann, H.J.; Goshen-Gottstein, Y.; Usher, M. Semantic similarity dissociates short from long-term recency effects: Testing a neurocomputational model of list memory. *Mem. Cogn.* **2006**, *34*, 323–334. [CrossRef]
28. Haarmann, H.J.; Usher, M. Maintenance of semantic information in capacity-limited item short-term memory. *Psychol. Bull. Rev.* **2001**, *8*, 568–578. [CrossRef]
29. Cowan, N. The magical number 4 in short-term memory: A reconsideration of mental storage capacity. *Behav. Brain Sci.* **2001**, *24*, 87–185. [CrossRef]
30. Raaijmakers, J.G.W.; Shiffrin, R.M. Search of associative memory. *Psychol. Rev.* **1981**, *88*, 93–134. [CrossRef]
31. Nelson, D.L.; McEvoy, C.L.; Schreiber, T.A. The University of South Florida word association, rhyme, and word fragment norms. Available online: http://www.usf.edu/FreeAssociation/ (accessed on 30 January 2008).
32. Bousfield, A.K.; Bousfield, W.A. Measurement of clustering and of sequential constancies in repeated free recall. *Psychol. Rep.* **1966**, *19*, 935–942. [CrossRef]
33. Delis, D.C.; Kramer, J.H.; Kaplan, E.; Ober, B. *California Verbal Learning Test: Adult Version Manual*, 1st ed.; The Psychological Corporation: San Antonio, TX, USA, 1987.
34. Sternberg, R.J.; Tulving, E. The measurement of subjective organization in free recall. *Psychol. Bull.* **1977**, *84*, 539–556. [CrossRef]
35. Naveh-Benjamin, M. Adult age differences in memory performance: Tests of an associative deficit hypothesis. *J. Exp. Psychol. Learn. Mem. Cogn.* **2000**, *26*, 1170–1187. [CrossRef]
36. Haarmann, H.J.; Ashling, G.E.; Davelaar, E.J.; Usher, M. Age-related declines in context maintenance and semantic short-term memory. *Q. J. Exp. Psychol.* **2005**, *58*, 34–53. [CrossRef] [PubMed]
37. Hirst, W.; Volpe, B.T. Memory strategies with brain damage. *Brain Cogn.* **1988**, *8*, 379–408. [CrossRef]

38. Tulving, E.; Kapur, S.; Craik, F.I.M.; Moscovitch, M.; Houle, S. Hemispheric encoding/retrieval asymmetry in episodic memory: Positron emission tomography findings. *Proc. Natl. Acad. Sci.* **1994**, *91*, 2016–2020. [CrossRef] [PubMed]
39. Becker, S.; Lim, J. A computational model of prefrontal control in free recall: Strategic memory use in the California Verbal Learning Task. *J. Cogn. Neurosci.* **2003**, *15*, 821–832. [CrossRef]
40. Moscovitch, M.; Winocur, G. Frontal lobes, memory and aging. *Ann. N. Y. Acad. Sci.* **1995**, *769*, 119–150. [CrossRef]

13

Thermotherapy Plus Neck Stabilization Exercise for Chronic Nonspecific Neck Pain in Elderly: A Single-Blinded Randomized Controlled Trial

Ho-Jin Shin [1,†], Sung-Hyeon Kim [1,†], Suk-Chan Hahm [2,*] and Hwi-Young Cho [1,3,*]

1 Department of Health Science, Gachon University Graduate School, Incheon 21936, Korea; sports0911@hanmail.net (H.-J.S.); 315201@hanmail.net (S.-H.K.)
2 Graduate School of Integrative Medicine, CHA University, Seongnam 13488, Korea
3 Department of Physical Therapy, Gachon University, Incheon 21936, Korea
* Correspondence: schahm@cha.ac.kr (S.-C.H.); hwiyoung@gachon.ac.kr (H.-Y.C.);

† These two authors contributed equally to this work as co-first authors.

Abstract: Neck pain is a serious problem for public health. This study aimed to compare the effects of thermotherapy plus neck stabilization exercise versus neck stabilization exercise alone on pain, neck disability, muscle properties, and alignment of the neck and shoulder in the elderly with chronic nonspecific neck pain. This study is a single-blinded randomized controlled trial. Thirty-five individuals with chronic nonspecific neck pain were randomly allocated to intervention ($n = 18$) or control ($n = 17$) groups. The intervention group received thermotherapy with a salt-pack for 30 min and performed a neck stabilization exercise for 40 min twice a day for 5 days (10 sessions). The control group performed a neck stabilization exercise at the same time points. Pain intensity, pain pressure threshold (PPT), neck disability index, muscle properties, and alignment of the neck and shoulder were evaluated before and after the intervention. Significant time and group interactions were observed for pain at rest ($p < 0.001$) and during movement ($p < 0.001$), and for PPT at the upper-trapezius ($p < 0.001$), levator-scapula ($p = 0.003$), and splenius-capitis ($p = 0.001$). The disability caused by neck pain also significantly changed between groups over time ($p = 0.005$). In comparison with the control group, the intervention group showed significant improvements in muscle properties for the upper-trapezius (tone, $p = 0.021$; stiffness, $p = 0.017$), levator-scapula (stiffness, $p = 0.025$; elasticity, $p = 0.035$), and splenius-capitis (stiffness, $p = 0.012$), and alignment of the neck ($p = 0.016$) and shoulder ($p < 0.001$) over time. These results recommend the clinical use of salt pack thermotherapy in addition to neck stabilization exercise as a complementary intervention for chronic nonspecific neck pain control.

Keywords: neck stabilization exercise; nonspecific neck pain; salt pack; thermotherapy

---

1. Introduction

Neck pain is a common health problem with a lifetime prevalence of 14.2% to 71% in the adult population and is considered a major problem for public health [1]. In particular, Korean women of middle and older age have a prevalence of 20.8% [2]. The common presentation of neck pain is nonspecific neck pain, defined as simple neck pain without a specific underlying disease causing the pain, which results from postural and mechanical causes [3,4]. Appropriate management of nonspecific neck pain is essential because chronic neck pain results in increased muscle tone, restricted cervical range of motion, functional impairments of activities of daily living, and decreased quality of life [4].

Nonspecific neck pain can be treated with a variety of interventions, such as medication, manual therapy, heat, and exercise [3–6]. In particular, exercise is an evidence-based practice to not only relieve pain in individuals with nonspecific neck pain, but also to improve muscle strength, motor function, and quality of life [7]. The efficacy of cervical-scapulothoracic stabilization exercise and neck stabilization exercise for the management of neck pain have been reported in previous studies [8–10].

Thermotherapy has been used to reduce chronic musculoskeletal pain and has been reported as a complementary intervention [11–19]. Since the application of thermotherapy to the skin increases the temperature and blood flow to the muscle and decreases muscle fatigue [14–16], it may be associated with an increase in muscle flexibility [17]. These effects of thermotherapy can also decrease muscle spasms [13]. Considering these findings, the application of thermotherapy followed by exercise during the rehabilitation process may strengthen the stability of neck muscles; thus, thermotherapy combined with neck stabilization exercise may be more effective than exercise alone for relieving nonspecific neck pain.

A hot pack is one of the most common methods of thermotherapy, and various heat transfer substances, such as silicate gel, polymer gel, and water, were used in the hot pack [20–23]. Salt can be an option for a heat transfer substance in hot packs. Considering that thermotherapy using salt have analgesic and anti-inflammatory effects [24,25], hot packs using salt can be used for management of musculoskeletal pain. However, no clinical trial has been specifically conducted to investigate the feasibility of salt packs in patients with nonspecific neck pain, and the efficacy of thermotherapy combined with neck stabilization exercise for nonspecific neck pain has not been investigated. Thus, the aim of this study was to investigate the efficacy of a combination of a salt pack with neck stabilization exercise on pain, pain pressure threshold (PPT), neck disability, and alignment in individuals with chronic nonspecific neck pain. To this end, we compared the effects of thermotherapy using a salt pack plus neck stabilization exercise versus a neck stabilization exercise alone for symptomatic relief from chronic nonspecific neck pain.

2. Methods

2.1. Study Design

This study was designed as a single-blinded, randomized controlled trial. The experimental protocol was approved by the Gachon University Institutional Review Board (1044396-201903-HR-040-01). The study was performed in accordance with the protocol, and all participants provided written informed consent prior to their enrollment in the study.

2.2. Participants and Sample Size

For this study, we enrolled elders (>60 years) with chronic nonspecific neck pain that had lasted longer than 6 months (visual analogue scale (VAS) > 3/10), who had not undertaken regular physical activity in the past year. Chronic nonspecific neck pain was defined as neck pain provoked by neck postures, movements, or pressure for at least 3 months without a known pathology (neurological, trauma-induced, etc.) as the cause of the complaints [26]. The exclusion criteria were neck pain associated with inflammatory, hormonal, and neurological disorders or structural deformity in the upper extremities; neck pain related to previous surgery; positive radicular signs consistent with nerve root compression; severe referred pain; severe psychological disorder; or pregnancy. In addition, participants were excluded if they were under anti-inflammatory, analgesic, anticoagulant, muscle relaxant, or antidepressant medication use 1 week before the study commenced [26].

The sample size was calculated using the computer software G-power (Heinrich-Heine-University Düsseldorf, version 3.1.9.4, Düsseldorf, Germany) In the present study, the effect size was set to 0.25 (medium effect size) [27], and the alpha level was 0.05. On the basis of these values, 34 participants (17 participants per group) were needed to achieve 80% power using a 2-sided test. Thus, with a 10% dropout rate, a total of 38 participants were required.

2.3. Experimental Procedures and Interventions

All participants were randomly assigned to treatment or control groups using a stratified randomization method [28]. Participants were stratified by age (60–69/70–79) and baseline VAS at rest (3–5/6–8) and randomization was performed within each stratum by using permuted block randomization (block size 4). The group allocation was concealed to the outcome assessor by blinding the group assignment, and primary and secondary variables were assessed before and after the intervention. Pre-test were performed on the morning (9 a.m. to 10 a.m.) before the first intervention, and post-tests were performed in the morning (9 a.m. to 10 a.m.) on the next day after the intervention. All assessments were conducted in a random order to exclude potential fatigue and order effects due to measurement order.

The intervention group performed neck stabilization exercise and thermotherapy using a salt pack, and the control group performed only neck stabilization exercises at Saesum Resort in Taean-gun. The neck stabilization exercise was applied by slightly modifying the exercise intervention performed in the previous study [10]. It consisted of a warm-up (5 min), main exercise (30 min), and cool-down (5 min), and was performed in both the intervention and control groups. The warm-up and cool-down consisted of neck and upper extremity stretching, and the main exercise was as follows: (1) Deep neck flexor isometric exercise in supine position; (2) Multi-directional isometric exercise (cervical flexion, extension, rotation, side bending) in a sitting position; (3) Upper extremity movement exercise; (4) Resistive exercise with Thera-band. The neck stabilization exercise was performed according to the therapist's instruction.

After the neck stabilization exercise, the intervention group performed additional thermotherapy using a salt pack. For thermotherapy, bay salt was used in packs. The salt was collected at Taean-gun, Chungcheongnam-do, Republic of Korea in April 2019 and then packed in cotton cloth. The far infrared radiation (FIR) emissivity of bay salt used in this study was 0.900 μm and the FIR emission power was 3.89×10^2 W/m^2·μm (Table A1 in Appendix A). The salt packs were kept in a warming cabinet (LH-1043G, Lassele Co., Ltd., Ansan, Korea) set at 60 °C until the start of the intervention. The participant was in a prone position. A salt pack set at 55 °C was applied to the neck and shoulder [29]; even after 30 min of application, it was maintained at about 40–50 °C. All interventions were conducted twice a day for 5 days, neck stabilization exercise was performed for 40 min and additional thermotherapy using salt pack was performed for 30 min.

2.4. Outcome Measures

2.4.1. Primary Variables

The visual analogue scale (VAS) [30] was used to assess pain intensity at rest and during movement. VAS at rest (resting pain) was defined as an unpleasant feeling or pain without movement, and VAS during movement (movement-induced pain) was defined as unpleasant feelings or pain incurred by neck movement (flexion, extension, lateral flexion, rotation) [31]. Patients marked their pain intensity at rest and during movement on a VAS table.

To assess the PPT of the neck, the PPT assessment method described in a previous study was used with a distal algometer (Somedic AB, Farsta, Sweden) containing a 1-cm^2 probe [11,32,33]. The pressure head of the algometer was applied to the upper trapezius, levator scapula, and splenius capitis of the neck and shoulder area, as in a previous study [34]. The assessor gradually increased the application pressure in 10-kPa/s increments until the participants expressed a pain response, such as a pain-induced vocalization and a gesture related to pain (hand grasp or eye blink) [32]. The measurement was repeated twice, and the measurement interval was 30 s. The mean threshold was calculated for the left- and right-side points.

The neck disability index (NDI) was used to assess functional disability due to neck pain; this assessment consists of 10 items describing the impact of pain on different daily living activities [33]. Each item is rated on a six-point Likert scale (range 0–5), with 0 indicating no limitation due to pain and 5 indicating that an activity is impossible to perform. The total score ranges from 0 to 50, with a higher score indicating a higher level of disability. The NDI is the most widely used tool for assessing functional outcomes in patients with neck pain and is recommended for evaluation of the effectiveness of neck pain treatment.

2.4.2. Secondary Variables

A handheld myotonometer (Myoton AS, Tallinn, Estonia) with excellent intra and inter-tester reliability (ICC = 0.97) was used to measure the mechanical properties of muscle (muscle tone, stiffness, and elasticity) [35]. The skeletal muscle assessments were performed at the same region where PPT was measured. Each time, the probe (3 mm diameter) of equipment was placed perpendicular to the skin's surface and five repeated measurements were obtained. The myofascial tissue oscillations were evoked with 5 brief (15 ms) mechanical impulses at 0.4 N force and frequency of 1 Hz. The mean threshold was calculated for the left- and right-side points. Muscle tone is a value expressing muscle tone in a passive or resting state without voluntary contraction. Muscle stiffness is a value representing the resistance of tissue to external mechanical impulse. Muscle elasticity is a value expressing the ability to recover to the initial shape after the disappearance of the external force of deformation.

Changes in cervical and shoulder alignments were assessed using the cervical angle and shoulder angle, respectively [36] (Figure A1). the cervical angle and shoulder angle were defined through three markers (tragus of ear, spinous process of the C7, acromion) attached to the participants' anatomical landmarks. Images were collected by a 16-megapixel camera (SM-N976N, Samsung, Suwon, Korea) with an acromion height of 1.5 m, located perpendicular to the ground by a spirit level. The collected images were processed through the MATLAB (version 2019b, Mathworks, Inc., Natick, MA, USA). The cervical angle is formed when a line drawn from the tragus of the ear to the C7 vertebra intersects a horizontal line, and the shoulder angle is formed when a horizontal line passing through the lateral shoulder meets the line drawn from C7 to the lateral shoulder.

2.5. Statistical Analysis

Data analyses were performed using IBM SPSS Statistics 25.0. (IBM-SPSS Inc, Chicago, IL, USA) The statistician was blinded to group allocation for all analyses. An independent *t*-test and the χ^2 test was performed in order to compare general characteristics between the two groups. Repeated measures ANOVA was used to analyze the changes in variables between groups over time and main effect comparisons were performed. Post-hoc analysis was performed through independent *t*-test and paired *t*-test using Bonferroni methods. A p-value of < 0.05 was considered statistically significant.

3. Results

3.1. Participant Characteristics

A total of 53 participants were recruited, all of whom were women. Fifteen individuals were excluded from participating; 13 did not meet the inclusion criteria and two declined to participate. Because individuals scheduled their problems, in the intervention group, one individual did not participate in the final assessment. In the control group, two individuals declined to participate after allocation. However, there were no complaints or dropout due to the intensity of the intervention except for those who were dropped out for the above reasons. A total of 35 patients completed the study. Figure 1 shows the participant flow through the enrollment, allocation, assessment, and analysis stages.

There were no significant differences between the intervention and control groups in terms of the general participant characteristics (age, height, weight, and body mass index) (Table 1). Additionally, there are no significant differences in the baseline values of the outcome variables assessed in this study between the two groups.

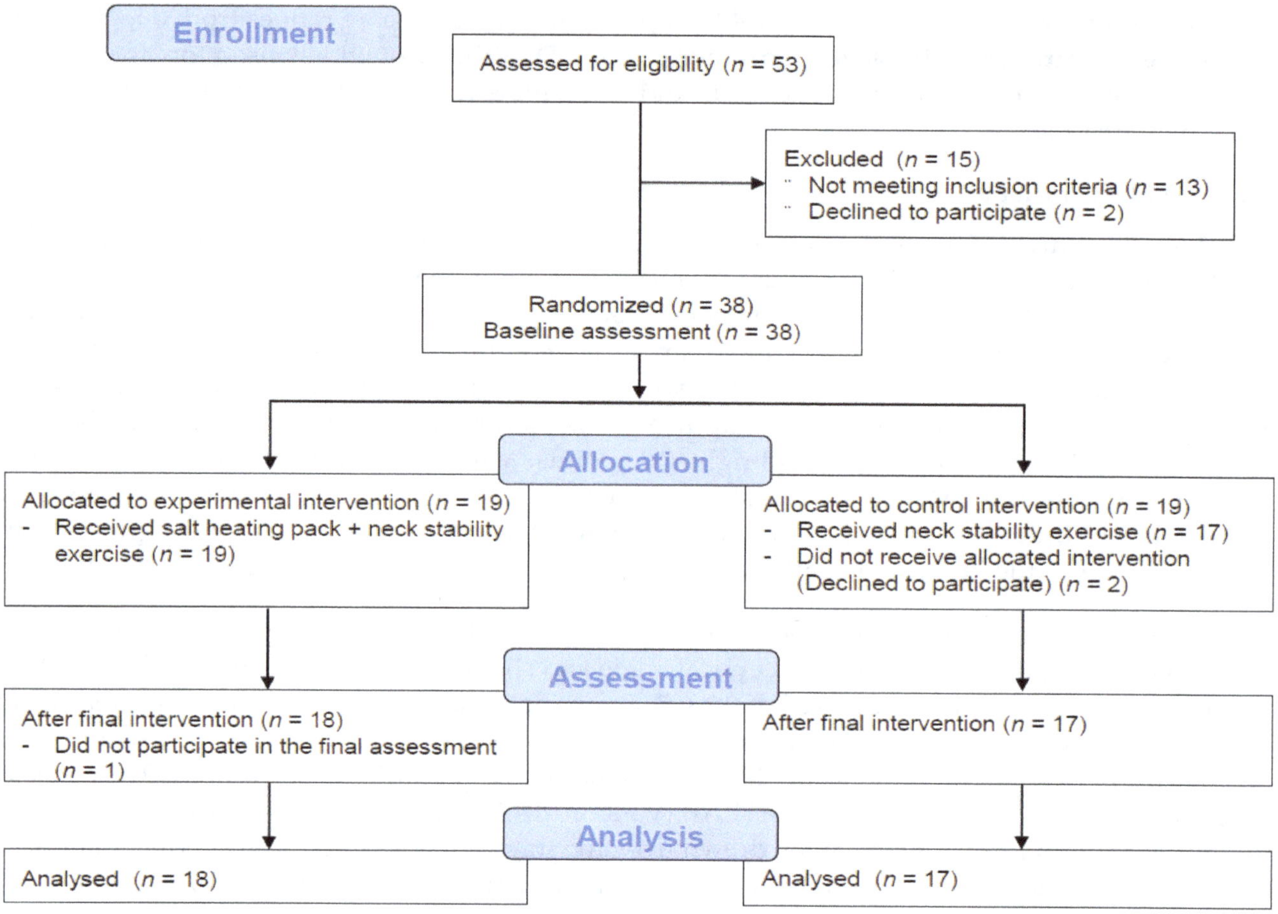

Figure 1. Flow diagram of study participants.

Table 1. General characteristics of the participants.

Variable	Intervention Group (n = 18)	Control Group (n = 17)	P
Age (years)	68.06 ± 4.71	66.24 ± 4.71	0.261
Height (m)	1.54 ± 0.04	1.53 ± 0.03	0.299
Weight (kg)	58.92 ± 7.52	57.34 ± 4.68	0.457
BMI (kg/m^2)	24.73 ± 2.93	24.5 ± 1.80	0.780
VAS at rest (cm)	4.78 ± 1.11	4.53 ± 1.37	0.560
Onset duration (month)	15.33 ± 7.76	14.29 ± 7.74	0.694
Job context †			
Working	13 (72.22)	11 (64.71)	0.632
Non-working	5 (27.78)	6 (35.29)	

Data are expressed as mean ± standard deviation or number (%) †. BMI, body mass index; P, p-value; VAS, visual analogue scale.

3.2. *Primary Outcomes*

3.2.1. Pain Intensity

As shown in Table 2, compared to neck stabilization exercise alone, salt pack therapy combined with neck stabilization exercise significantly improved pain intensity over time at rest ($p < 0.001$) and during movement ($p < 0.001$). The intervention group showed a significantly decreased pain intensity at rest ($p < 0.001$) and during movement ($p < 0.001$) after the intervention. The control group also showed a significantly decreased pain intensity at rest ($p = 0.009$) and during movement ($p = 0.001$).

Table 2. The changes in pain intensity, pain pressure threshold, and neck disability.

Outcome/Group	Baseline	Two Weeks Post-Treatment	P (Pairwise Comparison)	P (T * G)
VAS at rest(cm)				
Intervention group	4.78 ± 1.11	1.17 ± 1.04	<0.001	<0.001
Control group	4.53 ± 1.37	3.41 ± 1.28	0.009	
VAS during movement(cm)				
Intervention group	6.75 ± 1.06	2.28 ± 1.41	<0.001	<0.001
Control group	6.06 ± 1.14	4.53 ± 1.37	0.001	
PPT_Upper trapezius (kg)				
Intervention group	2.41 ± 0.50	4.28 ± 1.38	<0.001	0.002
Control group	2.56 ± 0.75	3.22 ± 0.87	0.014	
PPT_Levator scapula (kg)				
Intervention group	2.07 ± 0.51	4.12 ± 1.18	<0.001	<0.001
Control group	2.38 ± 0.89	2.99 ± 0.83	0.018	
PPT_Splenius capitis (kg)				
Intervention group	2.56 ± 0.93	4.52 ± 0.84	<0.001	0.001
Control group	2.90 ± 0.87	3.55 ± 0.78	0.015	
NDI (%)				
Intervention group	36.11 ± 12.88	16.56 ± 10.56	<0.001	0.005
Control group	33.65 ± 11.92	27.29 ± 10.79	0.052	

Data are expressed as mean ± standard deviation. P, *p*-value; T * G, time and group interaction; VAS, visual analog scale; PPT, pain pressure threshold; NDI, neck disability index.

3.2.2. Pain Pressure Threshold

A significant increase in the PPT for the upper trapezius ($p = 0.002$), levator scapula ($p < 0.001$), and splenius capitis ($p < 0.001$) was observed in the groups over time (Table 2). In comparison with the control, the intervention group showed a significant improvement in PPT for the upper trapezius ($p = 0.002$), levator scapula ($p < 0.001$), and splenius capitis ($p = 0.001$). Both thermotherapy with neck stabilization exercise (upper trapezius, $p < 0.001$; levator scapula, $p < 0.001$; splenius capitis, $p < 0.001$) and neck stabilization exercise alone (upper trapezius, $p = 0.014$; levator scapula, $p = 0.018$; splenius capitis, $p = 0.015$) significantly increased PPT after treatment.

3.2.3. Neck Disability

Significant improvement in disability due to neck pain was observed in groups over time ($p = 0.005$, Table 2). Interestingly, salt pack with neck stabilization exercise yielded significant improvements in disability due to neck pain in comparison with the improvements obtained with neck stability exercise alone ($p = 0.005$). The intervention group showed significant increases in NDI scores ($p < 0.001$). However, the control group did not show a significant change in NDI after neck stability exercise.

3.3. Secondary Outcomes

3.3.1. Muscle Properties

In comparison with the control group, the intervention group showed a significant improvement over time in muscle tone (upper trapezius, $p = 0.021$), stiffness (upper trapezius, $p = 0.017$; levator scapula, $p = 0.025$; splenius capitis, $p = 0.012$), and elasticity (levator scapula, $p = 0.035$) (Table 3). The intervention group also showed significant differences in muscle tone (upper trapezius, $p < 0.001$; levator scapula, $p = 0.003$; splenius capitis, $p = 0.006$), stiffness (upper trapezius, $p < 0.001$; levator scapula, $p < 0.001$; splenius capitis, $p < 0.001$), and elasticity (upper trapezius, $p = 0.001$; levator scapula, $p < 0.001$; splenius capitis, $p = 0.001$) after the intervention. However, the control group did not show significant improvements in muscle tone, stiffness, and elasticity after neck stabilization exercise.

Table 3. The changes in muscle characteristics.

Outcome/Group.	Baseline	Two Weeks Post-Treatment	P (Pairwise Comparison)	P (T * G)
Upper trapezius				
		Tone (Hz)		
Intervention group	13.71 ± 2.25	11.64 ± 0.91	<0.001	0.021
Control group	14.19 ± 2.72	13.88 ± 3.43	0.552	
		Stiffness (N/m)		
Intervention group	255.56 ± 19.25	229.83 ± 27.64	<0.001	0.017
Control group	260.94 ± 11.33	254.88 ± 32.14	0.288	
		Elasticity (logarithm)		
Intervention group	1.69 ± 0.26	1.97 ± 0.42	0.001	0.079
Control group	1.59 ± 0.23	1.67 ± 0.31	0.328	
Levator scapula				
		Tone (Hz)		
Intervention group	19.03 ± 1.89	17.04 ± 2.23	0.003	0.129
Control group	20.11 ± 2.66	19.48 ± 3.10	0.331	
		Stiffness (N/m)		
Intervention group	335.78 ± 48.50	280.06 ± 53.92	<0.001	0.025
Control group	345.00 ± 48.90	333.35 ± 54.75	0.393	
		Elasticity (logarithm)		
Intervention group	1.42 ± 0.17	1.65 ± 0.23	<0.001	0.035
Control group	1.38 ± 0.14	1.44 ± 0.25	0.325	
Splenius capitis				
		Tone (Hz)		
Intervention group	21.01 ± 1.65	19.07 ± 2.69	0.006	0.094
Control group	21.18 ± 2.47	20.88 ± 3.5	0.655	
		Stiffness (N/m)		
Intervention group	388.56 ± 48.13	332.22 ± 52.88	<0.001	0.012
Control group	395.24 ± 51.39	385.59 ± 59.32	0.449	
		Elasticity (logarithm)		
Intervention group	1.49 ± 0.15	1.64 ± 0.23	0.001	0.101
Control group	1.48 ± 0.15	1.53 ± 0.24	0.296	

Data are expressed as mean ± standard deviation. P, *p*-value; T * G, time and group interaction.

3.3.2. Cervical and Shoulder Alignments

In assessments of neck posture correction, cervical ($p = 0.016$) and shoulder ($p < 0.001$) alignments significantly improved in the groups over time (Table 4). As shown in Table 4, cervical ($p < 0.001$) and shoulder ($p < 0.001$) angles significantly improved after salt pack therapy with neck stabilization exercise. However, the control group did not show significant improvements in cervical and shoulder angles. Salt pack combined with neck stabilization exercise was not significantly more effective than neck stabilization exercise only.

Table 4. The changes in cervical and shoulder alignment.

Outcome/Group	Baseline	Two Weeks Post-Treatment	P (Pairwise comparison)	P (T * G)
		Cervical angle (degree)		
Intervention group	48.06 ± 6.31	50.26 ± 6.22	<0.001	0.016
Control group	50.12 ± 4.62	50.59 ± 5.43	0.352	
		Shoulder angle (degree)		
Intervention group	60.49 ± 4.57	65.86 ± 4.64	<0.001	<0.001
Control group	62.18 ± 5.49	62.97 ± 6.30	0.293	

Data are expressed as mean ± standard deviation. P, *p*-value; T * G, time and group interaction.

4. Discussion

This study aimed to compare the effects of thermotherapy combined with neck stabilization exercise to those of neck stabilization exercise alone on chronic nonspecific neck pain. This study is the first investigation to demonstrate that 10 sessions of salt pack thermotherapy plus neck stabilization exercise provide benefits that are superior to those of neck stability exercise alone on pain intensity, PPT, neck disability, muscle properties, and body alignment in individuals with chronic nonspecific neck pain. These results may provide evidence to use salt pack therapy plus neck stabilization exercise as a complementary intervention for relief from nonspecific neck pain.

Previous studies have reported the effects of therapeutic exercise, including neck stabilization exercise, with or without thermotherapy on nonspecific musculoskeletal pain and disability [8–12,34,37–39]. Our study also demonstrated that both thermotherapy using a salt pack plus neck stabilization exercise and neck stabilization exercise alone had significant effects in reducing pain intensity, increasing PPT, and improving disability. Interestingly, in comparison with neck stabilization exercise alone, the intervention group also showed significantly better neck pain control. In the study by Cramor et al. [12] both the thermotherapy and non-thermotherapy groups received their usual medication and physical therapy regimens during the study period, with the thermotherapy group receiving thermotherapy using mud packs; their findings suggested that the additional thermotherapy significantly alleviated nonspecific neck pain. Thermotherapy has been shown to effectively alleviate pain and improve somatosensory function in individuals with chronic neck pain [12]. The results of previous studies that applied thermotherapy with exercise for low back pain control support our findings [11]. In addition to the thermal effect, it appears that there is also the effect of FIR emitted from the bay salt. FIR can provide pain control and increased blood flow [40]. This effect of FIR may contribute to pain reduction and changes in muscle characteristics. The superiority of the intervention group may be explained by a reduction in pain intensity [11,12,37] and improvement in muscle flexibility [41] as a result of thermotherapy prior to neck stabilization exercise. These changes in pain intensity and PPT may have resulted in the decreased neck disability evidenced by the NDI results.

This study showed significant time and group interactions of PPT, and both intervention and control groups showed significant improvements in PPT. Prior studies have also reported that thermotherapy has a greater influence on PPT in comparison with other treatments for chronic neck pain [38,42]. However, a previous study [12] reported no significant change in PPT after thermotherapy application. That study explained that with hyperalgesia pressure is maintained by central sensitization in patients with chronic neck pain [43] and that thermotherapy had no effect on central sensitization. The discrepancies between the findings of our study and that study may be attributable to the alteration of pain memories associated with central sensitization in patients with chronic musculoskeletal pain via exercise [44]. A previous study [9] reported significant improvement in the PPT on the middle point of the upper trapezius in patients with nonspecific neck pain after neck stabilization exercise, which supports our results for PPT.

This study also examined the changes in muscle properties of the neck/shoulder in both groups. The intervention group demonstrated significantly decreased muscle tone, stiffness and elasticity, but the control group did not show significant changes in muscle properties. Thermotherapy increases the temperature of and blood flow to the muscle and reduces muscle fatigue [14–16], which may decrease muscle tone, stiffness, and elasticity. In addition, significant recovery of these muscle properties and neck pain may be associated with the significant differences in the effects on cervical and shoulder alignment between the two groups. Previous studies have reported that the high tone of the upper trapezius is associated with the forward neck [45,46], and that increased tone and stiffness of the neck and shoulder muscles can be a major physical factor for neck pain [47,48]. Our results showed a significant reduction in tone and stiffness of the neck and shoulder muscles, neck pain, and forward neck and round shoulder in the intervention group. These results showed that changes in muscle characteristics due to thermotherapy combined with neck stabilization exercise had a significant effect on neck and shoulder alignment and neck pain.

In the intervention group of this study, the intervention time for one session is more than one hour, which may be burdensome to the body. The participant's condition was continuously checked during and after the intervention, and there were no adverse symptoms such as pain, fatigue, and delayed onset muscle soreness. Moreover, there were no complaints about the interventions, and no participants dropped out due to problems with interventions. It seems that there was no problem because active intervention (neck stabilization exercise) was performed for only 40 min and then thermos-intervention was performed for 30 min.

There are some limitations to the present study. First, since the current study assessed the findings only after 10 sessions applied over 5 days, a thorough understanding of the effects of repeated thermotherapy with neck stability exercises over longer periods is necessary to evaluate the clinical use of salt pack interventions. Second, all participants in this study were women, even though sex was not an inclusion/exclusion criterion in this study. To obtain more generalizable conclusions relating to the efficacy of the salt pack combined with neck stabilization exercise for chronic nonspecific neck pain, further studies with suitable sex ratios may be needed. Third, although this feasibility study showed significant effects on pain intensity, PPT, muscle properties, and aliment in individuals with chronic nonspecific neck pain, the small sample size may limit the generalizability of these results.

5. Conclusions

According to the results of this study, salt pack thermotherapy combined with neck stabilization exercise is superior to neck stabilization exercise alone for chronic nonspecific neck pain control. However, to generalize the clinical use of this intervention for management of nonspecific neck pain, further studies with larger sample sizes and longer periods of application are needed.

Author Contributions: Conceptualization, S.-C.H., H.-Y.C.; Data curation, H.-J.S., S.-H.K.; Investigation, H.-J.S., S.-H.K.; Formal analysis, S.-C.H.; Funding acquisition, H.-Y.C.; Project administration, S.-C.H.; Methodology, S.-C.H., H.-J.S., S.-H.K.; Visualization, H.-J.S., S.-H.K.; Writing–original draft, H.-J.S., S.-H.K.; Writing–review and editing, S.-C.H. All authors have read and agreed to the published version of the manuscript.

Appendix A

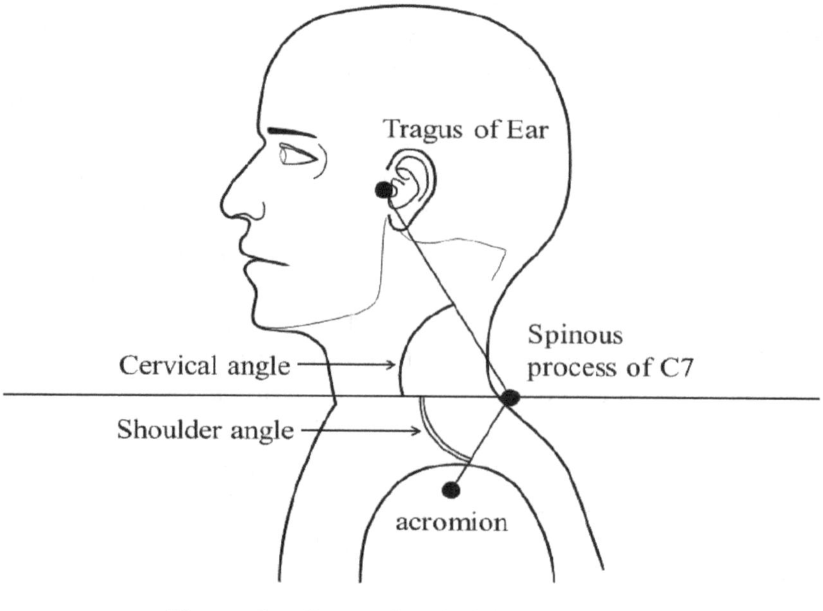

Figure A1. Cervical and shoulder angles.

Table A1. Emissivity and emission power of the far infrared radiation by 45 °C bay salt.

Emissivity (5~20 μm)	Emission Power ($W/m^2 \cdot \mu m$)
0.9000	3.89×10^2

References

1. Fejer, R.; Kyvik, K.O.; Hartvigsen, J. The prevalence of neck pain in the world population: A systematic critical review of the literature. *Eur. Spine J.* **2006**, *15*, 834–848. [CrossRef] [PubMed]
2. Son, K.M.; Cho, N.H.; Lim, S.H.; Kim, H.A. Prevalence and risk factor of neck pain in elderly Korean community residents. *J. Korean Med. Sci.* **2013**, *28*, 680–686. [CrossRef] [PubMed]
3. Binder, A. The diagnosis and treatment of nonspecific neck pain and whiplash. *Eur. Med.* **2007**, *43*, 79–89.
4. Tsakitzidis, G.; Remmen, R.; Peremans, L.; Van Royen, P.; Duchesnes, C.; Paulus, D.; Eyssen, M. Non-Specific neck pain: Diagnosis and treatment. *Good Clin. Pract.* **2009**. KCE Reports 119C. D/2009/10.273/56.
5. Gross, A.R.; Haines, T.; Goldsmith, C.H.; Santaguida, L.; McLaughlin, L.M.; Peloso, P.; Burnie, S.; Hoving, J. Knowledge to action: A challenge for neck pain treatment. *J. Orthop. Sports Phys. Ther.* **2009**, *39*, 351–363. [CrossRef] [PubMed]
6. Graham, N.; Gross, A.R.; Carlesso, L.C.; Santaguida, P.L.; Macdermid, J.C.; Walton, D.; Ho, E. An ICON Overview on Physical Modalities for Neck Pain and Associated Disorders. *Open Orthop. J.* **2013**, *7*, 440–460. [CrossRef] [PubMed]
7. O'Riordan, C.; Clifford, A.; Van De Ven, P.; Nelson, J. Chronic neck pain and exercise interventions: Frequency, intensity, time, and type principle. *Arch. Phys. Med. Rehabil.* **2014**, *95*, 770–783. [CrossRef]
8. Celenay, S.T.; Kaya, D.O.; Akbayrak, T. Cervical and scapulothoracic stabilization exercises with and without connective tissue massage for chronic mechanical neck pain: A prospective, randomised controlled trial. *Man. Ther.* **2016**, *21*, 144–150. [CrossRef]
9. Celenay, S.T.; Akbayrak, T.; Kaya, D.O. A Comparison of the Effects of Stabilization Exercises Plus Manual Therapy to Those of Stabilization Exercises Alone in Patients With Nonspecific Mechanical Neck Pain: A Randomized Clinical Trial. *J. Orthop. Sports Phys. Ther.* **2016**, *46*, 44–55. [CrossRef]
10. Dusunceli, Y.; Ozturk, C.; Atamaz, F.; Hepguler, S.; Durmaz, B. Efficacy of neck stabilization exercises for neck pain: A randomized controlled study. *J. Rehabil. Med.* **2009**, *41*, 626–631. [CrossRef]
11. Hahm, S.C.; Shin, H.J.; Lee, M.G.; Lee, S.J.; Cho, H.Y. Mud Therapy Combined with Core Exercise for Chronic Nonspecific Low Back Pain: A Pilot, Single-Blind, Randomized Controlled Trial. *Evid. Based Complement. Alternat. Med.* **2020**, *2020*, 7547452. [CrossRef] [PubMed]
12. Cramer, H.; Baumgarten, C.; Choi, K.E.; Lauche, R.; Saha, F.J.; Musial, F.; Dobos, G. Thermotherapy self-treatment for neck pain relief—A randomized controlled trial. *Eur. J. Integr. Med.* **2012**, *4*, e371–e378. [CrossRef]
13. Nadler, S.F.; Weingand, K.; Kruse, R.J. The physiologic basis and clinical applications of cryotherapy and thermotherapy for the pain practitioner. *Pain Physician* **2004**, *7*, 395–399. [PubMed]
14. Erasala, G.; Rubin, J.; Tuthill, T.; Fowlkes, J.; de Drue, S.; Hengehold, D.; Weingand, K.J. The effect of topical heat treatment on trapezius muscle blood flow using power Doppler ultrasound. *Phys. Ther.* **2001**, *81*, A5.
15. Nadler, S.F.; Deprince, M.L.; Stitik, T.P.; Hendgehold, D.; Weingand, K. Experimentally induced trapezius fatigue and the effects of topical heat on the EMG power density spectrum. *Am. J. Phys. Med. Rehab.* **1999**, *80*, 1123.
16. Mulkern, R.; McDannold, N.; Hynynen, K.; Fielding, J.; Panych, L.; Jolesz, F.; Weingand, K. Temperature Distribution Changes in Low Back Muscles during Applied Topical Heat: A Magnetic Resonance Thermometry Study. In Proceedings of the 7th Annual Meeting of the International Society of Magnetic Resonance, in Medicine, Philadelphia, PA, USA, 22–28 May 1999; p. 1054.
17. Strickler, T.; Malone, T.; Garrett, W.E. The effects of passive warming on muscle injury. *Am. J. Sports Med.* **1990**, *18*, 141–145. [CrossRef] [PubMed]
18. Petrofsky, J.; Laymon, M.; Lee, H. Local heating of trigger points reduces neck and plantar fascia pain. *J. Back Musculoskelet. Rehabil.* **2020**, *33*, 21–28. [CrossRef] [PubMed]

19. Petrofsky, J.S.; Laymon, M.; Alshammari, F.; Khowailed, I.A.; Lee, H. Use of low level of continuous heat and Ibuprofen as an adjunct to physical therapy improves pain relief, range of motion and the compliance for home exercise in patients with nonspecific neck pain: A randomized controlled trial. *J. Back Musculoskelet. Rehabil.* **2017**, *30*, 889–896. [CrossRef]
20. Robertson, V.J.; Ward, A.R.; Jung, P. The effect of heat on tissue extensibility: A comparison of deep and superficial heating. *Arch. Phys. Med. Rehabil.* **2005**, *86*, 819–825. [CrossRef]
21. Knight, C.A.; Rutledge, C.R.; Cox, M.E.; Acosta, M.; Hall, S.J. Effect of superficial heat, deep heat, and active exercise warm-up on the extensibility of the plantar flexors. *Phys. Ther.* **2001**, *81*, 1206–1214. [CrossRef]
22. Oshima-Saeki, C.; Taniho, Y.; Arita, H.; Fujimoto, E. Lower-limb warming improves sleep quality in elderly people living in nursing homes. *Sleep Sci.* **2017**, *10*, 87–91. [CrossRef] [PubMed]
23. Saeki, Y. Effect of local application of cold or heat for relief of pricking pain. *Nurs. Health Sci.* **2002**, *4*, 97–105. [CrossRef] [PubMed]
24. Vakilinia, S.R.; Vaghasloo, M.A.; Aliasl, F.; Mohammadbeigi, A.; Bitarafan, B.; Etripoor, G.; Asghari, M. Evaluation of the efficacy of warm salt water foot-bath on patients with painful diabetic peripheral neuropathy: A randomized clinical trial. *Complement. Ther. Med.* **2020**, *49*, 102325. [CrossRef] [PubMed]
25. Tishler, M.; Shoenfeld, Y. The medical and scientific aspects of spa therapy. *Isr. J. Med. Sci.* **1996**, *32*, S8–S10.
26. Cerezo-Téllez, E.; Torres-Lacomba, M.; Fuentes-Gallardo, I.; Perez-Muñoz, M.; Mayoral-Del-Moral, O.; Lluch-Girbés, E.; Prieto-Valiente, L.; Falla, D. Effectiveness of dry needling for chronic nonspecific neck pain: A randomized, single-blinded, clinical trial. *Pain* **2016**, *157*, 1905–1917. [CrossRef]
27. Cohen, J. *Statistical Power Analysis for the Behavioral Sciences*; Academic Press: New York, NY, USA, 2013.
28. Kim, J.; Shin, W. How to do random allocation (randomization). *Clin. Orthop. Surg.* **2014**, *6*, 103–109. [CrossRef]
29. Garra, G.; Singer, A.J.; Leno, R.; Taira, B.R.; Gupta, N.; Mathaikutty, B.; Thode, H.J. Heat or cold packs for neck and back strain: A randomized controlled trial of efficacy. *Acad. Emerg. Med.* **2010**, *17*, 484–489. [CrossRef]
30. Crichton, N. Visual analogue scale (VAS). *J. Clin. Nurs.* **2001**, *10*, 697–706.
31. Lauche, R.; Cramer, H.; Langhorst, J.; Michalsen, A.; Dobos, G.J. Reliability and validity of the pain on movement questionnaire (POM) in chronic neck pain. *Pain Med.* **2014**, *15*, 1850–1856. [CrossRef]
32. Hahm, S.-C.; Suh, H.R.; Cho, H.Y. The effect of transcutaneous electrical nerve stimulation on pain, muscle strength, balance, and gait in individuals with dementia: A double blind, pilot randomized controlled trial. *Eur. J. Integr. Med.* **2019**, *29*, 100932. [CrossRef]
33. Cleland, J.A.; Fritz, J.M.; Whitman, J.M.; Palmer, J.A. The reliability and construct validity of the Neck Disability Index and patient specific functional scale in patients with cervical radiculopathy. *Spine* **2006**, *31*, 598–602. [CrossRef] [PubMed]
34. Lluch, E.; Arguisuelas, M.D.; Coloma, P.S.; Palma, F.; Rey, A.; Falla, D. Effects of deep cervical flexor training on pressure pain thresholds over myofascial trigger points in patients with chronic neck pain. *J. Manip. Physiol. Ther.* **2013**, *36*, 604–611. [CrossRef] [PubMed]
35. Gapeyeva, H.; Vain, A. *Methodical Guide: Principles of Applying Myoton in Physical Medicine and Rehabilitation*; Muomeetria Ltd.: Tartu, Estonia, 2008.
36. Singla, D.; Veqar, Z.; Hussain, M.E. Photogrammetric Assessment of Upper Body Posture Using Postural Angles: A Literature Review. *J. Chiropr. Med.* **2017**, *16*, 131–138. [CrossRef] [PubMed]
37. Koyuncu, E.; Ökmen, B.M.; Özkuk, K.; Taşoğlu, Ö.; Özgirgin, N. The effectiveness of balneotherapy in chronic neck pain. *Clin. Rheumatol.* **2016**, *35*, 2549–2555. [CrossRef] [PubMed]
38. Cramer, H.; Lauche, R.; Hohmann, C.; Lüdtke, R.; Haller, H.; Michalsen, A.; Langhorst, J.; Dobos, G. Randomized-controlled trial comparing yoga and home-based exercise for chronic neck pain. *Clin. J. Pain* **2013**, *29*, 216–223. [CrossRef] [PubMed]
39. Lansinger, B.; Larsson, E.; Persson, L.C.; Carlsson, J.Y. Qigong and exercise therapy in patients with long-term neck pain: A prospective randomized trial. *Spine* **2007**, *32*, 2415–2422. [CrossRef]
40. Vatansever, F.; Hamblin, M.R. Far infrared radiation (FIR): Its biological effects and medical applications. *Photonics Lasers Med.* **2012**, *4*, 255–266. [CrossRef]
41. Lentell, G.; Hetherington, T.; Eagan, J.; Morgan, M. The use of thermal agents to influence the effectiveness of a low-load prolonged stretch. *J. Orthop. Sports Phys. Ther.* **1992**, *16*, 200–207. [CrossRef]
42. Hohmann, C.; Lauche, R.; Choi, K.E.; Saha, F.; Rampp, T.; Dobos, G.; Musial, F. Quantitative sensory testing in patients with chronic neck pain before and after the application of the acupressure pad—A randomized, controlled pilot study. *Eur. J. Integr. Med.* **2009**, *1*, 212–213. [CrossRef]

43. Sterling, M. Testing for sensory hypersensitivity or central hyperexcitability associated with cervical spine pain. *J. Manip. Physiol. Ther.* **2008**, *31*, 534–539. [CrossRef]
44. Nijs, J.; Lluch Girbés, E.; Lundberg, M.; Malfliet, A.; Sterling, M. Exercise therapy for chronic musculoskeletal pain: Innovation by altering pain memories. *Man. Ther.* **2015**, *20*, 216–220. [CrossRef] [PubMed]
45. Yip, C.H.; Chiu, T.T.; Poon, A.T. The relationship between head posture and severity and disability of patients with neck pain. *Man. Ther.* **2008**, *13*, 148–154. [CrossRef] [PubMed]
46. Fernández-de-Las-Peñas, C.; Cuadrado, M.L.; Pareja, J.A. Myofascial trigger points, neck mobility and forward head posture in unilateral migraine. *Cephalalgia* **2006**, *26*, 1061–1070. [CrossRef] [PubMed]
47. Ijmker, S.; Huysmans, M.A.; Blatter, B.M.; van der Beek, A.J.; van Mechelen, W.; Bongers, P.M. Should office workers spend fewer hours at their computer? A systematic review of the literature. *Occup. Environ. Med.* **2007**, *64*, 211–222. [CrossRef] [PubMed]
48. Wahlström, J. Ergonomics, musculoskeletal disorders and computer work. *Occup. Med.* **2005**, *55*, 168–176. [CrossRef]

14

Associations of Lifestyle Behaviour and Healthy Ageing in Five Latin American and the Caribbean Countries—A 10/66 Population-Based Cohort Study

Christina Daskalopoulou [1,*], Artemis Koukounari [2], José Luis Ayuso-Mateos [3,4,5], Martin Prince [1] and A. Matthew Prina [1]

1 Department of Health Service and Population Research, Institute of Psychiatry, Psychology and Neuroscience, King's College London, London SE5 8AF, UK; martin.prince@kcl.ac.uk (M.P.); matthew.prina@kcl.ac.uk (A.M.P.)

2 Department of Infectious Disease Epidemiology, London School of Hygiene & Tropical Medicine, Faculty of Epidemiology and Population Health, London WC1E 7HT, UK; Artemis.Koukounari@lshtm.ac.uk

3 Department of Psychiatry, Universidad Autónoma de Madrid, 28029 Madrid, Spain; joseluis.ayuso@uam.es

4 Instituto de Salud Carlos III, Centro de Investigación Biomedica en Red de Salud Mental (CIBERSAM), 28029 Madrid, Spain

5 Department of Psychiatry, Hospital Universitario de La Princesa, Instituto de Investigación Sanitaria Princesa (IIS-Princesa), 28006 Madrid, Spain

* Correspondence: christina.daskalopoulou@kcl.ac.uk

Abstract: Latin American and the Caribbean countries exhibit high life expectancy and projections show that they will experience the fastest growth of older people in the following years. As people live longer, it is important to maximise the opportunity to age healthily. We aimed to examine the associations of lifestyle behaviours with healthy ageing in Cuba, Dominican Republic, Peru, Mexico and Puerto Rico, part of the 10/66 study. Residents 65 years old and over (n = 10,900) were interviewed between 2003 and 2010. In the baseline survey, we measured four healthy behaviours: Physical activity, non-smoking, moderate drinking and fruits or vegetables consumption. Healthy ageing was conceptualised within the functional ability framework over a median of 4 years follow-up. Logistic models were calculated per country and then pooled together with fixed-effects meta-analysis. People engaging in physical activity and consuming fruits or vegetables had increased odds of healthy ageing in the follow-up (OR: 2.59, 95% CI: 2.20–3.03; OR: 1.24, 95% CI: 1.06–1.44, respectively). Compared with participants engaging in none or one healthy behaviour, the ORs of participants engaging in two, three or four healthy behaviours increased in a linear way (OR: 1.60, 95% CI: 1.40–1.84; OR: 2.29, 95% CI: 1.94–2.69; OR: 2.46, 95% CI: 1.54–3.92, respectively). Our findings highlight the importance of awareness of a healthy lifestyle behaviour among older people.

Keywords: older adults; healthy ageing; nutrition; physical activity; lifestyle behaviour

1. Introduction

The world population is ageing and by 2050 there will be more older than younger people [1]. Even though population ageing is a human achievement, there are still many health policy challenges to be addressed [2]. Increases in life expectancy have not been followed by relevant increases in disease-free years, meaning that people are living longer but are spending more years with illness and disability [3]. Living longer but in ill health could result in severe demand of public and health care resources [4]. As people experience ageing with great heterogeneity in their health pathways [5], it is crucial to identify those behaviours that are associated with a slower and healthier ageing process.

Until recently, healthy ageing research has been complicated by a lack of common definition and measurement of it [6,7]. However, the latest report on health and ageing from the World Health Organization (WHO) provided a common framework to conceptualise healthy ageing; the functional ability framework. Healthy ageing is now defined as the process of developing and maintaining the functional ability that enables well-being in older age [8]. Healthy lifestyle behaviours (for instance, never smoking, moderate alcohol consumption, physical activity and daily consumption of fruits and vegetables) have been consistently associated with better health outcomes in older people: successful ageing [9], increases in life-years spent in good health [10], a reduced risk of mortality [11,12], and of poor cognitive function [13]. Recent systematic reviews also indicated the beneficial effects of physical activity, non-smoking and of a healthy diet to healthy ageing [2,14,15].

The latter reviews also revealed the lack of evidence in low-and-middle income countries (LMICs) even though it is estimated that by 2050, 80% of the global population that is 60 years old and over will reside there [16]. Among those countries, Latin American and the Caribbean (LAC) are the ones that have been witnessing an increased life expectancy from 1990 to 2016 [17] and projections show that in the next 15 years they are to experience the fastest increase in the number of older people [1]. Dietary risk, physical inactivity, alcohol use and smoking are among the top leading factors of disability-adjusted life years (DALYs) in the area [18].

In this study, we aimed to examine the impact of four healthy lifestyle behaviours (i.e., physical activity, non-smoking, moderate alcohol consumption and consumption of fruits and vegetables), individually and in combination, on healthy ageing and survival in a cohort of people aged 65 years old and over living in five LAC countries after a follow-up period of 4 years.

2. Materials and Methods

2.1. Study Population

The 10/66 Dementia Research Group (10/66 DRG) population-based studies of ageing and dementia have been conducted in geographically defined catchment areas in LMICs (Cuba, Dominican Republic, Peru, Venezuela, Mexico, China, India and Puerto Rico) with a sample size between 1000 and 3000 (generally 2000). In this study, we used data from the baseline survey (2003–2008), including people 65 years old and over, and the follow-up assessments 3 to 5 years later (2008–2010) from Cuba (n = 3000), Dominican Republic, Peru, Mexico and Puerto Rico (n = 2000). Detailed description of the study settings is available elsewhere [19,20]. Access to the dataset can be obtained via the official website www.alz.co.uk/1066. Local ethical committees and the ethical committee of the Institute of Psychiatry of King's College London approved the studies: Cuba-Finlay Albarran Medical Faculty of Havana Medical University Ethical Committee (January 2003, September 2006); Dominican Republic-Consejo Nacional de Bioética y Salud (CONABIOS); Mexico-Instituto Nacional de Neurología y Neurocirugía Ethics Committee (Ref: 96/07; 78/07); Peru-El Instituto de la Memoria, Depresión y Enfermedades de Riesgo (IMEDER) Ethics Committee (August 2004, May 2007); Puerto Rico-Oficina para la Protección de Participantes Humanos en Investigación (OPPHI) (Ref: FWA00005561); King's College London-Institute of Psychiatry/SLAM NHS Trust Ethical Committee Research (ECR) (2004, Ref: 076/03), King's College Research Ethics Committee (KREC) (February 2007, Ref: CREC/06/07/38).

2.2. Baseline Measures

Lifestyle behaviours were assessed based on participants' responses to specific questionnaires. Physical activity was categorised as: "very physically active", "fairly", "not very", and "not at all". Smoking status was categorised as "current", "former" and "never smoker". Alcohol consumption was assessed by asking the units of alcohol drunk per week and then categorised as "no alcohol consumption", "moderate alcohol consumption" (1–14 units per week for women; 1–21 units per week for men) and "heavy alcohol consumption" ($\geq$15 units per week for women and $\geq$21 units per week for men) [21]. We assessed dietary habits by asking the number of fruit and vegetable servings in the last 3 days. In our analyses, we compared physically active participants ("very physically active" or "fairly") with non-physically active ("not very" or "not at all"); non-smokers with ever-smokers ("current" or "former"); moderate drinkers with abstainers (no alcohol consumption) or heavy drinkers; participants with "daily consumption" of fruits and vegetables (3 or more servings the last 3 days) with "non-daily consumption" (0–2 servings the last 3 days). We also adjusted our results for socioeconomic factors: age, sex and level of education (none, some, did not complete primary, completed primary, completed secondary, tertiary).

2.3. Outcome Assessment

In accordance with the WHO definition of healthy ageing, we conceptualised healthy ageing within the functional ability framework [8]. We created a healthy ageing index by employing information from 26 health related question-indicators which were either self-reported or were provided by key informants. Items included information on daily disabilities and difficulties, on pain and sleep problems and on cognition abilities among others (Supplementary File S1).

To create a measurement model for healthy ageing, we employed the framework of Exploratory Factor Analysis (EFA) and Confirmatory Factor Analysis (CFA) [22]. We initially identified the number of factors needed to reproduce the latent (unobserved) construct of healthy ageing (EFA) and then we used a bifactor model to represent a single general construct of it (CFA) [23]. To establish model fit, we examined the comparative fit index (CFI) and root mean square error of approximation (RMSEA) with 90% confidence intervals (CI). We considered a model to have an acceptable fit when CFI ≥ 0.90 and RMSEA values were close or less than 0.06 [24]. We also calculated omega hierarchical (ω_H) reliability coefficient of the bifactor structure; a high $\omega_H > 0.80$ indicates that the general factor is the dominant source of systematic variance [25]. Finally, we calculated healthy ageing (factor) scores by using the regression method [26].

We transformed scores in a scale of 0–100 with higher values indicating better health. We examined 3 categories for the outcome of interest: healthy ageing, normal ageing and death at follow-up. To create these categories, we calculated the quintiles of the baseline healthy ageing score distribution and participants belonging in the three lowest fifths (i.e., 0–67.92 scores) were characterised as "normal agers", whereas participants belonging in the two highest fifths (i.e., 67.93–100 scores) were characterised as "healthy agers".

We performed two separate logistic regression analyses: one to estimate the odds ratios (ORs) of healthy ageing (with normal ageing and death as the non-event) and another one to estimate the ORs for survival (in which death was the non-event). We did all analyses per country and we then provided a pooled result by performing fixed-effects meta-analysis. We also computed Higgin's I^2 to estimate the proportion of variability across countries that accounted mostly for heterogeneity rather than sampling error [27]. Heterogeneity up to 40% is conventionally considered negligible, whereas heterogeneity more than 50% is considered moderate to substantial [28].

We also performed sensitivity analyses to assess the robustness of our findings. Firstly, we examined whether the associations of lifestyle behaviours with healthy ageing were influenced by deaths. To do this, we excluded deaths from our sample. Secondly, we performed our analyses by including the non-dichotomised lifestyle variables. Finally, we investigated whether our findings were influenced by the way we categorised participants as healthy or normal agers and if there were differences between men and women. Our analyses were performed in STATA 14.1 and Mplus 7.4 [26].

3. Results

The EFA indicated a latent structure of four factors and the bifactor model ($\chi^2 = 4039.14$, df = 273, p-value < 0.001) exhibited good fit (CFI: 0.985; RMSEA: 0.040, 90%CI: 0.039–0.041). The psychometrically informative bifactor-derived statistics indicated that a strong percentage of the total score variance can be attributed to the general factor ($\omega_H = 0.85$). Hence, we proceeded by considering the score of the general factor only. More information about the EFA and CFA is provided in Supplementary File S2.

In our study there were 10,900 participants in the baseline assessment. In the follow-up survey 1648 were healthy agers, 5594 normal agers, 1734 died and 1924 were either untraceable or refused to be re-interviewed. We performed analyses per country and we checked if participants included in our analyses differ from those not available in the follow-up wave (*t*-test for continuous variables, χ^2 test for categorical). We found that participants included in our analyses in general did not differ with those excluded (Supplementary File S3). There were some statistically significant (i.e., *p*-value < 0.05) differences in Cuba and Peru regarding the dietary habits between those included in the follow-up wave and those excluded. A higher percentage of participants available in the follow-up wave endorsed daily consumption of fruits and vegetables compared to those not available (i.e., 75.4% versus 66.3% in Cuba; 82.5% versus 76.2% in Peru).

Table 1 presents the characteristics of participants characterised as healthy agers and those characterised as normal agers in the follow-up. Participants in the healthy ageing group, compared with the normal ageing group, were younger at baseline, had completed at least primary level education, were mostly physically active and endorsed daily consumption of fruits and vegetables.

The associations of each lifestyle behaviour with healthy ageing and survival at the end of the follow-up period are presented in Table 2. Compared with non-physically active participants, those who were physically active at baseline had 2.59 (95% CI: 2.20–3.03) times greater odds of being healthy agers and 2.23 (95% CI: 1.98–2.52) times greater odds of survival. Compared with people consuming two or less servings of fruits and vegetables in the last three days, people consuming three or more were more likely to experience healthy ageing (OR: 1.24, 95% CI: 1.06–1.44) and to survive at the end of the follow-up (OR: 1.13, 95% CI: 0.99–1.28). Non-smoking, compared to former or current smoking, was not associated with healthy ageing (OR: 0.95, 95% CI: 0.82–1.10) but it was positively associated with survival as never smokers had 1.17 (95% CI: 1.02–1.34) times greater odds of remaining alive in the follow-up assessment. Moderate drinking, compared to high or never drinking, was not associated with healthy ageing (OR: 1.04, 95% CI: 0.82–1.30) or survival (OR: 1.11, 95% CI: 0.90–1.37). Heterogeneity was not statistically significant in most cases (*p*-value < 0.05) indicating that the variation among countries was limited. The only significant heterogeneity was observed in the associations of physical activity with healthy ageing (I^2: 61.3%; *p*-value: 0.035). Further investigation concluded that Puerto Rico was the country exhibiting the highest point estimate (i.e., OR: 6.30; 95% CI: 3.43–11.56). We also reproduced the pooled estimates by excluding this country and the new pooled estimates did not change the direction or strength of associations between physical activity and healthy ageing (i.e., OR: 2.42; 95% CI: 2.05–2.86; I^2: 0.0%, *p*-value: 0.693).

Participants who engaged in two-four healthy lifestyle behaviours at baseline, compared with those who engaged in none or one, exhibited increased odds of healthy ageing (OR: 1.72, 95% CI: 1.45–2.05) (Figure 1a). Additionally, the association between number of healthy behaviours and odds of healthy ageing was positive linear. More specifically, compared with participants engaging in none or one healthy behaviour, those engaging in two had 1.46 times (95% CI: 1.22–1.76) the odds of healthy ageing, those engaging in three had 2.00 times (95% CI: 1.65–2.42) the odds and those in four had 2.46 times (95% CI: 1.54–3.92) the odds. A similar beneficial association was also observed in surviving (Figure 1b). Participants engaging in two or more healthy behaviours had 1.83 times (95% CI: 1.61–2.08) the odds of surviving compared with participants that engaged in none or one healthy behaviour. A positive linear relationship was also observed; two healthy behaviours OR: 1.60, 95% CI: 1.40–1.84; three healthy behaviours OR: 2.29, 95% CI: 1.94–2.69; four healthy behaviours OR: 2.64, 95% CI: 1.53–4.54 (Table 3). Heterogeneity was not statistically significant (*p*-value < 0.05) indicating that the variability among countries was limited.

Table 1. Baseline characteristics of participants in the healthy and normal ageing group * in the follow-up wave.

Country	Cuba		Dominican Republic		Mexico		Peru		Puerto Rico	
Characteristic	Healthy Ageing (n = 494)	Normal Ageing (n = 1513)	Healthy Ageing (n = 234)	Normal Ageing (n = 963)	Healthy Ageing (n = 153)	Normal Ageing (n = 1309)	Healthy Ageing (n = 579)	Normal Ageing (n = 732)	Healthy Ageing (n = 188)	Normal Ageing (n = 1077)
Age (mean, SD)	70.9 ± 4.61	74.87 ± 6.65 †	70.89 ± 5.17	74.7 ± 6.97 †	69.9 ± 4.00	74.2 ± 6.35 †	71.1 ± 5.20	76.7 ± 7.21 †	72.0 ± 4.56	75.7 ± 6.65 †
Gender-Female	291 (58.9%)	1041 (68.8%) †	140 (60.1%)	689 (71.6%) †	99 (64.7%)	845 (64.6%)	343 (59.2%)	474 (64.8%) †	141 (75.0%)	728 (67.8%)
Education Level-above primary	440 (89.4%)	1099 (72.7%) †	101 (43.2%)	259 (27.1%) †	87 (57.2%)	355 (27.1%) †	493 (86.2%)	559 (77.0%) †	164 (87.2%)	846 (78.9%) †
Never smoking	244 (49.6%)	589 (56.9%) †	124 (53.0%)	523 (54.4%)	91 (59.5%)	913 (69.7%) †	471 (81.8%)	625 (85.9%) †	150 (79.8%)	789 (73.5%)
Moderate alcohol consumption	53 (10.9%)	140 (9.4%)	19 (8.3%)	52 (5.4%)	30 (19.7%)	225 (17.3%)	21 (3.7%)	30 (4.2%)	21 (11.2%)	92 (8.6%)
Physical activity (very or fairly)	425 (86.6%)	1047 (69.4%) †	188 (80.7%)	626 (65.3%) †	133 (86.9%)	841 (64.6%) †	471 (81.6%)	462 (63.6%) †	176 (93.6%)	722 (67.3%) †
Fruits/vegetable consumption (≥3 servings in the last 3 days)	409 (83.1%)	1130 (74.8%) †	138 (59.0%)	460 (48.7%) †	116 (76.3%)	931 (71.5%)	477 (83.1%)	593 (82.4%)	156 (83.0%)	807 (75.3%) †

Notes: SD: standard deviation; †: *p*-value of the *t* test or the $\chi^2 < 0.05$. * healthy ageing group includes those participants who in the follow-up assessment were in the two highest fifths of the healthy ageing score distribution (i.e., better health level) and normal ageing group those who were in the three lowest fifths; percentages in the parentheses are calculated in the non-missing cases in the covariates.

Table 2. Associations between lifestyle behaviours, healthy ageing and survival.

Country/Lifestyle Behaviour	Physical Activity (Very or Fairly vs. Not Very or Never)	Smoking (Never vs. Former or Current)	Drinking Behaviour (Moderate Drinking vs. Never or Heavy Drinking)	Fruits/Vegetables Consumption (≥3 Servings in the Last Three Days vs. <3)
			Healthy Ageing * Adjusted OR † (95% CI)	
Cuba	2.56 (1.93–3.41)	0.97 (0.77–1.24)	0.83 (0.57–1.20)	1.41 (1.06–1.87)
Dominican Republic	2.11 (1.46–3.04)	1.03 (0.75–1.40)	1.21 (0.68–2.17)	1.35 (0.99–1.83)
Mexico	2.98 (1.81–4.93)	0.58 (0.37–0.90)	1.09 (0.66–1.81)	1.11 (0.73–1.68)
Peru	2.32 (1.75–3.08)	0.90 (0.62–1.30)	0.70 (0.34–1.44)	0.92 (0.66–1.29)
Puerto Rico	6.30 (3.43–11.56)	1.30 (0.85–1.97)	1.80 (1.02–3.17)	1.44 (0.94–2.21)
Pooled Effect	2.59 (2.20–3.03)	0.95 (0.82–1.10)	1.04 (0.82–1.30)	1.24 (1.06–1.44)
I^2; *p*-value	61.3%; 0.035	44.7%; 0.124	38.0%; 0.168	16.6%; 0.309
			Survival * Adjusted OR † (95% CI)	
Cuba	2.29 (1.86–2.82)	1.16 (0.92–1.45)	1.04 (0.74–1.46)	1.15 (0.92–1.44)
Dominican Republic	1.82 (1.43–2.30)	1.18 (0.93–1.50)	1.36 (0.78–2.37)	0.94 (0.75–1.19)
Mexico	2.08 (1.50–2.86)	0.94 (0.61–1.44)	1.16 (0.74–1.80)	1.17 (0.84–1.64)
Peru	2.75 (1.90–3.63)	1.20 (0.70–2.04)	0.72 (0.33–1.60)	1.06 (0.66–1.73)
Puerto Rico	2.71 (2.02–3.63)	1.34 (0.95–1.89)	1.24 (0.73–2.09)	1.45 (1.08–1.96)
Pooled Effect	2.23 (1.98–2.52)	1.17 (1.02–1.34)	1.11 (0.90–1.37)	1.13 (0.99–1.28)
I^2; *p*-value	34.4%; 0.192	0.0%; 0.807	0.0%; 0.737	21.9%; 0.275

Notes: CI: confidence interval; OR: Odds ratio; I^2: heterogeneity. *: healthy ageing compared to normal ageing or death; survival (healthy or normal ageing) compared to death; number of participants per country: Cuba: 2557, Dominican Republic: 1608, Mexico: 1633, Peru: 1392, Puerto Rico: 1554. †: models are adjusted for age, gender, education level and all other lifestyle behaviour variables.

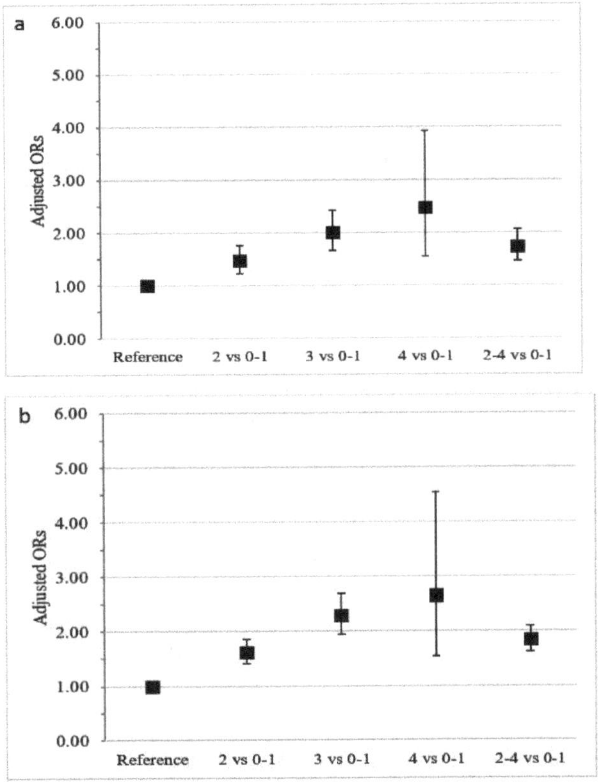

Figure 1. Associations of (**a**) healthy ageing and (**b**) survival with the number of healthy behaviours. Notes: ORs: Odds Ratios (pooled effects of the fixed-effects meta-analysis); models are adjusted for sex, age and education level and for all behaviours at baseline. Associations are given per individual number of healthy behaviours (two, three, four) and for two-four compared to no or one healthy behaviour (reference category). Error bars indicate 95% confidence intervals.

Further sensitivity analysis showed that when we excluded deaths from our sample, the associations of lifestyle behaviour with healthy ageing did not substantially change (i.e., fairly or very physically active OR: 2.28, 95% CI: 1.93–2.69; never smoking OR: 0.95, 95% CI: 0.81–1.10; moderate drinking OR: 1.05, 95% CI:0.83–1.32; daily consumption of fruits and vegetables OR: 1.22, 95% CI: 1.04–1.42). In addition, supplementary analysis showed that the higher the level of physical activity the more increased the ORs of healthy ageing compared to normal ageing or death (very physically active OR: 9.64, 95% CI: 5.62–16.55; fairly OR: 8.20, 95% CI: 4.77–14.12; not very OR: 4.20, 95% CI: 2.42–7.31; not at all: reference category). The same trend was also observed for the vegetable and fruits consumption (more than six servings OR: 1.51, 95% CI: 1.23–1.85; three to six servings OR: 1.16, 95% CI: 0.99–1.36; less than two servings: reference category). Smoking and alcohol consumption had no significant associations.

To examine whether our findings differed between men and women, we also performed our analyses separately for these two subpopulations. The observed relationships between lifestyle behaviours and healthy ageing compared to normal ageing or death did not change (Supplementary File S4). In addition, to examine whether our conclusions were influenced by the categorisation of participants as healthy agers based on the two highest quintiles of the healthy ageing score, we also performed our analyses by using a different categorisation. We performed our analyses by considering participants scoring in the three highest quintiles of the healthy ageing score distribution as healthy agers (i.e., 59.70–100 scores) and compared them against normal agers (i.e., 0–59.69 scores) or dead participants. Our conclusions regarding the protective effect of physical activity and daily consumption of fruits and vegetables did not alter (Supplementary File S5).

Table 3. Associations between number of healthy behaviours, healthy ageing and survival.

Country	Healthy Ageing * Adjusted OR † (95% CI) Number of Healthy Behaviours Compared to Zero or One			
	Two	Three	Four	Two-Four
Cuba	1.67 (1.23–2.29)	2.12 (1.54–2.92)	1.74 (0.77–3.96)	1.86 (1.39–2.49)
Dominican Republic	1.64 (1.16–2.32)	1.98 (1.32–2.96)	2.48 (0.78–7.86)	1.77 (1.28–2.43)
Mexico	1.29 (0.74–2.24)	1.31 (0.74–2.33)	2.75 (1.04–7.26)	1.35 (0.80–2.29)
Peru	0.98 (0.64–1.51)	1.64 (1.08–2.49)	1.14 (0.21–6.22)	1.31 (0.88–1.96)
Puerto Rico	1.63 (0.84–3.17)	4.21 (2.25–7.87)	4.93 (1.77–13.71)	2.92 (1.60–5.36)
Pooled Effect	1.46 (1.22–1.76)	2.00 (1.65–2.42)	2.46 (1.54–3.92)	1.72 (1.45–2.05)
I^2; *p*-value	16.0%; 0.313	53.0%; 0.074	0.0%; 0.509	31.5%; 0.211
	Survival * Adjusted OR † (95% CI)			
Cuba	1.57 (1.24–2.00)	2.17 (1.66–2.85)	3.53 (1.21–10.28)	1.80 (1.44–2.24)
Dominican Republic	1.45 (1.13–1.88)	1.71 (1.22–2.40)	1.80 (0.48–6.72)	1.53 (1.21–1.93)
Mexico	1.79 (1.24–2.60)	2.19 (1.42–3.36)	2.13 (0.79–5.68)	1.94 (1.37–2.75)
Peru	1.52 (0.90–2.55)	2.91 (1.66–5.12)	1.80 (0.26–12.22)	2.02 (1.22–3.34)
Puerto Rico	1.84 (1.33–2.54)	3.44 (2.34–5.05)	4.11 (1.18–14.28)	2.35 (1.73–3.18)
Pooled Effect	1.60 (1.40–1.84)	2.29 (1.94–2.69)	2.64 (1.53–4.54)	1.83 (1.61–2.08)
I^2; *p*-value	0.0%; 0.790	50.3%; 0.090	0.0%; 0.840	22.0%; 0.274

Notes: CI: confidence interval; OR: Odds ratio; I^2: heterogeneity. *: healthy ageing compared to normal ageing or death; survival (healthy or normal ageing) compared to death; number of participants per country: Cuba: 2557, Dominican Republic: 1608, Mexico: 1633, Peru: 1392, Puerto Rico: 1554. †: models are adjusted for age, gender, education level and all other lifestyle behaviour variables.

4. Discussion

In this study, we investigated the associations of four healthy lifestyle behaviours with healthy ageing and survival from a large dataset (n = 10,900) of five LAC countries (Dominican Republic, Cuba, Peru, Puerto Rico and Mexico). Participants engaging in physical activity and in a diet with daily consumption of fruits and vegetables were individually associated with increased odds of healthy ageing and survival. In addition, we found that the more physically active the participants and the higher the number of fruits and vegetables servings, the higher the odds of ageing healthily. Never smoking and moderate alcohol consumption were not individually associated with healthy ageing but all these four behaviours in combination had a positive effect both for healthy ageing and survival.

The world's older population is increasing at a higher pace than the total population, and the region of LAC exhibits the highest growth rate of the 60-and-older population from 2015 to 2020 [29]. Although research on healthy ageing has been growing, there is still limited research available for LAC [2]. Our study is among the first reporting a beneficial association of lifestyle habits with healthy ageing or survival in a LAC dataset. These findings are in accordance with those from other studies, which examined lifestyle behaviours and adverse health outcomes in older age, in datasets from high-and-middle income countries [9,14,30]. Physical activity seems to be related with an increased healthy life expectancy by preventing many chronic diseases (i.e., arterial hypertension, diabetes mellitus type 2, store, cancer) [31], and/or age-related diseases (i.e., dementia and Alzheimer's disease) [32]. The complex biophysiological pathway between physical activity and healthy ageing and survival is yet to be solved. However, this could be partly explained by the favourable biomarker profile of physically active people; higher cell endurance, muscle tissue functionality and energy metabolism [33], reduced fat mass and adipose tissue inflammation [34]. Other studies have also reported a beneficial association of fruits and vegetables consumption with healthy ageing [35,36]. Research has shown that adherence to Mediterranean diet, which includes high consumption of fruits and vegetables, is associated with decreased risk of all-cause mortality, better health outcomes in older people and a reduced risk of frailty [37]. The high antioxidant capacity of fruits and vegetables along with their high fibre and vitamins content could possibly explain this beneficial association [38]. In addition, fruits and vegetables are sources of phytochemicals—the bioactive non-nutrient plant compound—which could contribute to the prevention or minimization of oxidative stress caused by free radicals and thus decrease the risk of chronic diseases [39]. For instance, carotenoids, polyphenols, saponins and phytoestrogens are among those phytochemicals which have shown anticarcinogenic, antioxidative and immunomodulatory effects among others [40].

In regards to moderate alcohol consumption and never smoking, our study did not indicate an individual significant association with healthy ageing. A recent meta-analysis has shown that moderate alcohol consumption seems to be positively associated with healthy ageing but in general associations are mixed [15]. The latest report on the alcohol burden of disease also did not replicate the finding that moderate consumption of alcohol is beneficial; a zero level of alcohol consumption constitutes the level that minimises health loss in the total population [41]. Nevertheless, other studies have found a protective effect of light-to-moderate alcohol consumption against functional health decline among middle-aged people [42]. However these findings should be interpreted with caution, as the beneficial effects of the low to moderate drinking groups (compared with non-drinkers) could be biased by the poor health of former drinkers that are also included in the non-drinkers group in many studies [43,44]. The non-significant result of smoking could be attributed to the limited period of follow-up time (i.e., 4 years) or the relatively older cohort. Studies, which include an older sample, are biased towards those smoking and surviving compared to those that have never smoked and died (survival bias) [45]. Previous meta-analysis also confirms that the negative effects of smoking are more pronounced in younger cohorts [15]. When considering all behaviours in combination, we found that the higher the number of healthy lifestyle behaviours that a participant engaged in during the baseline, the more increased the likelihood of healthy ageing and survival in the follow-up. This comes in agreement with previous research within a high-income setting [9].

A prolonged life longevity is accompanied by multimorbidity [46] which as a consequence poses an extra burden in health systems. As LAC area already exhibits high life expectancy and is the one with the fastest estimated ageing growth, major concerns are raised about the need for early non-pharmacological measures and interventions in older adults to promote healthy ageing. Our findings reflect the importance of healthy lifestyle behaviours and point out the public health actions that must be preserved and prioritised. Adoption of healthy behavioural habits could contribute to the improvement of well-being of the older populations in LACs. Nevertheless, other socioeconomic factors should also be considered when healthy ageing interventions are suggested. For instance, a study with data from 32 countries indicated that overall economic development of the region, public health expenditure and sanitation facilities considerably relate to healthy ageing [47].

Strengths and Limitations

Based on our knowledge, this is the first study, including a large sample, which examined healthy ageing within the functional ability framework and lifestyle behaviour in LAC countries. Our results contribute to the advance of healthy ageing knowledge in under-examined areas and especially in LMICs as current research has mostly focused on other countries [2]. The limited attrition between baseline assessment and follow-up together with our further analyses, which indicated that in most of the cases participants included in the study did not differ with those excluded, limit any potential information bias. In addition, the observed heterogeneity (I^2) was minimal in most cases, reflecting the limited variability in point estimates among countries.

In our study, we created a healthy ageing index within the functional ability framework, as it is the latest recommendation from the WHO [8]. Previous research has mostly focused on the presence or not of some disease/illness as a recent review indicated [7]. Yet, the functioning framework is considered more useful for effective public-health responses than considering specific diseases [8]. For this reason, we created this healthy ageing index by not taking into account specific conditions (i.e., depression, cardiovascular diseases, etc.). Furthermore, we did not consider other domains of healthy ageing (i.e., psychological well-being and social well-being) [48] since the healthy ageing model provided by WHO also incorporates "resilience" as an ability to maintain or improve the level of functioning during challenging periods. This suggests that older people could use psychological/physiological resources and environmental characteristics (i.e., social relationships) to maintain or improve their functional ability. However, these domains were not included in our index, as our ultimate intention was to build an index focusing on the final observed outcome -functional ability-.

Our findings should be interpreted within the context of this study limitations. Lifestyle behaviours were all assessed via self-reported questionnaires. Therefore, potential measurement error could have occurred. Furthermore, questions were too broad not allowing to holistically assess the impact of different frequencies and intensities in physical activity, or of specific fruits and vegetables that were consumed. In addition, even though interviewers underwent substantial training to ensure consistency in the way surveys were conducted in the various settings, we cannot exclude the bias of cross-cultural differences among countries in the conceptualisation of some questions. Another limitation of our study could be the quite arbitrary way of categorising participants who are in the two highest fifths of the baseline healthy ageing score distribution as healthy agers and all others as normal agers. Nevertheless, supplementary analyses (Supplementary File S5) indicated that our conclusions were not influenced by a different categorisation of participants in the health and normal ageing groups. In addition, we characterised healthy behaviour when participants were "very" or "fairly" physically active and when they consumed fruits and vegetables on a daily basis. These categorisations constitute assumptions of our study and consequently our findings should be interpreted within the limitations caused by these. The limited follow-up time inherited with these data also made it impossible to examine the impact of lifestyle behaviours in a more prolonged time. Finally, our sample included participants 65 years old and over. Hence, we were unable to assess lifestyle behaviour and examine healthy ageing within a life course perspective approach [49].

5. Conclusions

Physical activity and a diet rich in fruits and vegetables seem to be associated with healthy ageing and survival. Even though never smoking and moderate alcohol consumption were not significantly associated, once we combine all four healthy behaviours their effect is substantial. Furthermore, the more the healthy lifestyle behaviours adopted, the higher the odds of being old and maintaining well-being. Our results could help in the establishment of policies promoting a healthy lifestyle in LAC countries. Future studies evaluating physical activity, nutritional and other lifestyle interventions within the LAC area are needed to attain a better ageing process for these populations.

Author Contributions: C.D. made the study conception and design, analysed the data and wrote the paper; A.K. supervised the data analyses and contributed to paper writing; J.L.A.-M. contributed to paper writing; M.P. provided insight in the 10/66 cohort and contributed to paper writing; A.M.P. provided insight in the 10/66 cohort, supervised the data analyses, contributed to data interpretation and to paper writing.

Acknowledgments: The authors would like to thank the ATHLOS (Ageing Trajectories of Health: Longitudinal Opportunities and Synergies) project, funded by the European Union's Horizon 2020 Research and Innovation Programme under grant agreement number 635316.

References

1. United Nations. *World Population Ageing 2015*; United Nations, Department of Economic and Social Affairs, Population Division: New York, NY, USA, 2015.
2. Kralj, C.; Daskalopoulou, C.; Rodríguez-Artalejo, F.; García-Esquinas, E.; Cosco, T.D.; Prince, M.; Prina, A.M. *Healthy Ageing: A Systematic Review of Risk Factors*; ATHLOS Consortium: London, UK, 2018.
3. GBD 2013 DALYs and HALE Collaborators; Murray, C.J.; Barber, R.M.; Foreman, K.J.; Abbasoglu Ozgoren, A.; Abd-Allah, F.; Abera, S.F.; Aboyans, V.; Abraham, J.P.; Abubakar, I. Global, regional, and national disability-adjusted life years (DALYs) for 306 diseases and injuries and healthy life expectancy (HALE) for 188 countries, 1990–2013: Quantifying the epidemiological transition. *Lancet* **2015**, *386*, 2145–2191. [CrossRef]

4. Prina, A.M. Ageing, resilience and depression: Adding life to years as well as years to life. *Epidemiol. Psychiatr. Sci.* **2017**, *26*, 571–573. [CrossRef] [PubMed]
5. Lowsky, D.J.; Olshansky, S.J.; Bhattacharya, J.; Goldman, D.P. Heterogeneity in Healthy Aging. *J. Gerontol. Ser. A Boil. Sci. Med. Sci.* **2014**, *69*, 640–649. [CrossRef] [PubMed]
6. Depp, C.A.; Jeste, D.V. Definitions and predictors of successful aging: A comprehensive review of larger quantitative studies. *Am. J. Geriatr. Psychiatry Off. J. Am. Assoc. Geriatr. Psychiatry* **2006**, *14*, 6–20. [CrossRef] [PubMed]
7. Cosco, T.D.; Prina, A.M.; Perales, J.; Stephan, B.C.; Brayne, C. Operational definitions of successful aging: A systematic review. *Int. Psychogeriatr.* **2014**, *26*, 373–381. [CrossRef] [PubMed]
8. World Health Organization. *World Report on Ageing and Health*; World Health Organization: Geneva, Switzerland, 2015.
9. Sabia, S.; Singh-Manoux, A.; Hagger-Johnson, G.; Cambois, E.; Brunner, E.J.; Kivimaki, M. Influence of individual and combined healthy behaviours on successful aging. *CMAJ* **2012**, *184*, 1985–1992. [CrossRef] [PubMed]
10. Stenholm, S.; Head, J.; Kivimaki, M.; Kawachi, I.; Aalto, V.; Zins, M.; Goldberg, M.; Zaninotto, P.; Magnuson Hanson, L.; Westerlund, H.; et al. Smoking, physical inactivity and obesity as predictors of healthy and disease-free life expectancy between ages 50 and 75: A multicohort study. *Int. J. Epidemiol.* **2016**, *45*, 1260–1270. [CrossRef] [PubMed]
11. Knoops, K.T.; de Groot, L.C.; Kromhout, D.; Perrin, A.E.; Moreiras-Varela, O.; Menotti, A.; van Staveren, W.A. Mediterranean diet, lifestyle factors, and 10-year mortality in elderly European men and women: The HALE project. *JAMA* **2004**, *292*, 1433–1439. [CrossRef] [PubMed]
12. Kvaavik, E.; Batty, G.D.; Ursin, G.; Huxley, R.; Gale, C.R. Influence of individual and combined health behaviors on total and cause-specific mortality in men and women: The United Kingdom health and lifestyle survey. *Arch. Intern. Med.* **2010**, *170*, 711–718. [CrossRef] [PubMed]
13. Sabia, S.; Nabi, H.; Kivimaki, M.; Shipley, M.J.; Marmot, M.G.; Singh-Manoux, A. Health behaviors from early to late midlife as predictors of cognitive function: The Whitehall II study. *Am. J. Epidemiol.* **2009**, *170*, 428–437. [CrossRef] [PubMed]
14. Daskalopoulou, C.; Stubbs, B.; Kralj, C.; Koukounari, A.; Prince, M.; Prina, A.M. Physical activity and healthy ageing: A systematic review and meta-analysis of longitudinal cohort studies. *Ageing Res. Rev.* **2017**, *38*, 6–17. [CrossRef] [PubMed]
15. Daskalopoulou, C.; Stubbs, B.; Kralj, C.; Koukounari, A.; Prince, M.; Prina, A.M. Associations of smoking and alcohol consumption with healthy ageing: A systematic review and meta-analysis of longitudinal studies. *BMJ Open* **2018**, *8*, e019540. [CrossRef] [PubMed]
16. World Health Organization. Ageing and Health. 2015. Available online: http://www.who.int/mediacentre/factsheets/fs404/en/ (accessed on 16 March 2018).
17. Institute for Health Metrics and Evaluation. Global Burden of Disease (GBD) Data. 2016. Available online: http://ghdx.healthdata.org/gbd-results-tool (accessed on 30 August 2018).
18. Institute for Health Metrics and Evaluation; Human Development Network; The World Bank. *The Global Burden of Disease: Generating Evidence, Guiding Policy—Latin America and Caribbean Regional Edition*; IHME: Seattle, WA, USA, 2013.
19. Prince, M.; Ferri, C.P.; Acosta, D.; Albanese, E.; Arizaga, R.; Dewey, M.; Gavrilova, S.I.; Guerra, M.; Huang, Y.; Jacob, K.S.; et al. The protocols for the 10/66 dementia research group population-based research programme. *BMC Public Health* **2007**, *7*, 165. [CrossRef] [PubMed]
20. Prina, A.M.; Acosta, D.; Acosta, I.; Guerra, M.; Huang, Y.; Jotheeswaran, A.T.; Jimenez-Velazquez, I.Z.; Liu, Z.; Llibre Rodriguez, J.J.; Salas, A.; et al. Cohort Profile: The 10/66 study. *Int. J. Epidemiol.* **2017**, *46*, 406–406i. [CrossRef] [PubMed]
21. Royal College of Physicians. *Alcohol Guidelines*; Authority of the House of Commons; House of Commons Science and Technology Committee: London, UK, 2011.
22. Brown, T.A. *Confirmatory Factor Analysis for Applied Research*, 2nd ed.; The Guilford Press: New York, NY, USA, 2015.
23. Reise, S.P. Invited Paper: The Rediscovery of Bifactor Measurement Models. *Multivar. Behav. Res.* **2012**, *47*, 667–696. [CrossRef] [PubMed]

24. Hair, J.F.; Black, W.C.; Babin, B.J.; Anderson, R.E. *Multivariate Data Analysis*, 7th ed.; Pearson: New York, NY, USA, 2010.
25. Rodriguez, A.; Reise, S.P.; Haviland, M.G. Evaluating bifactor models: Calculating and interpreting statistical indices. *Psychol. Methods* **2016**, *21*, 137–150. [CrossRef] [PubMed]
26. Muthén, L.K.; Muthén, B.O. *Mplus User's Guide*, 7th ed.; Muthén & Muthén: Los Angeles, CA, USA, 1998–2015.
27. Higgins, J.P.; Thompson, S.G.; Deeks, J.J.; Altman, D.G. Measuring inconsistency in meta-analyses. *BMJ* **2003**, *327*, 557–560. [CrossRef] [PubMed]
28. Deeks, J.J.; Higgins, J.P.T.; Altman, D.G. Analysing data and undertaking meta-analyses. In *Cochrane Handbook for Systematic Reviews of Interventions*; Higgins, J.P.T., Green, S., Eds.; Version 5.1.0; The Cochrane Collaboration, 2011; Available online: www.handbook.cochrane.org (accessed on 22 October 2018).
29. National Academies of Sciences, Engineering, Medicine. Strengthening the Scientific Foundation for Policymaking to Meet the Challenges of Aging in Latin America and the Caribbean: Summary of a Workshop. Committee for the Workshop on Strengthening the Scientific Foundation, Caribbean. In *Committee on Population, Division of Behavioral and Social Sciences and Education*; Kinsella, K., Steering, R., Eds.; The National Academies Press: Washington, DC, USA, 2015.
30. Ford, E.S.; Zhao, G.; Tsai, J.; Li, C. Low-risk lifestyle behaviors and all-cause mortality: Findings from the National Health and Nutrition Examination Survey III Mortality Study. *Am. J. Public Health* **2011**, *101*, 1922–1929. [CrossRef] [PubMed]
31. Reimers, C.D.; Knapp, G.; Reimers, A.K. Does physical activity increase life expectancy? A review of the literature. *J. Aging Res.* **2012**, *2012*, 243958. [CrossRef] [PubMed]
32. Reiner, M.; Niermann, C.; Jekauc, D.; Woll, A. Long-term health benefits of physical activity–a systematic review of longitudinal studies. *BMC Public Health* **2013**, *13*, 813. [CrossRef] [PubMed]
33. Radak, Z.; Hart, N.; Sarga, L.; Koltai, E.; Atalay, M.; Ohno, H.; Boldogh, I. Exercise plays a preventive role against Alzheimer's disease. *J. Alzheimer's Dis.* **2010**, *20*, 777–783. [CrossRef] [PubMed]
34. Woods, J.A.; Wilund, K.R.; Martin, S.A.; Kistler, B.M. Exercise, Inflammation and Aging. *Aging Dis.* **2012**, *3*, 130–140. [PubMed]
35. Hodge, A.M.; O'Dea, K.; English, D.R.; Giles, G.G.; Flicker, L. Dietary patterns as predictors of successful ageing. *J. Nutr. Health Aging* **2014**, *18*, 221–227. [CrossRef] [PubMed]
36. Kiefte-de Jong, J.C.; Mathers, J.C.; Franco, O.H. Nutrition and healthy ageing: The key ingredients. *Proc. Nutr. Soc.* **2014**, *73*, 249–259. [CrossRef] [PubMed]
37. Sofi, F.; Abbate, R.; Gensini, G.F.; Casini, A. Accruing evidence on benefits of adherence to the Mediterranean diet on health: An updated systematic review and meta-analysis. *Am. J. Clin. Nutr.* **2010**, *92*, 1189–1196. [CrossRef] [PubMed]
38. Slavin, J.L.; Lloyd, B. Health Benefits of Fruits and Vegetables. *Adv. Nutr.* **2012**, *3*, 506–516. [CrossRef] [PubMed]
39. Liu, R.H. Health benefits of fruit and vegetables are from additive and synergistic combinations of phytochemicals. *Am. J. Clin. Nutr.* **2003**, *78* (Suppl. 3), 517s–520s. [CrossRef] [PubMed]
40. Leitzmann, C. Characteristics and Health Benefits of Phytochemicals. *Complement. Med. Res.* **2016**, *23*, 69–74. [CrossRef] [PubMed]
41. Griswold, M.G.; Fullman, N.; Hawley, C.; Arian, N.; Zimsen, S.R.M.; Tymeson, H.D.; Venkateswaran, V.; Tapp, A.D.; Forouzanfar, M.H.; Salama, J.S.; et al. Alcohol use and burden for 195 countries and territories, 1990–2016, a systematic analysis for the Global Burden of Disease Study 2016. *Lancet* **2018**, *392*, 1015–1035. [CrossRef]
42. Chen, L.Y.; Hardy, C.L. Alcohol Consumption and Health Status in Older Adults:A Longitudinal Analysis. *J. Aging Health* **2009**, *21*, 824–847. [CrossRef] [PubMed]
43. Hu, Y.; Pikhart, H.; Malyutina, S.; Pajak, A.; Kubinova, R.; Nikitin, Y.; Peasey, A.; Marmot, M.; Bobak, M. Alcohol consumption and physical functioning among middle-aged and older adults in Central and Eastern Europe: Results from the HAPIEE study. *Age Ageing* **2015**, *44*, 84–89. [CrossRef] [PubMed]
44. Stockwell, T.; Greer, A.; Fillmore, K.; Chikritzhs, T.; Zeisser, C. How good is the science? *BMJ* **2012**, *344*, e2294. [CrossRef] [PubMed]
45. Hernan, M.A.; Alonso, A.; Logroscino, G. Cigarette smoking and dementia: Potential selection bias in the elderly. *Epidemiology* **2008**, *19*, 448–450. [CrossRef] [PubMed]

46. Divo, M.J.; Martinez, C.H.; Mannino, D.M. Ageing and the epidemiology of multimorbidity. *Eur. Respir. J.* **2014**, *44*, 1055–1068. [CrossRef] [PubMed]
47. Kim, J.I.; Kim, G. Factors affecting the survival probability of becoming a centenarian for those aged 70, based on the human mortality database: Income, health expenditure, telephone, and sanitation. *BMC Geriatr.* **2014**, *14*, 113. [CrossRef] [PubMed]
48. Lu, W.; Pikhart, H.; Sacker, A. Domains and Measurements of Healthy Aging in Epidemiological Studies: A Review. *Gerontologist* **2018**, gny029. [CrossRef] [PubMed]
49. Kuh, D.; Richards, M.; Cooper, R.; Hardy, R.; Ben-Shlomo, Y. Life course epidemiology, ageing research, and maturing cohort studies: A dynamic combination for understanding healthy ageing. In *A Life Course Approach to Healthy Ageing*; Oxford University Press: Oxford, UK, 2014.

15

Investigating Age-Related Neural Compensation During Emotion Perception Using Electroencephalography

Tao Yang [1,2,*], Caroline Di Bernardi Luft [3], Pei Sun [1], Joydeep Bhattacharya [2] and Michael J. Banissy [2]

[1] Department of Psychology, Tsinghua University, Beijing 100084, China; peisun@tsinghua.edu.cn

[2] Department of Psychology, Goldsmiths, University of London, London SE14 6NW, UK; j.bhattacharya@gold.ac.uk (J.B.); m.banissy@gold.ac.uk (M.J.B.)

[3] School of Biological and Chemical Sciences, Queen Mary University of London, London E1 4NS, UK; luft@qmul.ac.uk

* Correspondence: t_yang@tsinghua.edu.cn

Abstract: Previous research suggests declines in emotion perception in older as compared to younger adults, but the underlying neural mechanisms remain unclear. Here, we address this by investigating how "face-age" and "face emotion intensity" affect both younger and older participants' behavioural and neural responses using event-related potentials (ERPs). Sixteen young and fifteen older adults viewed and judged the emotion type of facial images with old or young face-age and with high- or low- emotion intensities while EEG was recorded. The ERP results revealed that young and older participants exhibited significant ERP differences in two neural clusters: the left frontal and centromedial regions (100–200 ms stimulus onset) and frontal region (250–900 ms) when perceiving neutral faces. Older participants also exhibited significantly higher ERPs within these two neural clusters during anger and happiness emotion perceptual tasks. However, while this pattern of activity supported neutral emotion processing, it was not sufficient to support the effective processing of facial expressions of anger and happiness as older adults showed reductions in performance when perceiving these emotions. These age-related changes are consistent with theoretical models of age-related changes in neurocognitive abilities and may reflect a general age-related cognitive neural compensation in older adults, rather than a specific emotion-processing neural compensation.

Keywords: emotion perception; ageing; neural compensation; electroencephalogram

---

1. Introduction

The perception of emotional facial expression plays an important role in interpersonal communication [1,2]. Emotional expression can alter the meaning of speech and the ability to accurately identify emotional content is particularly important in social interactions [2]. Difficulties with emotion perception are associated with specific types of social impairment, including poor interpersonal interaction, reduced social competence and loneliness (e.g., [3,4]). These outcomes can have negative impacts on health and wellbeing (e.g., [5]), thus establishing how the capacity for emotion perception is affected as a function of normal adult aging is an important challenge.

Most studies have consistently demonstrated that older adults appear to have declined perception of some negative facial expressions of emotions, such as anger, sadness, fear and surprise (e.g., [6–10]). In contrast, age-related decline in the perception of happiness is less consistent: early studies suggested similar performance levels for young and older adults when using prototypical emotions [8,11,12] (see [1] for a review), but recent work suggests that there may be differences when more subtle emotional stimuli are used [13].

In addition, one issue involved in previous studies comparing both young and older people's face perceptual abilities is the other-age effect—participants tend to show superior performance in the perception of own versus other age faces [14–17]. Therefore, the decline in the performance of older adults might be due to the use of young adult actors in the task, which favours young adult participants. It is also known that irrespective of the age of the perceiver, processing different age faces expressing the emotion can also influence emotion perception more broadly. For instance, in some studies, emotion perceptual accuracy of older faces was reported to be lower than young faces, as the wrinkles and folds of older faces can reduce the signal clarity of facial expressions [18–20]. Further, some researchers proposed that smile/happiness was easier to be perceived in young faces than older faces (e.g., [21]), whereas decoding facial expression of anger was higher in older faces than younger faces [22].

Age-Related Neural Compensation in Emotion Perception

Functional neuroimaging studies have found that older participants exhibit a different neural activation pattern from younger participants during emotion perception [23–26]. Generally, older people tend to recruit more frontal cortical regions during emotion perception. For example, Gunning-Dixon, Gur, and Perkins [23] investigated age-related neural activations in cortical and limbic regions using functional magnetic resonance imaging (fMRI) by presenting facial stimuli of a mixture of negative emotions to both young and older participants. They observed neural activation in the amygdala and surrounding temporolimbic regions in younger participants, whereas older participants showed neural activations in left inferior and middle frontal regions. Similar results were found by Tessitore and colleagues [24] who compared older and younger participants' neural processing of fearful and threatening stimuli using fMRI and found older participants were associated with increased prefrontal cortical neural responses and lower neural responses in the amygdala and posterior fusiform gyri relative to younger adults.

These studies have uncovered important age-related neural correlates of emotion processing; however, there are limitations. Firstly, most neuroimaging studies have typically investigated facial displays of only negative emotions [23–26]; therefore, it is not entirely clear whether the age-related compensation patterns reflect older people's general emotion processing or processing of negative emotions only. Second, perceptual biases may have influenced previous neuroimaging results, since most have only used younger faces, which may lead to the other-age effect influencing performance [14,17]. Another set of issues that have largely been overlooked in most previous studies is the variation of emotional intensity or task difficulty. Previous studies have found that older adults have more difficulty than younger adults at labelling facial emotion with less intensity [27]. Further, recent work has suggested that age-related differences in emotion matching might be limited to low-intensity expressions [28]. However, high-intensity facial emotions displays that are typically linked with high performance have been used in most neuroimaging studies. This may potentially mask group differences in performance (e.g., see [13]), which leads to two issues: (1) it is unclear how older people's perception of subtle/low-intensity facial expressions are linked with brain activity; and (2) it is unclear how task difficulty/face emotion intensity interacts with age-related neural activation changes.

In addition, much prior work using neuroimaging to investigate emotion processing in ageing has used fMRI [23–36]. Electroencephalography (EEG) has better temporal resolution than fMRI and enables inference about the neural time course of emotional facial expression processing. However, most previous ERP studies focused on studying young people's ERPs during perceiving emotions (e.g., [20,29]). Those ERP studies that have compared young versus older neural activation differences mostly investigated neural activations within specific emotion-related ERP components that were previously defined by studying younger people (e.g., early posterior negativity (EPN)). For example, in one study, the late positive potentials (LPP) amplitudes were investigated as a function of age (between 18–81 years) and revealed that the LPP for negative images decreases linearly with age, but LPP for positive images is age-invariant across most of the adult life span [31]. Wieser et al. [32]

compared young and older people's early posterior negativity (EPN, an index of early emotion discrimination) during emotion (neutral, positive and negative) discrimination tasks. They found that EPN (168–232 ms) was delayed in older adults compared to younger adults, but a later component (232–296 ms) was unaffected. This study suggested an age-related delay of early visual emotion discrimination, but the delay does not seem to influence the discrimination of emotional stimuli. Tsolaki et al. [33] compared older and younger adults' neural responses within face-selective ERP component N170 during viewings of facial images of anger and fear. They found that the N170 early component was modulated by the type of emotions and tends to have larger amplitudes in the elderly than the young during the viewing of negative stimuli (such as "anger" and "fear"). Although these studies have revealed important age-related neural activation differences during emotion processing, it is still not clear: (1) whether older people also recruit additional frontal neural regions during the perception of neutral emotion, and (2) what the effects of face emotion intensity and face-age are in modulating the neural compensation patterns.

With these in mind, the aim of this study is to compare older and young adults' neural activation patterns and behavioral responses during the perception of both low- and high- emotional intensities of anger and happiness facial emotions. In particular, the present study seeks to compare older and young people's compensation patterns at neutral (baseline), easy (high emotional intensities) and hard (low emotional intensities) conditions of anger and happiness emotion perception. By doing so, we seek to learn more about older adults' neural compensation patterns in processing positive (happiness) and negative (anger) facial emotions with different task difficulties, which could speak to contemporary theoretical models. One model of interest is the compensation-related utilization of the neural circuits hypothesis (CRUNCH) model [37]. This model suggests that older people's processing inefficiencies lead the ageing brain to recruit additional neural resources to perform at the level of younger adults: at lower levels of task demand, older adults exhibit a region-specific neural overactivation pattern but they can achieve similar or equivalent behavioural performance as younger adults (successful neural compensation); however, beyond a certain level of task demand, the older adult brain falls short of sufficient neural activation and their behavioural performance declines compared to younger people (neural compensation failure). Based on the predictions of the CRUNCH model, we expect to find that different task demands (face emotion images with low- and high- emotional intensities) might require different levels of neural compensation in older adults.

2. Materials and Methods

2.1. Participants

Thirty-one adult human volunteers participated in our study. Participants were divided into two groups: younger adults ($N = 16$, 12 female, mean ± SD of age: 24 ± 6 years), and older adults ($N = 15$, 12 female, mean ± SD of age: 69 ± 9 years). The study was conducted in the U.K., and all participants were native English speakers, with no known history of neurological problems, dyslexia or other language-related problems. They had normal or corrected-to-normal vision (self-reported). They gave written informed consent prior to beginning the experiment. The experimental protocol was approved by the local ethics committee of the Department of Psychology at Goldsmiths.

Level of education, premorbid intelligence (National Adult Reading Test, NART) [34], handedness, screening tests of working memory (digit span) [35], and alexithymia trait [36] were recorded for all participants. Further, we also administered the Mini-Mental State Examination (MMSE) as screening for possible dementia in the older adults group [38]; all participants had scores higher than 24, a usual cut-off limit for dementia [39].

2.2. Stimuli

The stimuli used in this study consisted of computer-generated human faces created by the FaceGen software ((www.facegen.com/products.htm), [40]), which were used in previous studies on emotion perception [18,41,42]. The facial stimuli had no hair or facial hair to avoid gender cues other than facial structure and features. All images were three-dimensional, greyscale, front profile Caucasian faces. Faces of thirty young (18–40 years; 15 female) and thirty old (65 years and above; 15 female) individuals were used. Each facial stimulus displayed anger or happiness in five emotional intensities: 0%, 15%, 30%, 60% and 75%. For both angry and happy faces, we formed two groups: faces with high intensities (60% and 75%), faces with low intensities (15% and 30%), corresponding to easy and difficult trials, respectively (see Figure 1 for examples). Faces with zero intensity correspond to neutral trials. Therefore, we had ten conditions in total (young/old face × angry/happy emotion × low/high intensity, and young/old face × neutral). Each condition comprised 60 experimental trials.

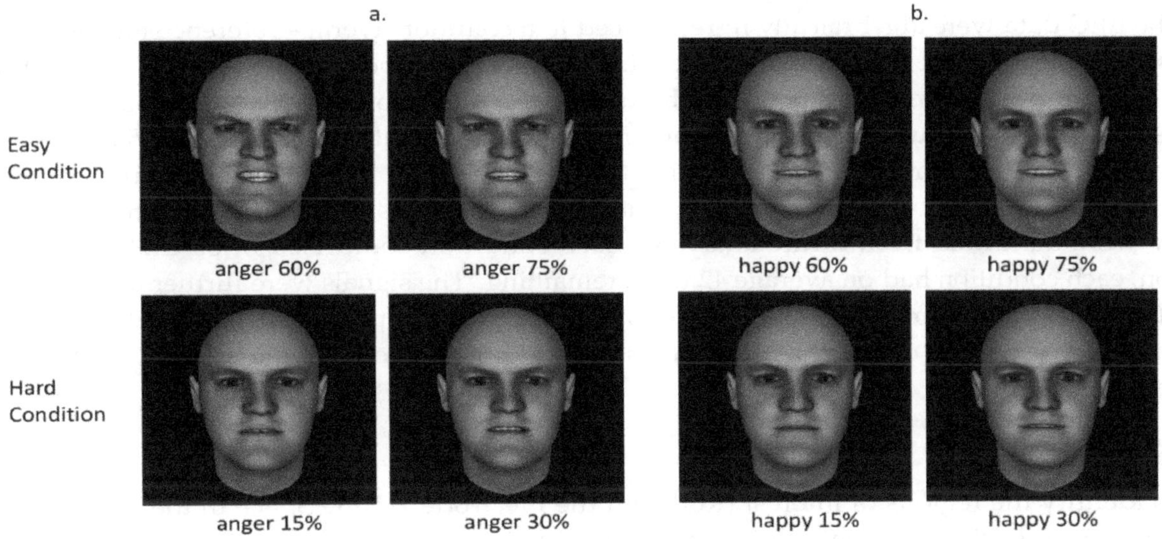

Figure 1. Example of emotional facial stimuli of anger (**a**) and happiness (**b**) used in the experiment. Hard task conditions contain facial stimuli with lower emotional intensities (15% and 30%), and easy task conditions contain facial stimuli with higher emotional intensities (60% and 75%).

2.3. Experimental Procedure

Participants were seated approximately 50 cm in front of a computer screen in a dimly lit, sound-attenuated room, and completed an emotion perception task. In each trial (Figure 2), a face was briefly presented for 500 ms, followed by a fixation cross for 500 ms, and then participants reported emotional category of the earlier face by pressing a key out of three options (anger, happiness, and neutral). The next trial started 1500 ms after the response (see Figure 2). At the beginning of the experiment, participants were informed that some facial expressions were subtle. There was a practice block (30 trials) before the experiment.

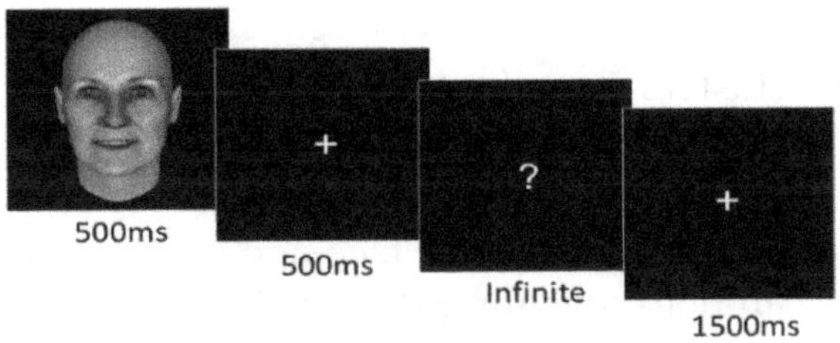

Figure 2. An outline of a trial. In each trial, a face was presented for 500 ms, followed by a blank screen with a fixation cross for 500 ms, and then followed by a prompt, asking participants to provide a response on the emotion category, happy or angry or neutral. The inter-trial interval was 1500 ms.

2.4. EEG Recording and Analysis

EEG signals were recorded with sixty-four Ag-AgCl electrodes placed according to the extended 10–20 electrode placement system, and amplified by a BioSemi ActiveTwo amplifier (www.biosemi.com). Four additional electrodes were placed above and below each eye, and at the outer canthus of each eye, to record vertical and horizontal eye movements, respectively. The sixty-four EEG signals were recorded with a sampling frequency of 512 Hz, bandpass filtered between 0.16–100 Hz. For the sixty-four EEG signals, MATLAB toolbox EEGLAB [43] was used for data preprocessing, and FieldTrip [44] for data analysis and statistical comparisons.

2.5. Preprocessing

The EEG data were algebraically re-referenced to a common average reference for ERP analyses because it is a less biased reference for comparing across scalp topographies [45,46]. The continuous data were high-pass filtered at 0.5 Hz and subsequently epoched from −1500 to 1500 ms time-locked to the onset of a face stimulus. The artifacts were treated in a semi-automated fashion. Visual inspection was initially made to remove any large artifacts, followed by an independent component analysis for correcting the eye blink-related artifacts. Subsequently, epochs containing amplitudes exceeding ±75 μV were discarded from future analysis. Each condition comprised of 60 trials; after artifact rejection, each condition had on average 42 trials remaining. The signals were further low-pass filtered at 35 Hz and epoched from −200 to 1000 ms following the stimulus presentation. The EEG signal of the epochs were averaged to obtain the ERP signals per condition. The ERPs were subsequently baseline corrected (−200 to 0 ms).

2.6. ERP Analysis

To identify the regions of interest (ROIs) on the Electrode x Time Space in the ERP differences between groups (old vs. young) while perceiving happy or angry emotion, we used a data-driven exploratory approach using a neutral emotion condition as a baseline. The ERPs of older and younger adults while perceiving neutral faces were compared by a non-parametric cluster-based permutation test [47], which is hypothesis-free, that controls the Type I error rate, and is widely used to analyse multidimensional EEG/MEG data [48–50]. The method consists of two steps as follows. First, the multidimensional (time, amplitude and electrode) clusters were detected by grouping neighboring data points that showed a significant effect ($p < 0.05$) of group (young vs. old) by independent t-tests, and a cluster-level statistic was subsequently calculated by summing the t-values in each cluster. Here, we considered electrodes with a distance of less than 5 cm as neighbors, yielding on average 4.2 neighbors per electrode. Second, Monte Carlo randomisation was used to calculate the exact probability that a cluster with the maximum cluster-level statistic was observed under the assumption that the ERP values of the two compared groups or conditions were not significantly different. A histogram of maximum cluster-level statistics was obtained by calculating the cluster-level statistic by repeating the entire analysis a large number of times (=500 in the current study) on random permutation of the pooled data of the two groups or conditions; this histogram was subsequently used to calculate the exact p-value for that cluster, and these procedures were subsequently carried out for the lower ranking cluster-level statistics [48]. The clusters thus obtained were subsequently used as the ROIs to find the main differences between the younger and older adults by standard factorial mixed ANOVA on the mean ERP amplitudes at these ROIs. By choosing a neutral condition as the baseline, this method can show the role of emotion type, task difficulty and face-age in modulating the same spatiotemporal brain profiles. Specifically, it can help revealing the participants' neural changes from baseline to easy and hard emotion conditions, which provides the evidence for validating the age-related neural compensation hypothesis.

3. Results

3.1. Participants' Characteristics

Demographic characteristics of the two groups are listed in Table 1. The two groups did not significantly differ ($p > 0.05$) in level of education, premorbid intelligence (NART), handedness, working memory (digit span), or Toronto Alexithymia Scale (TAS-20).

Table 1. Basic demographic and descriptive characteristics of the two study groups.

	Old (n = 15)	*Young (n = 16)*
Gender (male/female)	3/12	4/12
Age (years)	69.20 (8.809)	24.19 (5.576)
Education (years)	15 (3)	16 (2)
Handedness (right/left)	14/1	15/1
Premorbid IQ (NART)	120.07 (8.430)	115.44 (10.295)
Working memory (digit-span)	105.27 (16.867)	106.63 (12.209)
TAS-20 score	43.00 (7.329)	44.75 (9.692)

3.2. Behavioral Results

Prior to data analysis, accuracy outliers were excluded from further analysis (using a criteria of >3 standard deviations from the mean on any individual variable of interest and significance using Grubb's test). Specifically, two datasets from *older face_neutral* condition, one dataset from *older face_anger_easy* condition, one dataset from *younger face_neutral* condition, one dataset from *younger face_anger_easy* condition, and two datasets from *younger face_happy_easy* condition were identified as outliers and excluded from further analysis. No RT outliers were found. Participants' perceptual performance (accuracy and RTs) on each task were analysed.

3.2.1. Perception of Neutral Facial Expression

Perceptual performance on neutral emotion condition was analysed by a 2 × 2 mixed factorial ANOVA with group (young, old) as a between-participants factor and face-age (young, old) as a within-participants factor. Older adults showed marginally higher accuracy on recognizing neutral emotion than younger adults ($F(1, 26) = 4.195$, $p = 0.051$, $\eta^2 = 0.139$; Figure 3). No other significant main effect or interaction was found (see Supplementary Material).

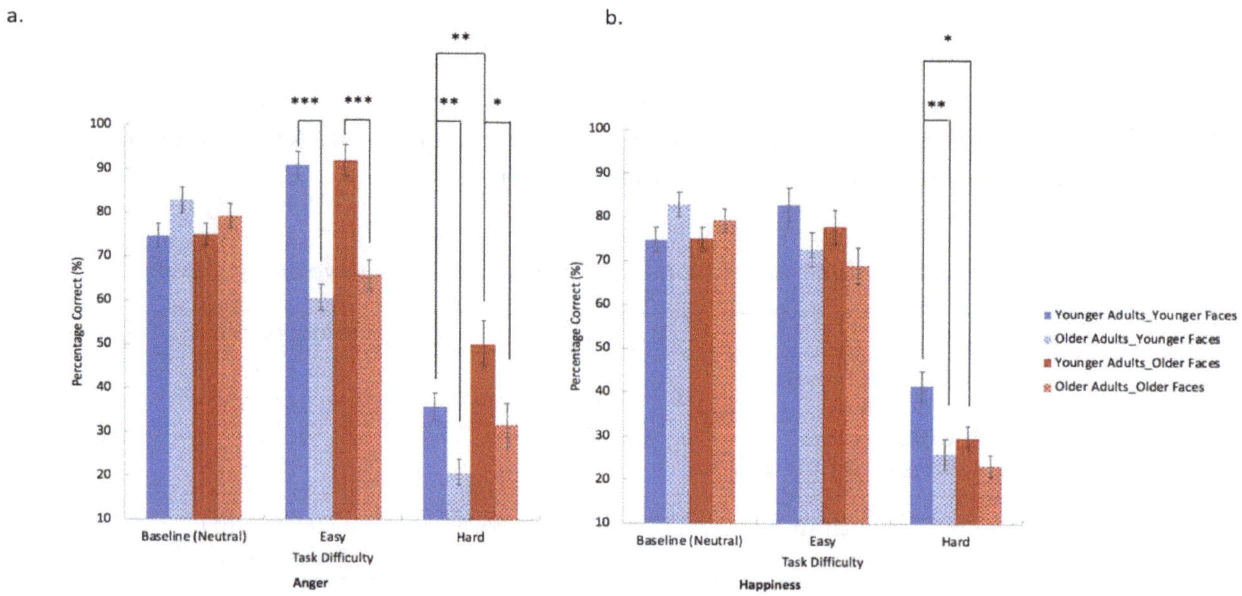

Figure 3. Older (patterned bars) and younger (solid bars) participants' perceptual performance (accuracy) in anger (**a**) and happiness (**b**) experimental trials at different task difficulties (neutral (baseline), easy and hard). Bars in red represent trials with older face stimuli, bars in blue represent trials with younger face stimuli. (1) Anger perception (**a**): older group performed worse than younger group in both easy (old face stimuli condition and young face stimuli condition) and hard (old face stimuli condition and young face stimuli condition) levels. (2) Happiness perception (**b**): older adults performed poorer in hard condition using younger face stimuli, but not in other conditions. (3) In addition, within-group comparison revealed that younger participants' performance on young and old face stimuli were significantly different for only hard level of anger and happiness perception tasks, with superior performance on younger face stimuli in happiness perceptual tasks and superior performance on older face stimuli in anger perceptual tasks. Error bars represents S.E. (*** represents $p < 0.001$. ** represents $p < 0.01$. * represents $p < 0.05$).

3.2.2. Perception of Anger and Happiness Facial Expressions

Perceptual performance on anger and happiness trials were analysed by a $2 \times 2 \times 2 \times 2$ mixed ANOVA with group (young, old) as the between-participants factor, and emotion type (anger, happiness), face-age (young, old), and task difficulty (easy, hard) as within-participants factors. Younger adults showed overall better performance than the older adults ($F(1, 26) = 30.357$, $p < 0.001$, $\eta^2 = 0.539$; Figure 3). The main effect of task difficulty was also significant ($F(1, 26) = 381.512$, $p < 0.001$, $\eta^2 = 0.936$), which was due to the overall accuracy for easy trials being significantly higher than hard trials. The main effects of emotion type and face-age were not significant. The interaction of emotion type × face-age was significant ($F(1, 26) = 24.495$, $p < 0.001$, $\eta^2 = 0.485$). Pairwise comparisons (with Bonferroni correction) revealed that this was due to the overall accuracy for older face stimuli being significantly higher than younger face stimuli for anger emotion (anger: $p < 0.001$; $d = 1.699$). For the happy facial emotion, the overall accuracy for younger face stimuli was significantly higher than for older face stimuli (happiness: $p = 0.008$, $d = 1.441$, Bonferroni corrected).

The interaction of emotion type × face-age × task difficulty was also significant ($F(1, 26) = 15.085$, $p = 0.001$, $\eta^2 = 0.367$). Pairwise comparison (Bonferroni-corrected) revealed that participants' overall accuracy for older face stimuli was significantly higher than younger face stimuli in the hard level of anger perceptual tasks ($p < 0.001$, $d = 1.744$). In the hard level of happiness perceptual tasks, participants' overall accuracy for younger face stimuli was significantly higher than older face stimuli ($p < 0.001$, $d = 1.538$).

The interaction of emotion type × face-age × task difficulty × group was also significant ($F(1, 26) = 4.893$, $p = 0.036$, $\eta^2 = 0.158$). Pairwise comparison (Bonferroni-corrected) revealed that the older group performed worse than the younger group at anger perception in both easy (old face stimuli condition: $p < 0.001$, $d = 1.608$; young face stimuli condition: $p < 0.001$, $d = 1.865$) and hard (old face stimuli condition: $p = 0.032$, $d = 1.203$; young face stimuli condition: $p = 0.008$, $d = 1.463$) levels (Figure 3a). Older adults also performed poorer in hard condition of happiness perception using younger face stimuli ($p = 0.008$, $d = 1.443$), but not in other conditions (Figure 3b). In addition, within-group comparison revealed that younger participants' performance on young and old face stimuli were significantly different for only the hard level of anger and happiness perception tasks (anger: $p = 0.008$, $d = 1.438$; happiness: $p < 0.001$, $d = 1.512$), with superior performance on younger face stimuli in happiness perceptual tasks and superior performance on older face stimuli in anger perceptual tasks. In contrast, older participants' performances on younger and older face stimuli were not significantly different in both easy and hard levels of anger and happiness perception tasks.

3.3. *ERP Analysis*

3.3.1. Selections of ERP Clusters that Showed Difference between Old and Young Group

In order to select the ROIs, we compared young and older participants' ERPs (young vs. old) on neutral emotion condition by using the non-parametric cluster permutation tests (ERPs corresponding to the old and young faces stimuli trials of neural condition were merged). The significant clusters are shown in Figure 4. We identified two significant clusters: the first cluster was a left-frontal and centromedial cluster between 100–200 ms (Figure 4a), and the second cluster was over the frontal region between 250–900 ms (Figure 4b). These two spatiotemporally distinct clusters served as our two ROIs.

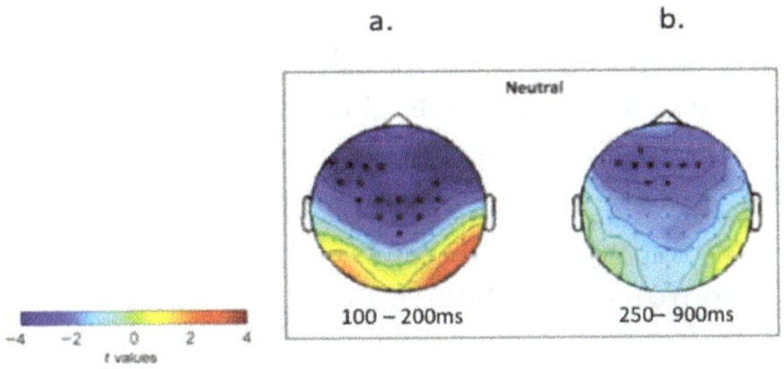

Figure 4. Significant clusters of the nonparametric cluster randomisation test comparing the two groups (young minus old) on neutral condition. First cluster time window: 100–200 ms, left-frontal and centromedial area (F1, F3, F5, F7, Fc5, Fc5, C1, C3, Cp1, Pz, Cpz, Fc4, Cz, C2, C4); second cluster time window: 250–900 ms; frontal area (AF3 F1, F3, F5, Fc1, Fz, F2, F4, Fcz).

3.3.2. The Effect of Emotion, Face-age and Task Difficulty in Modulating ERPs

For each cluster, we computed individual participant mean ERP amplitudes, and the data were subsequently analyzed by a mixed 2 × 2 × 2 × 2 ANOVA with emotions (anger, happiness), face-age (young and old), task difficulty (easy, hard) as within-participants factors, and group (young, old) as a between-participants factor.

Cluster one

The results revealed that older participants exhibited significantly higher overall mean ERP amplitudes than younger group (main effect of group, $F(1, 26) = 20.273$, $p < 0.001$, $\eta^2 = 0.438$; Figure 5). In addition, the easy condition (high-intensity facial expressions) elicited significantly higher overall mean ERP amplitudes in left frontal and centromedial regions (100–200 ms) than the hard condition (low-intensity facial expression) [the main effect of task difficulty, $F(1, 26) = 4.974$, $p = 0.035$, $\eta^2 = 0.161$]. The main effects of emotion type and face-age were not significant.

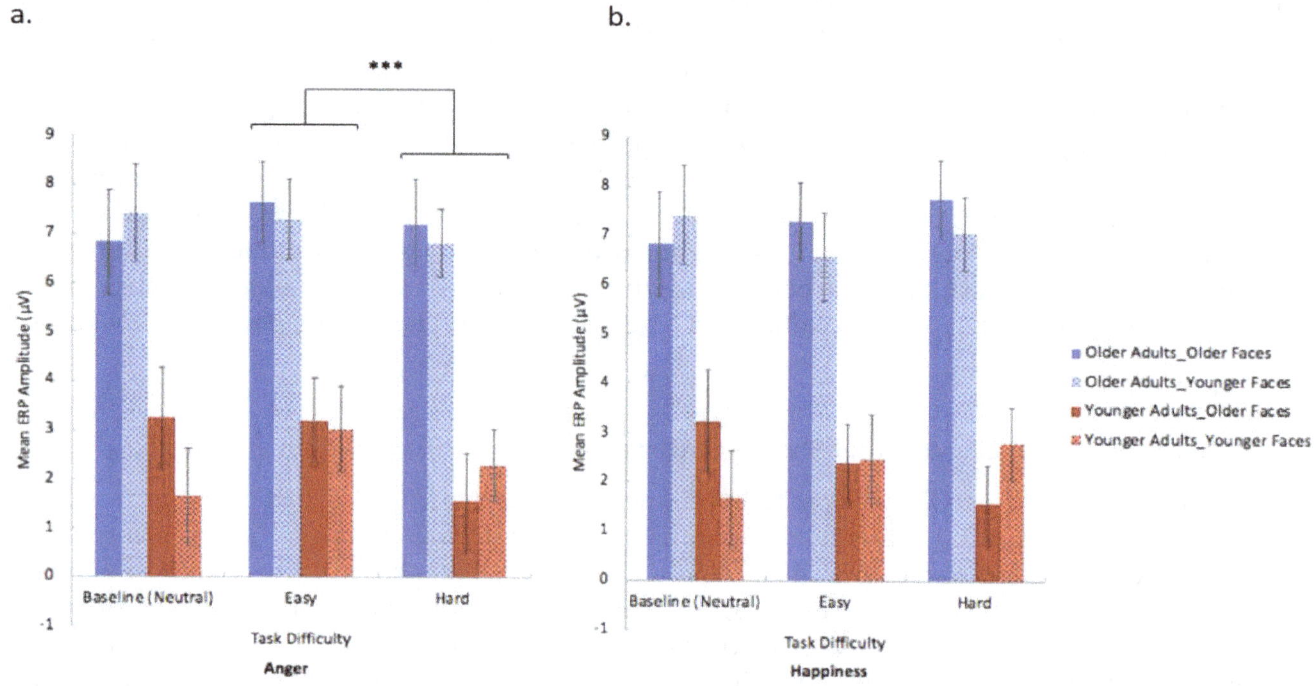

Figure 5. Older (bars in blue) and younger (bars in red) participants' cluster one mean ERP amplitude for anger (**a**) and happiness (**b**) experimental trials at different task difficulties (neutral (baseline), easy and hard). Solid bars represent trials with older face stimuli; patterned bars represent trials with younger face stimuli. The overall left-frontal and centromedial mean ERP amplitude (100–200 ms) of easy condition was significantly higher than the hard condition in anger task, regardless of group. Error bars represents S.E. (*** represents $p < 0.001$).

The interaction of face-age × group was significant [$F(1, 26) = 5.775, p = 0.024, \eta^2 = 0.182$]. Pairwise comparison (with Bonferroni correction) revealed that older participants exhibited significantly higher mean ERP amplitudes in left frontal and centromedial regions (100–200 ms) than younger participants in both older and younger face stimuli conditions (older face stimuli, $p < 0.001$, $d = 1.764$; younger face stimuli, $p < 0.001$, $d = 1.583$). No significant results was found in within-group comparisons (old group: $p = 0.054$ and young group: $p = 0.172$; with Bonferroni correction; Figure 5). The interaction of emotion type × difficulty was significant ($F(1, 26) = 6.632, p = 0.017, \eta^2 = 0.201$). Pairwise comparison revealed that the mean left-frontal and centromedial ERP amplitude (100–200 ms) of the easy condition was significantly higher than the hard condition in anger task ($p < 0.001$, $d = 1.537$) (Figure 5).

Cluster two

A 2 (emotion type) × 2 (task difficulty) × 2 (face-age) × 2 (group) mixed ANOVA on the ERP amplitudes of the second cluster (250–900 ms) revealed significant main effect of group ($F(1, 26) = 17.051, p < 0.001, \eta^2 = 0.396$), which was due to older participants exhibiting significantly higher overall mean ERP amplitudes than younger group (Figure 6). The main effect of task difficulty was significant ($F(1, 26) = 6.813, p = 0.015, \eta^2 = 0.208$), which was due to the easy condition (high-intensity facial expressions) eliciting significantly higher overall mean ERP amplitudes in frontal regions (250–900 ms) than the hard condition (low-intensity facial expression) (Figure 6). The main effects of emotion type and face-age were not significant.

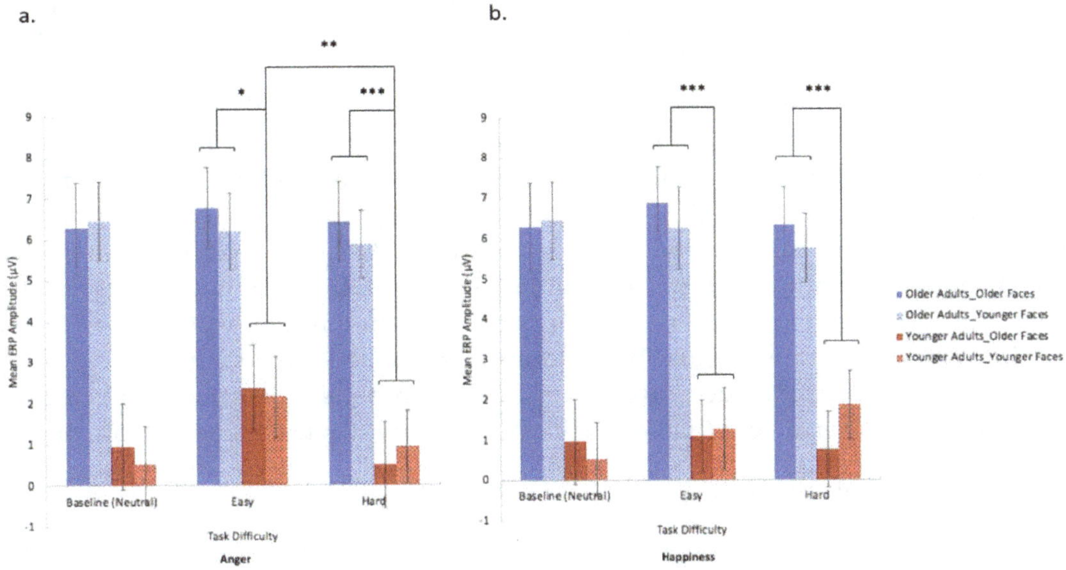

Figure 6. Older (bars in blue) and younger (bars in red) participants' cluster two mean ERP amplitude for anger (**a**) and happiness (**b**) experimental trials at different task difficulties (neutral (baseline), easy and hard). Solid bars represent trials with older face stimuli; patterned bars represent trials with younger face stimuli. (1) Older participants exhibited significantly higher frontal ERP amplitudes (250–900 ms) in both easy and hard levels of anger and happiness perceptual tasks compared to younger participants. (2) Within-group comparison revealed that younger participants' mean frontal ERP amplitudes (250–900 ms) for the easy condition was significantly higher than the hard condition in anger perception, but not significantly different in the happiness perceptual tasks; whereas older participants did not show significant different ERPs across easy and hard task conditions in both the happiness and anger perceptual tasks. Error bars represents S.E. (significances are marked by *** $p < 0.001$, ** $p < 0.01$, and * $p < 0.05$).

The interaction of face-age × group was significant, $F(1, 26) = 5.468, p = 0.027, \eta^2 = 0.174$, which was due to older adults exhibiting significantly higher ERPs than younger adults in both older ($p < 0.001$, $d = 1.641$) and younger ($p = 0.008$, $d = 1.428$, Bonferroni corrected) face stimuli (Figure 6). In addition, within-group comparison revealed that the older group's mean ERP amplitude for younger faces was significantly lower than for older faces ($p = 0.047$, $d = 0.216$), whereas the younger group's mean ERP for young and old face stimuli did not differ ($p = 0.221$).

The interaction of emotion type × task difficulty × group was significant ($F(1, 26) = 5.781, p = 0.024$, $\eta^2 = 0.182$). Pairwise comparison (with Bonferroni correction) revealed that older participants exhibited significantly higher frontal ERP amplitudes (250–900 ms) in both easy and hard levels of anger (easy: $p = 0.048$, $d = 1.367$; hard: $p < 0.001$, $d = 1.766$) and happiness (easy: $p < 0.001$, $d = 1.540$; hard: $p < 0.001$, $d = 1.511$) perceptual tasks. In addition, the within-group comparison revealed that younger participants' mean frontal ERP amplitudes (250–900 ms) for the easy condition was significantly higher than the hard condition in anger perception ($p = 0.008$, $d = 1.487$), but not significantly different in the happiness perceptual tasks, whereas older participants did not show significant different ERPs across easy and hard task conditions in both the happiness and anger perceptual tasks (Figure 6).

4. Discussion

The aim of the present study is to examine age-related changes in emotion perception and to further reveal the underlying neural mechanisms. Our study contributes to the current literature in two main ways. First, most neuroimaging studies have typically investigated people's emotion perception by using facial displays of (1) only negative emotions, (2) only young faces, or (3) only high-emotional intensity. To overcome these limitations, we used an integrative approach by considering how "emotion type", "face-age" and "face emotion intensity" affect younger and older participants' emotion perception, all in the same study. Second, one of the main strengths and novelty of our study is related to our data-driven approach. We used an entirely data-driven approach to explore the age-related neural differences during emotion perception—this is an important contribution as we did not limit ourselves to the known ERP components (e.g., [29,30]). Our study provides additional insights by showing that: (1) older participants exhibited neural differences in the left frontal and centromedial region (100–200 ms stimuli onset) and frontal region (250–900 ms stimuli onset) at neutral condition, which suggests that older people's neural compensation may start at the neutral (baseline) condition; (2) within the same neural clusters, older participants also exhibited similar patterns of neural activity during anger and happiness emotion perceptual tasks; (3) older people's compensation was successful in processing neutral emotion as they exhibited similar behavioural performance as younger participants; however, this was not enough for them to successfully apply the compensation strategy in processing facial expressions of anger and happiness (hard condition). We now discuss these in more detail below.

4.1. *Age-Related Behavioural Perceptual Performance Differences*

For the perception of anger, older participants' mean accuracy was significantly lower than younger participants in both hard and easy conditions. This finding suggests that older participants show declined abilities in processing both low- and high-intensities of anger facial expressions. This finding adds confirmation to prior work indicating that older participants show declined perception of anger (see [1] for review). For the perception of happiness, older participants showed poorer performance than younger participants in perceiving low-intensity/subtle happiness from younger faces; however, their perception of high-intensity happiness remain intact. This is consistent with previous findings that older participants exhibit significantly poorer performance in perceiving low-intensity happiness from older faces (e.g., [13]), but relatively intact performance on prototypical emotions displayed by younger adults [7–9,51]. Furthermore, it has recently been found that older adults are associated with larger congruency sequence effect [52,53] in the Stroop task compared to younger adult controls [54]. In future studies, it will be interesting to investigate the trial-to-trial carryover effect in emotion perception and to see how typical aging affects this interference effect.

4.2. *Effect of Face-Age on Behavioural Perceptual Performance*

For anger, younger participants' accuracy for perceiving anger from old face stimuli was significantly higher than from younger faces in the hard condition, which is consistent with Hühnel et al.'s [22] finding that facial expression of anger is easier to detect from older faces than from young faces. This might suggest that some facial features (e.g., winkles around eyes and mouths) of older faces may exaggerate subtle expressions of anger. However, the superior performance in perceiving subtle anger from older faces was not found in older participants, as their performance on younger and older face stimuli was not significantly different in easy or hard levels of anger. It will be important to explore this question further in future work using alternative stimuli to those used in the current design.

For happy emotion, within-group comparison revealed that the younger participants' performance in perceiving low-intensity happiness from younger faces was significantly better than from older faces, which is consistent with Murphy et al.'s finding [21] that smile/happiness is easier to perceive in young than older faces, whereas, older participants' performance in perceiving happiness from younger and older faces did not significantly differ in either low or high intensity. Younger participants' superior performance on younger faces trials (in low emotion intensity condition) might reflect "own-age bias" where people are better at perceiving faces of their own ages [55]. However, this "own-age bias" was not shown in older participants. Younger participants' superior performance in perceiving subtle happiness from younger faces might partially account for the perceptual performance gap between younger and older participants. In other words, the reported poorer performance of older participants might not be entirely due to their perceptual decline, but younger participants' superior perception of their own-age faces.

4.3. Facial Emotion Perception and Neural Compensation in Older People Revealed by ERPs

Previous ERP studies have revealed three major facial emotion-related components, which are early frontocentral positivity (around 120 ms stimulus onset), a later broadly distributed sustained positivity beyond 250 ms post-stimulus, and enhanced negativity at lateral posterior sites (EPN) [30,56,57]. The results of the current study revealed that older participants showed significantly higher early frontal and centromedial ERP positivity (100–200 ms) and a later sustained positivity beyond 250 ms post-stimulus across all facial emotions types including neutral emotion.

Based on earlier studies of Eimer et al. [29,30], the early and late frontal and centromedial positivity can be interpreted to reflect a non-automatic and attentive approach of emotion processing, which do not appear to be modulated by emotion type. Older people's significantly higher early (100–200 ms) and late (250–900 ms) frontal and centromedial positivities compared to younger participants during emotion processing may be interpreted as evidence to suggest that older adults require more cortical neural resources than younger people in all types of emotion perception. This additional recruitment of frontal regions during processing facial emotional expression is in parallel with previous fMRI studies, which also found that older people showed significantly higher frontal neural activations compared to younger adults during emotion perception tasks (e.g., [24,25]).

One aim of the present study is to examine the relationship between emotion task difficulty (emotional intensity) and older participants' age-related neural compensation patterns. The ERP results revealed that older participants exhibited significantly higher activations in the left frontal and centromedial regions (100–200 ms stimuli onset) and frontal region (250–900 ms stimuli onset) compared to young participants when perceiving neutral facial expression. This might suggest that neural differences between young and old participants may start at the neutral (baseline) condition in order to compensate for cortical processing inefficiency. In addition, older participants also exhibited similar patterns during perceiving easy- and hard- levels of anger and happiness facial expressions. When combined with the behavioural results, the findings seem to suggest efficient processing of neutral emotion as they performed equally well as younger participants on neutral emotion perceptual trials. A similar level of neural resources was not enough for older adults to successfully process facial expressions of anger (both easy and hard conditions) and happiness (hard condition), where they showed significantly poorer perceptual performance on both happiness (only hard condition) and anger (both easy and hard conditions) perceptual trials. This pattern of results seems in line with the CRUNCH model [37], which proposes that at a lower level of task demand, older participants exhibit a region-specific neural overactivation pattern, but they can achieve similar or equivalent behavioural as younger participants (successful neural compensation). However, beyond a certain level of task demand, there is insufficient neural activation and their behavioural performance declines compared to the young people (neural compensation failure).

It should be noted that the neural overactivation in left frontal and central regions (100–200 ms stimuli onset) and frontal region (250–900 ms stimuli onset) might not reflect emotion-specific neural compensation. Other aging studies have also shown that older people tend to recruit more frontal cortical regions than younger people when performing identical cognitive tasks, especially effortful tasks [58,59]. This has been found in other brain imaging studies, including melodic expectancy processing [60], attention [61–63], working memory [64,65] and executive functioning [66]. Therefore, the neural overactivation in frontal-centro regions might reflect a top-down and controlled neural compensation to suppress or inhibit irrelevant information rather than emotion-specific neural compensation (e.g., [67]). It is also important to note that we only compared the ERP amplitudes of the same clusters (young–old neural activation difference extracted from neutral condition), which might potentially ignore some emotion-specific neural compensation patterns.

4.4. Effects of "Emotion Type", "Task Difficulty" and "Face-Age" on ERPs

The results showed that the effect of emotion type (happiness and anger) did not significantly modulate younger and older participants' early (100–200 ms) or late (250–900 ms) positivities during facial emotion perceptual tasks. These findings are in line with previous studies that claimed the early and late positivities are not modulated by emotion type [29,30]. The effect of face-age seems to modulate older people's frontal region ERP between 250–900 ms. Older group's mean ERP amplitude for older faces was significantly higher than for younger faces, which might be due to that the facial expressions portrayed by older faces are harder to be processed compared to those portrayed by younger faces [18–20], whereas younger group mean ERP for young and old face stimuli did not differ, which might suggest that younger people's neural processing for young and older emotional faces is similar and they need to recruit more neural regions to process older emotional faces. This finding is novel and awaits further replication.

In contrast, the effect of task difficulty (or facial emotional intensities) significantly modulated the overall ERP amplitudes of both early (100–200 ms) frontal and centromedial and late (250–900 ms) frontal brain regions in anger tasks, but not in happiness tasks. Specifically, the overall mean left-frontal and centromedial ERP amplitudes (100–200 ms) of easy condition (high emotion intensity) was significantly higher than hard condition (low emotion intensity) in anger task, regardless of group and face-age. In other words, higher intensities of anger elicited significantly higher early (100–200 ms) frontal and centromedial positivities in participants, regardless of group and face-age. Furthermore, younger participants' mean frontal ERP amplitudes (250–900 ms) for the easy condition was significantly higher than the hard condition (low emotion intensity) in anger perception, but this pattern was not shown in the happiness condition. Whereas, older participants did not show significant different ERPs across easy and hard conditions in both happiness and anger perceptual tasks. In other words, higher intensities of anger elicited significantly higher late (250–900 ms) frontal positivities in younger participants only. These findings suggest that higher intensities of anger can trigger higher early (100–200 ms) frontal and centromedial positivities and late (250–900 ms, only in younger participants) frontal positivities. These findings seem consistent with Eimer et al.'s [29,30] interpretation that these two positivity components may contribute to attention-regulated emotional processing, as higher intensities of anger signal potential threat and they are normally associated with a higher level devotion of attention [68]. In addition, a recent study has also shown that anger elicits significantly higher late P3 component (350–450 ms at temporo-occipital and parieto-occipital channel locations) compared to happiness in both younger and older adults [69]. The present finding also partially agrees with a previous proposal suggesting high intensities of emotional images elicited larger late positive potentials than lower intensities of emotional images [70], as it is not the case for happiness perception in the present study.

4.5. Limitations and Future Avenues

Most of the emotion-related ERP components were conceptualized by observing younger adults' ERPs (e.g., [29,30]). Later EEG studies that investigated older people's emotion processing only compared young–old neural differences within these previously defined electrodes and time windows (e.g., [32,33]). However, ageing can lead to older people recruiting additional neural regions during emotion processing (neural compensation), that may extend beyond these already defined EEG neural sites. Recently, some ageing studies started to investigate how ageing affects the previously defined emotion-related components [31–33], but fewer studies have investigated how ageing and other factors (task difficulty, emotion type) affect the ERPs of other neural sites during perceiving facial emotions. In this study, instead of focusing on specific ERP components a priori, we adopted a data-driven approach and selected the ROIs based on the differences between younger and older adults for the neutral condition; therefore, the neutral condition serves as a baseline and helps to reveal the changes in participants' neural responses from baseline to easy and hard emotion conditions. By using the neutral condition, we can examine the effects of emotion type and task difficulty in modulating participants' age-related neural compensation patterns when processing facial expressions, which provides the evidence to demonstrate the age-related neural compensation. There is some evidence that even neutral is processed as an expression [71,72], therefore contrasting the ERP responses between young and older participants on neutral condition gave us the signal differences related to age when trying to recognize emotion in general. In addition, contrasting young and old neural responses to neutral faces enabled us to compare their responses to emotional faces which makes the analyses non-circular to avoid the danger of double-dipping as we tested the differences between the groups on data that we did not use to explore the age-related differences [73]. This is our second reason—as by doing this, we were able to use a data-driven approach to explore the data as a first step (using appropriate methods taking into account the multiple comparison problem) and to test these differences, an unseen dataset when stronger emotions of high and low intensity were being presented.

While useful to address this question, our approach might have ignored the group ERP differences in response to specific emotions, as prior studies have suggested that neutral, anger and happiness facial emotions are processed by different neural regions (e.g., [74,75]). In addition, our selections might have neglected emotion-specific neural compensation in other brain areas, which awaits further neuroimaging studies (e.g., fMRI) to investigate in depth.

Author Contributions: T.Y., M.J.B., and J.B. contributed to the study conception and design. T.Y. carried out data collection. Data were analysed and interpreted by C.D.B.L. and T.Y. The drafting of manuscript was written by T.Y. and was critically revised by M.J.B., J.B., C.D.B.L. and P.S. All authors have read and agreed to the published version of the manuscript.

Acknowledgments: We would like to thank Amna Ghani, Danying Wang, and Bin Chen for their assistance and support.

References

1. Ruffman, T.; Henry, J.D.; Livingstone, V.; Phillips, L.H. A meta-analytic review of emotion recognition and aging: Implications for neuropsychological models of aging. *Neurosci. Biobehav. Rev.* **2008**, *32*, 863–881. [CrossRef]
2. Ryan, M.; Murray, J.; Ruffman, T. Aging and the perception of emotion: Processing vocal expressions alone and with faces. *Exp. Aging Res.* **2009**, *36*, 1–22. [CrossRef]
3. Spell, L.A.; Frank, E. Recognition of nonverbal communication of affect following traumatic brain injury. *J. Nonverbal Behav.* **2000**, *24*, 285–300. [CrossRef]
4. Kanai, R.; Bahrami, B.; Duchaine, B.; Janik, A.; Banissy, M.J.; Rees, G. Brain structure links loneliness to social perception. *Curr. Biol.* **2012**, *22*, 1975–1979. [CrossRef] [PubMed]
5. Holt-Lunstad, J.; Smith, T.B.; Baker, M.; Harris, T.; Stephenson, D. Loneliness and social isolation as risk factors for mortality: A meta-analytic review. *Perspect. Psychol. Sci.* **2015**, *10*, 227–237. [CrossRef] [PubMed]
6. McDowell, C.L.; Harrison, D.W.; Demaree, H.A. Is right hemisphere decline in the perception of emotion a function of aging? *Int. J. Neurosci.* **1994**, *79*, 1–11. [CrossRef]
7. Phillips, L.H.; MacLean, R.D.; Allen, R. Age and the understanding of emotions neuropsychological and sociocognitive perspectives. *J. Gerontol. Ser. B Psychol. Sci. Soc. Sci.* **2002**, *57*, 526–530. [CrossRef]
8. Calder, A.J.; Keane, J.; Manly, T.; Sprengelmeyer, R.; Scott, S.; Nimmo-Smith, I.; Young, A.W. Facial expression recognition across the adult life span. *Neuropsychologia* **2003**, *41*, 195–202. [CrossRef]
9. Sullivan, S.; Ruffman, T. Emotion recognition deficits in the elderly. *Int. J. Neurosci.* **2004**, *114*, 403–432. [CrossRef]
10. Mill, A.; Allik, J.; Realo, A.; Valk, R. Age-related differences in emotion recognition ability: A cross-sectional study. *Emotion* **2009**, *9*, 619. [CrossRef]
11. Moreno, C.; Borod, J.C.; Welkowitz, J.; Alpert, M. The perception of facial emotion across the adult life span. *Dev. Neuropsychol.* **1993**, *9*, 305–314. [CrossRef]
12. Orgeta, V.; Phillips, L.H. Effects of age and emotional intensity on the recognition of facial emotion. *Exp. Aging Res.* **2007**, *34*, 63–79. [CrossRef] [PubMed]
13. Yang, T.; Penton, T.; Köybaşı, Ş.L.; Banissy, M.J. Social perception and aging: The relationship between aging and the perception of subtle changes in facial happiness and identity. *Acta Psychol.* **2017**, *179*, 23–29. [CrossRef] [PubMed]

14. Anastasi, J.S.; Rhodes, M.G. An own-age bias in face recognition for children and older adults. *Psychon. Bull. Rev.* **2005**, *12*, 1043–1047. [CrossRef] [PubMed]
15. Ebner, N.C.; He, Y.I.; Johnson, M.K. Age and emotion affect how we look at a face: Visual scan patterns differ for own-age versus other-age emotional faces. *Cogn. Emot.* **2011**, *25*, 983–997. [CrossRef] [PubMed]
16. Ebner, N.C.; Johnson, M.K. Young and older emotional faces: Are there age group differences in expression identification and memory? *Emotion* **2009**, *9*, 329. [CrossRef]
17. Wright, D.B.; Stroud, J.N. Age differences in lineup identification accuracy: People are better with their own age. *Law Hum. Behav.* **2002**, *26*, 641. [CrossRef]
18. Hess, U.; Adams, R.B., Jr.; Simard, A.; Stevenson, M.T.; Kleck, R.E. Smiling and sad wrinkles: Age-related changes in the face and the perception of emotions and intentions. *J. Exp. Soc. Psychol.* **2012**, *48*, 1377–1380. [CrossRef]
19. Courgeon, M.; Buisine, S.; Martin, J.C. Impact of expressive wrinkles on perception of a virtual character's facial expressions of emotions. In *International Workshop on Intelligent Virtual Agents*; Springer: Berlin/Heidelberg, Germany, 2009; pp. 201–214.
20. Richter, D.; Dietzel, C.; Kunzmann, U. Age differences in emotion recognition: The task matters. *J. Gerontol. Ser. B Psychol. Sci. Soc. Sci.* **2010**, *66*, 48–55. [CrossRef]
21. Murphy, N.A.; Isaacowitz, D.M. Age effects and gaze patterns in recognising emotional expressions: An in-depth look at gaze measures and covariates. *Cogn. Emot.* **2010**, *24*, 436–452. [CrossRef]
22. Hühnel, I.; Fölster, M.; Werheid, K.; Hess, U. Empathic reactions of younger and older adults: No age related decline in affective responding. *J. Exp. Soc. Psychol.* **2014**, *50*, 136–143. [CrossRef]
23. Gunning-Dixon, F.M.; Gur, R.C.; Perkins, A.C.; Schroeder, L.; Turner, T.; Turetsky, B.I.; Chan, R.M.; Loughead, J.W.; Alsop, D.C.; Maldjian, J.; et al. Age-related differences in brain activation during emotional face processing. *Neurobiol. Aging* **2003**, *24*, 285–295. [CrossRef]
24. Tessitore, A.; Hariri, A.R.; Fera, F.; Smith, W.G.; Das, S.; Weinberger, D.R.; Mattay, V.S. Functional changes in the activity of brain regions underlying emotion processing in the elderly. *Psychiatry Res. Neuroimaging* **2005**, *139*, 9–18. [CrossRef] [PubMed]
25. Fischer, H.; Nyberg, L.; Bäckman, L. Age-related differences in brain regions supporting successful encoding of emotional faces. *Cortex* **2010**, *46*, 490–497. [CrossRef]
26. Fischer, H.; Sandblom, J.; Gavazzeni, J.; Fransson, P.; Wright, C.I.; Bäckman, L. Age-differential patterns of brain activation during perception of angry faces. *Neurosci. Lett.* **2005**, *386*, 99–104. [CrossRef] [PubMed]
27. West, J.T.; Horning, S.M.; Klebe, K.J.; Foster, S.M.; Cornwell, R.E.; Perrett, D.; Burt, D.M.; Davis, H.P. Age effects on emotion recognition in facial displays: From 20 to 89 years of age. *Exp. Aging Res.* **2012**, *38*, 146–168. [CrossRef] [PubMed]
28. Mienaltowski, A.; Groh, B.; Secula, D.; Rinne, A.; Rogers, C. Impact of expressive intensity on age differences in fear and anger detection in the periphery. *J. Vis.* **2018**, *18*, 568. [CrossRef]
29. Eimer, M.; Holmes, A. Event-related brain potential correlates of emotional face processing. *Neuropsychologia* **2007**, *45*, 15–31. [CrossRef]
30. Eimer, M.; Holmes, A.; McGlone, F.P. The role of spatial attention in the processing of facial expression: An ERP study of rapid brain responses to six basic emotions. *Cogn. Affect. Behav. Neurosci.* **2003**, *3*, 97–110. [CrossRef]
31. Kisley, M.A.; Wood, S.; Burrows, C.L. Looking at the sunny side of life: Age-related change in an event-related potential measure of the negativity bias. *Psychol. Sci.* **2007**, *18*, 838–843. [CrossRef]
32. Wieser, M.J.; Mühlberger, A.; Kenntner-Mabiala, R.; Pauli, P. Is emotion processing affected by advancing age? An event-related brain potential study. *Brain Res.* **2006**, *1096*, 138–147. [CrossRef] [PubMed]
33. Tsolaki, A.C.; Kosmidou, V.E.; Kompatsiaris, I.Y.; Papadaniil, C.; Hadjileontiadis, L.; Tsolaki, M. Age-induced differences in brain neural activation elicited by visual emotional stimuli: A high-density EEG study. *Neuroscience* **2017**, *340*, 268–278. [CrossRef] [PubMed]
34. Nelson, D.B. Conditional heteroskedasticity in asset returns: A new approach. *Econom. J. Econom. Soc.* **1991**, *59*, 347–370. [CrossRef]
35. Turner, M.; Ridsdale, J. The digit memory test. *Dyslexia Int.* **2004**.
36. Bagby, R.M.; Parker, J.D.; Taylor, G.J. The twenty-item Toronto Alexithymia Scale—I. Item selection and cross-validation of the factor structure. *J. Psychosom. Res.* **1994**, *38*, 23–32. [CrossRef]

37. Reuter-Lorenz, P.A.; Cappell, K.A. Neurocognitive aging and the compensation hypothesis. *Curr. Dir. Psychol. Sci.* **2008**, *17*, 177–182. [CrossRef]
38. Folstein, M.F.; Folstein, S.E.; McHugh, P.R. "Mini-mental state": A practical method for grading the cognitive state of patients for the clinician. *J. Psychiatr. Res.* **1975**, *12*, 189–198. [CrossRef]
39. Chayer, C. The neurologic examination: Brief mental status. *Can. J. Geriatr. Care* **2002**, *1*, 265–267.
40. Roesch, E.B.; Tamarit, L.; Reveret, L.; Grandjean, D.; Sander, D.; Scherer, K.R. FACSGen: A tool to synthesize emotional facial expressions through systematic manipulation of facial action units. *J. Nonverbal Behav.* **2011**, *35*, 1–16. [CrossRef]
41. Oosterhof, N.N.; Todorov, A. Shared perceptual basis of emotional expression and trustworthiness impression from faces. *Emotion* **2009**, *9*, 128–133. [CrossRef]
42. Penton, T.; Bate, S.; Dalrymple, K.; Reed, T.; Kelly, M.; Godovich, S.; Tamm, M.; Duchaine, B.; Banissy, M.J. Using high frequency transcranial random noise stimulation to modulate face memory performance in younger and older adults: Lessons learnt from mixed findings. *Front. Neurosci.* **2018**, *12*, 863. [CrossRef] [PubMed]
43. Delorme, A.; Makeig, S. EEGLAB: An open source toolbox for analysis of single-trial EEG dynamics including independent component analysis. *J. Neurosci. Methods* **2004**, *134*, 9–21. [CrossRef] [PubMed]
44. Oostenveld, R.; Fries, P.; Maris, E.; Schoffelen, J.M. FieldTrip: Open source software for advanced analysis of MEG, EEG, and invasive electrophysiological data. *Comput. Intell. Neurosci.* **2011**, *1*, 1–9. [CrossRef] [PubMed]
45. Picton, T.W.; van Roon, P.; Armilio, M.L.; Berg, P.; Ille, N.; Scherg, M. Blinks, saccades, extraocular muscles and visual evoked potentials (Reply to Verleger). *J. Psychophysiol.* **2000**, *14*, 210–217. [CrossRef]
46. Pfurtscheller, G.; Da Silva, F.L. Event-related EEG/MEG synchronization and desynchronization: Basic principles. *Clin. Neurophysiol.* **1999**, *110*, 1842–1857. [CrossRef]
47. Maris, E.; Oostenveld, R. Nonparametric statistical testing of EEG-and MEG-data. *J. Neurosci. Methods* **2007**, *164*, 177–190. [CrossRef]
48. Lindsen, J.P.; Jones, R.; Shimojo, S.; Bhattacharya, J. Neural components underlying subjective preferential decision making. *Neuroimage* **2010**, *50*, 1626–1632. [CrossRef]
49. Luft, C.D.B.; Takase, E.; Bhattacharya, J. Processing graded feedback: Electrophysiological correlates of learning from small and large errors. *J. Cogn. Neurosci.* **2014**, *26*, 1180–1193. [CrossRef]
50. Sandkühler, S.; Bhattacharya, J. Deconstructing insight: EEG correlates of insightful problem solving. *PLoS ONE* **2008**, *3*, 1459. [CrossRef]
51. MacPherson, S.E.; Phillips, L.H.; Sala, S.D. Age-related differences in the ability to perceive sad facial expressions. *Aging Clin. Exp. Res.* **2006**, *18*, 418–424. [CrossRef]
52. Gratton, G.; Coles, M.G.; Donchin, E. Optimizing the use of information: Strategic control of activation of responses. *J. Exp. Psychol. Gen.* **1992**, *121*, 480. [CrossRef] [PubMed]
53. Schmidt, J.R. Questioning conflict adaptation: Proportion congruent and Gratton effects reconsidered. *Psychon. Bull. Rev.* **2013**, *20*, 615–630. [CrossRef] [PubMed]
54. Aschenbrenner, A.J.; Balota, D.A. Dynamic adjustments of attentional control in healthy aging. *Psychol. Aging* **2017**, *32*, 1–15. [CrossRef] [PubMed]
55. Lamont, A.C.; Stewart-Williams, S.; Podd, J. Face recognition and aging: Effects of target age and memory load. *Mem. Cogn.* **2005**, *33*, 1017–1024. [CrossRef]
56. Eimer, M.; Holmes, A. An ERP study on the time course of emotional face processing. *Neuroreport* **2002**, *13*, 427–431. [CrossRef]
57. Balconi, M.; Pozzoli, U. Face-selective processing and the effect of pleasant and unpleasant emotional expressions on ERP correlates. *Int. J. Psychophysiol.* **2003**, *49*, 67–74. [CrossRef]
58. Raz, N. Aging of the brain and its impact on cognitive performance: Integration of structural and functional findings. In *The Handbook of Aging and Cognition*; Craik, F.I.M., Salthouse, T.A., Eds.; Lawrence Erlbaum Associates Publishers: Mahwah, NJ, USA, 2000; pp. 1–90.
59. Grady, C.L. Functional brain imaging and age-related changes in cognition. *Biol. Psychol.* **2000**, *54*, 259–281. [CrossRef]
60. Halpern, A.R.; Zioga, I.; Shankleman, M.; Lindsen, J.; Pearce, M.T.; Bhattacharya, J. That note sounds wrong! Age-related effects in processing of musical expectation. *Brain Cogn.* **2017**, *113*, 1–9. [CrossRef]

61. Johannsen, P.; Jakobsen, J.; Bruhn, P.; Hansen, S.B.; Gee, A.; Stødkilde-Jørgensen, H.; Gjedde, A. Cortical sites of sustained and divided attention in normal elderly humans. *Neuroimage* **1997**, *6*, 145–155. [CrossRef]
62. Madden, D.J.; Turkington, T.G.; Provenzale, J.M.; Hawk, T.C.; Hoffman, J.M.; Coleman, R.E. Selective and divided visual attention: Age-related changes in regional cerebral blood flow measured by H2 15O PET. *Hum. Brain Mapp.* **1997**, *5*, 389–409. [CrossRef]
63. Anderson, N.D.; Iidaka, T.; Cabeza, R.; Kapur, S.; McIntosh, A.R.; Craik, F.I. The effects of divided attention on encoding-and retrieval-related brain activity: A PET study of younger and older adults. *J. Cogn. Neurosci.* **2000**, *12*, 775–792. [CrossRef] [PubMed]
64. Hartley, A.A.; Speer, N.K.; Jonides, J.; Reuter-Lorenz, P.A.; Smith, E.E. Is the dissociability of working memory systems for name identity, visual-object identity, and spatial location maintained in old age? *Neuropsychology* **2001**, *15*, 3. [CrossRef] [PubMed]
65. Mitchell, K.J.; Johnson, M.K.; Raye, C.L.; Mather, M.; D'esposito, M. Aging and reflective processes of working memory: Binding and test load deficits. *Psychol. Aging* **2000**, *15*, 527. [CrossRef] [PubMed]
66. Smith, E.E.; Geva, A.; Jonides, J.; Miller, A.; Reuter-Lorenz, P.; Koeppe, R.A. The neural basis of task-switching in working memory: Effects of performance and aging. *Proc. Natl. Acad. Sci. USA* **2001**, *98*, 2095–2100. [CrossRef] [PubMed]
67. Gazzaley, A.; Cooney, J.W.; Rissman, J.; D'Esposito, M. Top-down suppression deficit underlies working memory impairment in normal aging. *Nat. Neurosci.* **2005**, *8*, 1298–1300. [CrossRef] [PubMed]
68. Phelps, E.A.; Ling, S.; Carrasco, M. Emotion facilitates perception and potentiates the perceptual benefits of attention. *Psychol. Sci.* **2006**, *17*, 292–299. [CrossRef]
69. Houston, J.R.; Pollock, J.W.; Lien, M.C.; Allen, P.A. Emotional arousal deficit or emotional regulation bias? An electrophysiological study of age-related differences in emotion perception. *Exp. Aging Res.* **2018**, *44*, 187–205. [CrossRef]
70. Schupp, H.T.; Cuthbert, B.N.; Bradley, M.M.; Cacioppo, J.T.; Ito, T.; Lang, P.J. Affective picture processing: The late positive potential is modulated by motivational relevance. *Psychophysiology* **2000**, *37*, 257–261. [CrossRef]
71. Van der Gaag, C.; Minderaa, R.B.; Keysers, C. Facial expressions: What the mirror neuron system can and cannot tell us. *Soc. Neurosci.* **2007**, *2*, 179–222. [CrossRef]
72. Jabbi, M.; Keysers, C. Inferior frontal gyrus activity triggers anterior insula response to emotional facial expressions. *Emotion* **2008**, *8*, 775. [CrossRef]
73. Kriegeskorte, N.; Simmons, W.K.; Bellgowan, P.S.; Baker, C.I. Circular analysis in systems neuroscience: The dangers of double dipping. *Nat. Neurosci.* **2009**, *12*, 535. [CrossRef] [PubMed]
74. Fusar-Poli, P.; Placentino, A.; Carletti, F.; Landi, P.; Allen, P.; Surguladze, S.; Benedetti, F.; Abbamonte, M.; Gasparotti, R.; Barale, F.; et al. Functional atlas of emotional faces processing: A voxel-based meta-analysis of 105 functional magnetic resonance imaging studies. *J. Psychiatry Neurosci.* **2009**, *34*, 418–432. [PubMed]
75. Kesler, M.L.; Andersen, A.H.; Smith, C.D.; Avison, M.J.; Davis, C.E.; Kryscio, R.J.; Blonder, L.X. Neural substrates of facial emotion processing using fMRI. *Cogn. Brain Res.* **2001**, *11*, 213–226. [CrossRef]

16

Cytoplasmic and Mitochondrial NADPH-Coupled Redox Systems in the Regulation of Aging

Patrick C. Bradshaw

Department of Biomedical Sciences, James H. Quillen College of Medicine, East Tennessee State University, Johnson City, TN 37614, USA; bradshawp@etsu.edu

Abstract: The reduced form of nicotinamide adenine dinucleotide phosphate (NADPH) protects against redox stress by providing reducing equivalents to antioxidants such as glutathione and thioredoxin. NADPH levels decline with aging in several tissues, but whether this is a major driving force for the aging process has not been well established. Global or neural overexpression of several cytoplasmic enzymes that synthesize NADPH have been shown to extend lifespan in model organisms such as *Drosophila* suggesting a positive relationship between cytoplasmic NADPH levels and longevity. Mitochondrial NADPH plays an important role in the protection against redox stress and cell death and mitochondrial NADPH-utilizing thioredoxin reductase 2 levels correlate with species longevity in cells from rodents and primates. Mitochondrial NADPH shuttles allow for some NADPH flux between the cytoplasm and mitochondria. Since a decline of nicotinamide adenine dinucleotide (NAD^+) is linked with aging and because $NADP^+$ is exclusively synthesized from NAD^+ by cytoplasmic and mitochondrial NAD^+ kinases, a decline in the cytoplasmic or mitochondrial NADPH pool may also contribute to the aging process. Therefore pro-longevity therapies should aim to maintain the levels of both NAD^+ and NADPH in aging tissues.

Keywords: NADPH; aging; redox; lifespan; longevity; mitochondrial; NADP; nicotinamide adenine dinucleotide phosphate; glutathione; thioredoxin; *Drosophila*; *C. elegans*

---

1. NADPH and the Redox Theories of Aging

The reduced form of nicotinamide adenine dinucleotide phosphate, NADPH, protects cells from redox stress and is required for the synthesis of fatty acids, cholesterol, and deoxynucleotides. NADPH is also required for steroid biosynthesis and protects cells from toxic metabolites by providing reducing power to cytochrome P450 enzymes. NADPH levels decrease with age [1,2] due to both aging-related loss of nicotinamide adenine dinucleotide (NAD^+) [3], a precursor for its synthesis, and to the aging related increase in the $[NADP^+]/[NADPH]$ ratio that occurs as a result of oxidative stress due to increased mitochondrial electron transport chain dysfunction [4] and inflammation [5]. Therapies that increase NAD^+ levels combined with therapies that increase NADPH levels could greatly benefit subjects with aging-related disorders. This type of combination therapy has already been shown to be better than either monotherapy alone in an animal model of ischemic stroke [6]. The major objectives of this review are to discuss the mechanisms contributing to the aging-related loss of NADPH, to detail the mechanisms regulating the cytoplasmic and mitochondrial $[NADP^+]/[NADPH]$, and to give an update on enzymes of the NADPH-powered redox systems that have been identified to modulate lifespan.

The mitochondrial free radical theory of aging (MFRTA) has been a leading theory of aging for nearly 50 years [7] and states that increased levels of mitochondrial reactive oxygen species (ROS) stimulate aging. It therefore suggests that antioxidants and NADPH, which is used for the recycling of many antioxidants, will protect cells from mitochondrial generated ROS to delay tissue and organismal aging. Over the past two decades data has shown that ROS-mediated signaling events in young and healthy organisms can lead to lifespan extension, instead of lifespan decline as was originally proposed by the MFRTA [8]. There are also many experimental results that appear to refute the MFRTA [9]. For example, overexpression of antioxidant enzymes, such as superoxide dismutase (SOD) [10] or catalase [11], or administration of antioxidant supplements, such as vitamins C (ascorbate) [12] or E (tocopherols) [13], do not extend lifespan in several model organisms, although there are exceptions to this statement [14–16], the most notable being expression of mitochondrial-targeted catalase extending the lifespan of mice [17].

The fact that many supplemented antioxidants or overexpression of SODs or catalase do not generally extend lifespan could be explained if the activities of the NADPH-fueled redox systems are limiting factors for the protection against lifespan-shortening redox stress and that the activities of SODs and catalase are not limiting. However, it is acknowledged that SOD1 or SOD2 must first detoxify the superoxide produced from the mitochondrial electron transport chain (ETC) to H_2O_2 before the NADPH-linked redox systems can detoxify the H_2O_2 to water. In addition it is evident that SOD2 plays an essential role in ROS detoxification in newborns due to the death of SOD2 knockout mice shortly after birth [18]. NADPH is required for optimal catalase activity as it binds and stabilizes the catalase tetramer [19]. Antioxidant vitamins such as vitamins C or E that rely upon NADPH to be recycled to their active reduced forms would be expected to provide little longevity benefit in aged organisms where NADPH levels have declined to such an extent to prevent their efficient recycling. The Redox Stress Theory of Aging [20] and the Redox Theory of Aging [21] suggest that lifespan is regulated by redox changes, including alterations in the [$NADP^+$]/[NADPH], GSSG/GSH (oxidized glutathione disulfide/reduced glutathione), and oxidized thioredoxin/reduced thioredoxin ratios. These theories also highlight the ability of redox changes to influence aging by not only altering oxidative damage, but by altering cell signaling. Examples of this include the activation of the lifespan-extending transcriptional regulators DAF-16/FOXO and SKN-1/Nrf2 in *C. elegans* by compounds that stimulate ROS production [22,23].

Much data obtained over the past two decades greatly support the MFRTA-derived redox-based theories of aging including the strong negative correlation between the rate of mitochondrial superoxide generation and lifespan in closely related species [24], the strong positive correlation between phospholipid fatty acid saturation levels and lifespan, and the negative correlation between the frequency of cysteine residues in mitochondrial electron transport chain transmembrane spanning regions and lifespan [25]. The higher fatty acid saturation in longer lived species likely evolved to prevent the ROS-mediated oxidation of fatty acid double bonds [26], while the depletion of mitochondrial inner transmembrane cysteine residues likely evolved to prevent thiyl radical formation and potentially lifespan shortening protein crosslinking that can occur when superoxide reacts with protein sulfhydryl groups [27]. The mitochondrial inner membrane is enriched with the phospholipid cardiolipin, which is essential for ETC function and ADP/ATP transport and due to its high degree of fatty acid unsaturation is especially vulnerable to ROS-mediated damage [28].

2. Loss of NAD^+ as a Major Cause for Loss of NADPH With Aging

One cause for the aging-related loss of NADPH and increase in oxidative stress with aging is the decrease in the levels of cellular NAD^+ [3], the immediate precursor for the synthesis of $NADP^+$ by NAD^+ kinases. NAD^+ levels decline with aging in mammals for several reasons, one of which is the aging-related decrease in the salvage pathway of NAD^+ synthesis as a result of decreased expression of nicotinamide phosphoribosyl transferase (NAMPT) [29], a committed step in this pathway. There is also an increase in NAD^+ degradation with aging. The decreased NAD^+ levels may be a cause of sirtuin protein deacetylase-dependent [30,31] or sirtuin-independent alterations in mitochondrial ETC activity that results in increased ROS production and increased nuclear DNA damage that activates poly-ADP-ribose polymerase (PARP) in several aged tissues including liver, heart, kidney, and lung [32]. This PARP activation together with the aging-related increase in expression and activity of the NAD^+ and $NADP^+$ hydrolyzing enzyme CD38 [33] lead to increased hydrolysis of NAD^+ and $NADP^+$ in aged tissues. CD38 was shown to have greater activity (6-fold lower K_m and 2-fold higher V_{max}) using $NADP^+$ as a substrate than NAD^+ [34,35]. PARP activation also leads to decreased NADPH levels as PARP inhibits hexokinase, the first enzyme of glycolysis also required for glucose flux into the NADPH-generating pentose phosphate pathway (PPP) [36].

In brain, SARM1 is another NADase that contributes to the loss of NAD^+ under pathological conditions [37]. But whether or not SARM1 is activated in aged brain has yet to be studied in mammals. There are no homologs of CD38 present in the genomes of the aging models *Drosophila* or *C. elegans*, but both genomes encode homologs of PARP and SARM1 [38]. Expression of the *Drosophila* homolog of SARM1 increased during aging or mitochondrial ETC inhibition and was shown to play a role in inducing a pro-inflammatory state [39]. $NADP^+$ phosphatase activities, resulting in the degradation of $NADP^+$ to NAD^+, have also been observed in rat liver mitochondrial and Golgi extracts [40,41], but the proteins responsible these activities or any aging-related changes in enzyme activity levels have yet to be identified.

Nematodes and insects, as with other invertebrates, lack NAMPT homologs and the two-step NAD^+ salvage pathway present in vertebrates, but instead possess a four-step salvage pathway. In this pathway, nicotinamide is first deaminated to nicotinic acid by a nicotinamidase and then the 3-step Preiss–Handler pathway for NAD^+ salvage synthesis from nicotinic acid is employed [42,43]. In addition, like mammals, *C. elegans* can synthesize NAD^+ through a de novo pathway from tryptophan [44]. The *Drosophila* genome lacks a 3-hydroxyanthanilic acid dioxygenase gene encoding an enzyme that synthesizes quinolinic acid in the de novo NAD^+ synthesis pathway [45]. Therefore *Drosophila* appears to strictly rely upon the salvage pathway for NAD^+ synthesis.

Several lines of evidence suggest that loss of NAD^+ and NADPH may play a role in the aging of *Drosophila* and *C. elegans*. The NAD^+/NADH ratio declines with aging in both species [46,47], while in *C. elegans* this loss was driven almost entirely by a decrease in NAD^+ levels. Since greater than 80% of pyridine nucleotides are bound to proteins and not free in solution [48], the (free) $[NAD^+]/[NADH]$ as measured by the pyruvate/lactate ratio is a much better functional indicator than measuring total levels. In aging *C. elegans* a loss of (free) $[NAD^+]/[NADH]$ also paralleled the loss in total NAD^+/NADH [46]. Addition of NAD^+ (10 μM–1 mM) [49], nicotinamide (0.2 mM), or nicotinamide riboside (0.5 mM) [50] to the culture medium extended lifespan in *C. elegans*, even though the *C. elegans* genome apparently lacks a nicotinamide riboside kinase gene to convert nicotinamide riboside to nicotinamide mononucleotide. But *C. elegans* possesses homologs to purine nucleoside phosphorylase (PNP) and methylthioadenosine phosphorylase (MTAP) that can likely catabolize nicotinamide riboside to nicotinamide for synthesis of NAD^+ synthesis through the salvage pathway [51].

The decreased nuclear NAD^+ levels with aging in mouse muscle lead to stabilization of hypoxia inducible factor-1α (HIF-1α) and decreased c-Myc-induced expression of mitochondrial targeted genes, including mitochondrial transcription factor A (TFAM), required for mitochondrial ETC function [52]. Decreased ETC complex I function with aging increases mitochondrial NADH and decreases mitochondrial NAD^+ levels, which likely results in decreased phosphorylation of NAD^+ to $NADP^+$ by mitochondrial NAD^+ kinase 2 (NADK2). Decreased ETC function with aging also reduces the proton-motive force across the mitochondrial inner membrane, which decreases mitochondrial nicotinamide nucleotide transhydrogenase (NNT)-mediated synthesis of NADPH and NAD^+ from $NADP^+$ and NADH in the matrix space.

The increase in cytoplasmic and mitochondrial $[NADP^+]/[NADPH]$ with aging decreases the activities of cytoplasmic and mitochondrial glutathione reductase (GSR) and thioredoxin reductases (cytoplasmic TXNRD1 and mitochondrial TXNRD2), which lead to more oxidized states of the glutathione redox couple (GSSG/GSH) and thioredoxins (cytoplasmic TXN and mitochondrial TXN2), resulting in decreased activities of glutathione peroxidases (GPX) and peroxiredoxins (also called thioredoxin peroxidases). See Figure 1 for an overview of the cytoplasmic and mitochondrial NADPH-linked redox systems. This oxidation of the NADPH-linked redox systems with aging also causes the oxidation of glutaredoxins, ascorbate (vitamin C), and tocopherols (vitamin E) [53] and eventually leads to oxidation of lipids, nucleic acids, and amino acids and the cell and tissue dysfunction that accompanies the aging process.

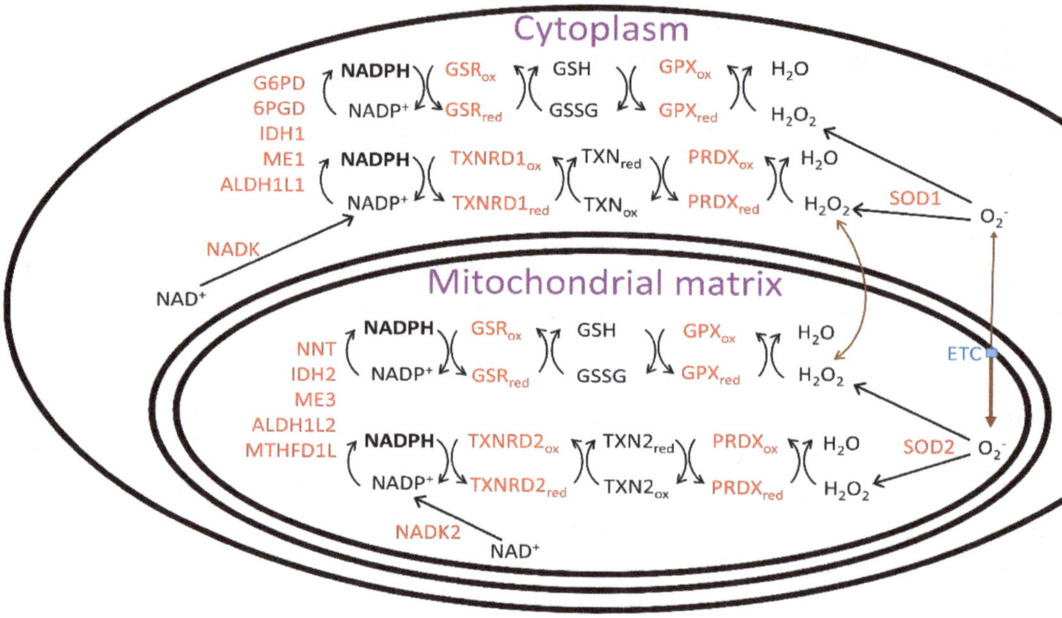

Figure 1. Cytoplasmic and mitochondrial reduced nicotinamide adenine dinucleotide phosphate (NADPH)-linked redox systems. NADK: nicotinamide adenine dinucleotide (NAD^+) kinase; ETC: electron transport chain; GSR: glutathione reductase; GSH: reduced glutathione; GSSG: oxidized glutathione disulfide; GPX: glutathione peroxidase; TXN: thioredoxin; TXNRD: thioredoxin reductase; PRDX: peroxiredoxin; H_2O_2: hydrogen peroxide; O_2^-: superoxide; G6PD: glucose-6-phosphate dehydrogenase; 6PGD: 6-phosphogluconate dehydrogenase; IDH: isocitrate dehydrogenase; ME: malic enzyme ALDH: aldehyde dehydrogenase; MTHFD: methylenetetrahydrofolate dehydrogenase; NNT: nicotinamide nucleotide transhydrogenase.

3. Aging is Associated with Redox Imbalance

All multicellular organisms that have been studied thus far, with the possible exception of extremely long-lived naked mole rats [54], show oxidizing redox changes with aging accompanied by oxidative damage to macromolecules. Redox stress appears to contribute to almost all aging-related disorders including diabetes, heart disease, and neurodegenerative disease. The [$NADP^+$]/[NADPH] redox couple is the most important redox couple in the fight against aging-induced cellular oxidation. The redox potentials of the free cytoplasmic and mitochondrial [$NADP^+$]/[NADPH] are roughly −400 to −20 mV and are the most negative redox potentials in the cell [55,56]. The cytoplasmic and the mitochondrial [NAD^+]/[NADH] couples [57], which are roughly 99.9% and 87% oxidized, respectively, in healthy cells [56,58] become more reduced with aging, while the cytoplasmic and most likely also the mitochondrial [$NADP^+$]/[NADPH] couple, which are both roughly 99% reduced in healthy cells [56,58] become more oxidized with aging. For example, the energy of the cytoplasmic $NADP^+$/NADPH couple became 35 mV less negative with aging corresponding to a 23% loss of brain NADPH levels from 10 to 21 months of age in mice [2]. The initial mechanisms involved in this redox imbalance remain unclear, but at least in the brain the aging-induced redox imbalances may result from the decreased expression of NAMPT and NNT [2].

The GSH/GSSG ratio in cells depends heavily on the [$NADP^+$]/[NADPH], but appears not to be in equilibrium due to the moderate expression level of glutathione reductase, the enzyme that links these couples. The GSH/GSSG is approximately 20:1 to 100:1 (95–99% reduced) [59], while during times of oxidative stress this ratio may drop to 5:1 (80% reduced) or even 1:1 (50% reduced) [60]. Cytoplasmic and mitochondrial GSH levels are 1 to 10 mM, two to three orders of magnitude higher than cytoplasmic and mitochondrial [NADPH] [61,62], due in part to the fact that the vast majority of cellular NADP(H) is bound and not free [63]. In addition in rat liver 59% of the total cellular NADP(H) was reported to be present in mitochondria [58], although mitochondria only make up 10–15% of the cell volume. Therefore it may take many hours to days for cells to completely recover from oxidation of GSH if the cells are able to recover at all [64].

Opposite to the oxidizing effects of aging on the plasma GSSG/GSH and cystine/cysteine ratios [65], the $NADP^+$/NADPH ratio in human plasma has been reported to become more reduced with aging due to increased levels of NADPH, even though $NADP^+$ levels declined [66]. Inhibiting cellular export or stimulating cellular uptake of different forms of vitamin B3 (niacin) may be a strategy to maintain cell and tissue NADPH levels with aging. In this regard supplementation with nicotinamide riboside has been shown to be beneficial to increase plasma NAD^+ levels [67]. No reports of plasma membrane transport of NADP(H) could be found, but intraperitoneal or tail vain injection of NADPH in mice was shown to increase the levels of NADPH in plasma and brain, respectively [68].

In *Drosophila* the $NADP^+$/NADPH increased in late adulthood in parallel with the decline in the NAD^+/NADH [47]. To the best of our knowledge total $NADP^+$ and NADPH levels have not been measured in young and aged *C. elegans*. The isocitrate/alpha-ketoglutarate ratio as a measure of the cytoplasmic [$NADP^+$]/[NADPH] in young and old worms has also yet to be determined. As only one malic enzyme gene is present in *C. elegans* and it contains a mitochondrial targeting signal [69], measurement of the nematode malate/pyruvate ratio will likely not be indicative of the cytoplasmic [$NADP^+$]/[NADPH] as it is in mammals, which possess a cytoplasmic $NADP^+$-dependent malic enzyme (ME1) [56].

4. Reductive Stress Can Influence the Rate of Aging

Although the study of oxidative stress is common, the study of reductive stress is somewhat rare, especially as it pertains to aging. The terms oxidative and reductive stress are somewhat unclear [70] as they do not specifically refer to the [$NADP^+$]/[NADPH] or [NAD^+]/[NADH] couple. Most investigators utilize the term oxidative stress to refer to a state where the [$NADP^+$]/[NADPH], GSSG/GSH, and protein cysteine thiols are more oxidized than the normal healthy condition and reductive stress to mean that these redox couples are more reduced than normal.

Quantification of oxidative stress in lysed cell, tissue, or isolated mitochondrial extracts is frequently performed by measurements of GSSG/GSH. The cytoplasmic or mitochondrial [$NADP^+$]/[NADPH] is slightly more difficult to measure as one must either use a fluorescent probe in intact cells [71] or measure the ratios of specific metabolites that are in equilibrium with the [$NADP^+$]/[NADPH] in lysed cells or tissues [56,58]. Lysed cell measurements of total $NADP^+$/NADPH (or NAD^+/NADH) are not indicative of the free levels as bound nucleotides are released into solution upon lysis [56].

The oxidation state of protein thiols in live cells can be measured using the genetically encoded fluorescent probes roGFP or roGFP2 [72]. High levels of glutaredoxins can equilibrate roGFP or roGFP2 with the redox state of the glutathione pool. Therefore, a roGFP2-glutaredoxin fusion protein was developed and expressed in *Drosophila* to measure the GSSG/GSH with aging [73]. This probe showed a stable, highly reduced cytoplasmic GSSG/GSH with aging, while there was heterogeneous oxidation of the mitochondrial GSSG/GSH in both young and aged fat body, hemocytes, and Malpighian tubules, but a stable reduced GSSG/GSH in young and aged mitochondria from muscles and gut enterocytes [74]. Feeding N-acetylcysteine (NAC) to flies led to reductive stress characterized by slightly decreased cytoplasmic H_2O_2 in gut and increased mitochondrial H_2O_2 in fat, gut, and Malpighian tubules [74].

Further elegant studies using cytoplasmic and mitochondrial targeted roGFP have shown that increasing the reduction of cytoplasmic GSSG/GSH and protein thiols to induce reductive stress as measured by cytoplasmic roGFP leads to production of ROS in mitochondria and oxidative stress as evidenced by oxidation of mitochondrial roGFP [75]. Reducing power in the cytoplasm can be transmitted to the mitochondrial matrix by both the direct transport of GSH into the mitochondrial matrix [76,77] as well as by mitochondrial NADPH shuttles that can transfer NADPH reducing equivalents [78]. A major NADPH shuttle system uses cytoplasmic isocitrate dehydrogenase 1 (IDH1), the mitochondrial tricarboxylate (citrate) carrier, and mitochondrial isocitrate dehydrogenase 2 (IDH2). Once the reducing equivalents are transported into the matrix space, the reduced [$NADP^+$]/NADPH] in the matrix space activates glutathione reductase to reduce the GSSG/GSH and activates thioredoxin reductase to reduce thioredoxin. However, once the mitochondrial GSSG/GSH and thioredoxin pools become highly reduced, superoxide and hydrogen peroxide are generated by the mitochondrial glutathione reductase and thioredoxin reductase enzymes as flavins in these two enzymes produce ROS in the absence of their GSSG and oxidized thioredoxin substrates [79].

Adding 2-deoxyglucose to *C. elegans* culture medium or knocking down expression of the glycolytic enzyme glucose-6-phosphate isomerase, *gpi-1*, to inhibit glycolysis led to lifespan extension [23]. The mechanism of lifespan extension has not been fully established, but the authors showed a transient increase in respiration and ROS production following inhibition of glycolysis and showed that lifespan extension could be blocked by supplemented antioxidants [23]. Therefore, they concluded that a ROS signal mediates lifespan extension. However, others have suggested that the addition of antioxidants may have blocked lifespan extension by inducing reductive stress instead of by quenching ROS [80]. It has also been shown that inhibiting glycolysis stimulates metabolic flux through the PPP to increase NADPH production [81], so the lifespan extension by glycolytic inhibition may also have been due in part to a reduced cytoplasmic [$NADP^+$]/[NADPH] and increased redox defenses that followed the transient increase in ROS production. Studies using yeast where the glycolytic enzyme triose phosphate isomerase was deleted showed a reduced $NADP^+$/NADPH ratio likely due to increased PPP flux, but decreased replicative lifespan [82], perhaps in part due to reductive stress.

In mice reductive stress due to increased NADPH production by the PPP enzyme glucose-6-phosphate dehydrogenase (G6PD) has been shown to be associated with protein aggregation and cardiomyopathy [83]. Reductive stress could also potentially lower the already low levels of cytoplasmic [$NADP^+$] (1–100 nM) to decrease the activity of enzymes that rely upon it to drive metabolism. As cytoplasmic oxidative stress appears to be much more prevalent than reductive stress, especially in aged tissues, it does not appear likely that cytoplasmic reductive stress is a cause of mitochondrial oxidative stress in aging tissues or major aging-related diseases.

5. Could the Low Levels of Cytoplasmic Glutathione Peroxidase Activity in Long-Lived Species Function in the Preservation of [$NADP^+$]/[NADPH] and GSSG/GSH with Aging to Promote Longevity?

Since the redox theories of aging are gaining traction, more detailed studies of the roles of the cytoplasmic and mitochondrial NADPH-glutathione reductase and NADPH-thioredoxin reductase systems in aging are needed. There is also a dearth of knowledge on the mechanisms that cause the mitochondrial ETC of short-lived species to generate more superoxide than that of long-lived species and the mechanisms through which the ETC generates increased levels of superoxide with age [8]. Although compounds that block mitochondrial superoxide production from complex I [84] and complex III [85] without affecting oxidative phosphorylation have recently been identified as potential therapeutics, compounds that stabilize the cytoplasmic and mitochondrial [$NADP^+$]/[NADPH] redox couples to maintain redox defense systems with aging are also desperately needed for clinical trials for aging-related diseases.

Naked mole rats have a mean lifespan over 30 years, at least ten times longer than similarly sized mice, and surprisingly have 70-fold less cellular glutathione peroxidase activity than mice [86]. Glutathione peroxidase detoxifies hydrogen peroxide to water through the oxidation of GSH. Therefore, it is possible that increases in specific types of ROS, such as specific types of peroxides in the cytoplasm, are compatible with increased longevity [86]. An alternative to this hypothesis is that the NADPH-thioredoxin reductase-thioredoxin-peroxiredoxin detoxification system for peroxides is upregulated in naked mole rats to compensate for the low activity of the NADPH-glutathione reductase-GSH-glutathione peroxidase system.

The extremely low glutathione peroxidase activity of naked mole rats may even contribute to their extreme longevity through the preservation of reduced cytoplasmic GSSG/GSH and $[NADP^+]/[NADPH]$. If this is true, the maintained high energy of the $[NADP^+]/[NADPH]$ couple can then be used to stimulate longevity through increasing the activities of NADPH-utilizing enzymes such as glutathione reductase and thioredoxin reductase to combat other types of redox stress, such as that induced by peroxynitrite [87], which if left unchecked could decrease longevity. The increased lifespan of mice heterozygous for glutathione peroxidase-4 [88] and the strong inverse relationship between cellular glutathione peroxidase activity and lifespan in seven different rodent species [86] support a role for maintaining reduced cytoplasmic GSSG/GSH and $[NADP^+]/[NADPH]$ for increased longevity. If only cytoplasmic, but not mitochondrial glutathione peroxidase activity is low in long-lived species, mitochondrial shuttles and glutathione transporters could be used for the increased detoxification of mitochondrial peroxides as a mechanism responsible for the longevity of these species.

Unexpectedly, long lived *Drosophila* strains did not have more GSH than short-lived strains [89]. Likewise, in rodents and in birds there is no correlation between GSSG/GSH in liver and longevity and even a negative relationship was found between liver GSH and longevity [90]. This data suggests that the cytoplasmic NADPH-glutathione reductase-GSH redox system does not limit longevity. As possible compensation for their low GSH levels, liver from naked mole rats contain much higher levels of the cytoplasmically localized thioredoxin reductase (TXNRD1) and major peroxiredoxin (PRDX1) than short-lived guinea pigs [91]. This may be an indication of higher Nrf2 transcriptional activity in naked mole rats [92].

As mentioned above there is also a negative correlation between mitochondrial ETC-produced superoxide production and longevity [8]. Therefore, long-lived species appear to have evolved more efficient ETC machinery that plays an important role in maintaining a reduced intracellular environment. Consistent with this, it was also reported that naked mole rats have greatly decreased levels of proteins for ETC complex I, an important source of ROS, compared to short-lived guinea pigs [91]. However, another report indicated no difference in ETC complex I activity between naked mole rats and mice, but decreased ETC complex II activity in naked mole rats [93]. It was also shown that isolated mitochondria from naked mole rats have a greatly enhanced ability to detoxify hydrogen peroxide compared to those from mice, largely due to higher activity of the mitochondrial NADPH-glutathione reductase-GSH-glutathione peroxidase system [93].

To help resolve some of the current controversies in the field, future studies could focus on measurements of $[NADP^+]/[NADPH]$ and GSSG/GSH in hypothalamus and white adipose tissue in closely related species with different maximal lifespans. These tissues appear have a greater influence on organismal aging than tissues or cells where past measurements have been made [94,95]. Measurements using mitochondria isolated from these tissues would also be important, as only roughly 10–15% of cellular GSH is present in mitochondria [96]. Importantly NADPH has been shown to bind to the 39 kD subunit of ETC complex I to stabilize the complex [97,98] and ETC complex I activity declines with aging [99,100].

6. The NADPH-Thioredoxin Reductase Redox System and Aging

Thioredoxin reductases use NADPH to reduce oxidized thioredoxin. In the cytoplasm TXNRD1 reduces TXN and in mitochondria TXNRD2 reduces TXN2 [101]. Double heterozygous knock out mice ($TXN^{+/-}/TXN2^{+/-}$) were surprisingly long-lived [102] suggesting that TXN or TXN2 levels do not limit lifespan, although follow up studies should be performed to determine if compensatory reductions of other redox couples such as the $NADP^+/NADPH$ or GSSG/GSH are responsible for the increased longevity. Transgenic TXN or TXN2 mice show increased mean, but not maximal lifespan [102,103]. Overexpression of TXN and TXN2 together surprisingly led to decreased lifespan [101] suggesting that redox signaling occurs between the cytoplasmic and mitochondrial compartments.

Therapies that maintain a reduced [$NADP^+$]/[NADPH] in the cytoplasm or mitochondria of aged organisms, but without inducing excessive reductive stress are promising longevity therapies. Longevity studies using mice overexpressing TXNRD1 or TXNRD2 would aid our understanding of the role that these proteins play in mammalian longevity. Mitochondrial TXNRD2 is an especially promising candidate to overexpress or deplete in mice for aging studies because protein levels and activities in fibroblasts positively correlate with longevity across multiple rodent and primate species [104]. Overexpression of the *Drosophila* homolog of TXNRD2, Trxr-2, extended median lifespan [104], while overexpression of the mostly cytoplasmic, but partially mitochondrial *Drosophila* thioredoxin reductase Trxr-1 did not extend lifespan during normoxia [105], but it did during hyperoxia [106]. Further evidence for a role of the mitochondrial TXNRD2-TXN2 system in enhanced longevity is that growth hormone downregulates the expression of these two genes in liver and growth-hormone deficient Ames dwarf mice are long-lived [107].

In rat brain mitochondria that naturally lack catalase, roughly 75% of the hydrogen peroxide generated was shown to be detoxified by the NADPH-TXNRD2-TXN2-peroxiredoxin system, while only 25% was detoxified by the NADPH-glutathione reductase-GSH-glutathione peroxidase system [108]. This result was quite surprising given that GSH is present at roughly 100-1,000 fold higher levels than Txn2 in mitochondria [109]. In addition to reducing oxidized thioredoxin, thioredoxin reductases can reduce dehydroascorbate [110], ubiquinone [111], cytochrome c [112], lipoamide, lipoic acid, [113], and lipid hydroperoxides [114], which also may play a role in the regulation of lifespan.

Knockdown of *C. elegans* cytoplasmic thioredoxin reductase *trxr-1* [115,116] or mitochondrial thioredoxin reductase *trxr-2* [117] by RNA interference decreased lifespan. However, deletion of *trxr-1* did not affect lifespan [117], while deletion of *trx-2* decreased lifespan at 25 °C, a temperature at the high end of the normal culture range, but not at 20 °C, the most typical culture temperature [117]. TRXR-2 was found to be protective against beta-amyloid toxicity in a *C. elegans* Alzheimer's disease model [118], while TRXR-1 was found to be protective against 6-hydroxydopamine toxicity in a nematode Parkinson's disease model [119].

C. elegans peroxiredoxin *prdx-2*, homologous to human PRDX1, was required for the lifespan extension that occurs in *daf-2* insulin receptor-deficient worms [120] or when metformin was added to the culture medium [121]. The *prdx-2* gene was also required for the longevity that was induced by exposing *C. elegans* larvae to a 25 °C temperature when the culture temperature was otherwise kept at 15 °C [122]. However PRDX-2 did not become oxidized during the normal aging process in *C. elegans* [123], so its role in lifespan extension could be independent of redox changes.

Perhaps the redox enzyme with the strongest connection with longevity in invertebrates is methionine sulfoxide reductase A (MSRA). During oxidative stress, methionine is oxidized to methionine sulfoxide. MSRA catalyzes the reduction of methionine sulfoxide back to methionine. But MSRA must be reduced by the NADPH-thioredoxin reductase-thioredoxin system to be recycled for use [124]. There are two types of genes that encode isoforms of methione sulfoxide reductase, A and B, that each reduces one of the two isomers of methione sulfoxide. MSRA has been more closely linked with lifespan extension and uses both free methionine sulfoxide and the methionine sulfoxide present in proteins as substrates, while MSRB can only the use methionine-sulfoxide present in proteins [125]. MSRA is present in the cytoplasm, mitochondria and nucleus [126], while there are 3 genes in mammals encoding MSRBs, where the gene products localize to the cytoplasm, mitochondria, nucleus, and ER [126].

Knockdown of the *C. elegans* homolog of MSRA called *msra-1* decreased lifespan [127], likely due to an increase in protein unfolding and proteotoxicity when methionine sulfoxide cannot be repaired. *Msra-1* is induced by the pro-longevity transcription factor DAF-16/FOXO that becomes activated when insulin signaling is blocked. Knockdown of *msra-1* in long-lived *daf-2* insulin receptor mutant worms decreased lifespan. *Drosophila* that simultaneously lack both MSRA and MSRB are short-lived [128], while overexpression of the *Drosophila* homolog of MSRA, mostly in neurons, extended lifespan [129] and stimulated nuclear translocation of dFOXO [130]. However, in mice overexpression of MSRA in either the cytoplasm or mitochondria did not extend lifespan [131]. This may be due to the fact that *Drosophila* MSRA lacks methionine oxidase activity while mammalian MSRA contains methionine oxidase activity [132].

7. The NADPH-Glutathione Reductase Redox System and Aging

By analyzing data from multiple rodent and primate species, a positive association between glutathione reductase (GSR) protein levels (and activity) and lifespan in fibroblasts was found [104]. But a negative correlation between brain glutathione reductase activity and lifespan was found in another study [133]. *Drosophila* lacks a glutathione reductase gene and its function is replaced by the two thioredoxin reductase genes [134]. However, *C. elegans* studies of the NADPH-glutathione reductase redox system and aging have been performed. Like mammals *C. elegans* contain only one glutathione reductase gene *gsr-1* that generates both cytoplasmic and mitochondrial protein variants [135]. Lifespan extension of 18% occurred following overexpression [136]. Knockout of *gsr-1* was lethal as it is required for molting [137]. Transgenic overexpression of the cytoplasmic isoform but not the mitochondrial isoform rescued lethality [135]. Knockdown of *gsr-1* by RNAi resulted in decreased lifespan and increased sensitivity to the superoxide generator juglone. Decreased GSR-1 levels may decrease lifespan in part through decreasing autophagy and increasing proteotoxicity [138].

Global low level overexpression of the catalytic subunit of glutamate-cysteine ligase (GCL_C), the rate-limiting step in glutathione synthesis, or high level overexpression in neurons has also been shown to increase lifespan in *Drosophila* by up to 50%, while overexpression of the regulatory subunit of GCL increased lifespan by up to 24% [139,140]. Administering a recombinant glutaredoxin (small protein reduced by GSH) to *C. elegans* culture medium was shown to extend lifespan dependent upon upregulation of the pro-longevity transcriptional regulator heat shock factor-1 (HSF-1) [141]. Deletion of either of the yeast glutaredoxin genes Grx1 or Grx2 decreased chronological longevity by increasing ROS production that activated Ras-protein kinase A signaling. Therefore, altered redox status and glutaredoxin function modulates lifespan through the activation of longevity regulating signaling pathways.

Surprisingly, young naked mole rats have been shown to have a more oxidized liver GSSG/GSH than mice [142], even though the naked mole rats live much longer. But the naked mole rats did not show increased levels of oxidative damage with aging as was shown in mice [54]. In mice and rats, important redox couples have been shown to be maintained at distinct, non-equilibrium potentials in different subcellular compartments [143]. The mitochondrial [$NADP^+$]/[[NADPH] couple has been estimated to be around −419 mV compared to −400 mV for the cytoplasmic couple [58]. The mitochondrial GSSG/GSH couple was estimated to be between −280 and -330 mV [144–146], while the cytoplasmic couple was estimated to be between −200 and −260 mV [145]. So the existing data on GSSG/GSH ratios cannot be used to estimate cytoplasmic or mitochondrial [$NADP^+$]/[NADPH]. Therefore, the cytoplasmic and/or mitochondrial [$NADP^+$]/[NADPH] may not decline with aging in naked mole rats as they do in mice to drive longevity through maintaining thioredoxin and glutathione reductase activities in one or both of these compartments. Since several markers of oxidative damage, such as urinary isoprostanes (marker of lipid peroxidation) and liver malondialdehyde (marker of lipid damage) are higher in aged naked mole rats than in aged mice [54], naked mole rat redox potential is likely only maintained with aging in one or more specific subcellular compartments and not the entire cell as a whole.

Identifying the redox events that drive the aging process is a high priority. Measurements using isolated mitochondria may be required if the redox events that regulate aging are mostly confined to this organelle [107]. Some data suggest that the mitochondrial [$NADP^+$]/[NADPH] redox systems may play a role in longevity regulation, but further studies manipulating the mitochondrial [$NADP^+$]/[NADPH], GSSG/GSH, and oxidized thioredoxin/reduced thioredoxin ratios and monitoring lifespan are required to obtain a better understanding of how the activity of the NADPH-powered mitochondrial redox systems influence lifespan.

8. Evidence for the Regulation of Longevity by the NADPH-Powered Redox Systems in *Drosophila*

Data supporting the importance of the NADPH-powered redox networks in the regulation of *Drosophila* longevity include overexpression of glucose-6-phosphate dehydrogenase (G6PD), an NADPH-generating enzyme of the oxidative PPP, increasing lifespan by up to 50% [147]. Expression from a neuronal-specific promoter was able to extend lifespan by up to 40%. Longer-lived strains of *Drosophila* were shown to have higher G6PD activity than shorter-lived strains [148]. Knockdown of ribose-5-phosphate isomerase, an enzyme of the non-oxidative portion of the PPP, increased G6PD and NADPH levels and lifespan by over 30% [149]. Overexpression of the NADPH-generating cytoplasmic malic enzyme (Men) [150] extended lifespan in *Drosophila* as well [151,152]. Overexpression of Men, either throughout lifespan or only during larval development, was able to stimulate longevity, while adulthood only expression in the fat body did not extend lifespan. Surprisingly ROS production was increased when overexpression occurred during larval development that increased stress resistance during adulthood. The data suggest that cytoplasmic reductive stress may have been responsible for the increased mitochondrial ROS production during larval development resulting in the lifespan extension. Men, cytoplasmic isocitrate dehydrogenase (Idh), and G6PD have been shown to form a network maintaining cytoplasmic NADPH levels stable with Men having a slightly larger role than either of the other two enzymes [153].

It will be important to determine if overexpression of G6PD only during larval development increases cytoplasmic reductive stress and mitochondrial ROS production during this time period to increase lifespan. Also, it will be important to determine if overexpression of Pug/Pugilist, a cytoplasmic NADPH-generating methylenetetrahydrofolate dehydrogenase enzyme [154,155] extends lifespan. However, these results may be difficult to interpret as targeted overexpression of Nmdmc, a mitochondrial NADH-generating methylenetetrahydrofolate dehydrogenase gene, in the fat body also extended lifespan [156]. Lastly, much information could be gained by determining the effects of overexpression of *Drosophila* mitochondrial NADPH-generating malic enzyme (Men-b) on lifespan. The *Drosophila* genome also contains two other uncharacterized malic enzyme-like genes Menl-1 and Menl-2 whose gene products also likely have a mitochondrial localization [157].

Further data linking NADPH levels with increased lifespan in *Drosophila* include the association between longevity and a specific allele of the cytoplasmic NADPH-generating isocitrate dehydrogenase gene Idh [158] and flies that were selected for a long lifespan showing increased activities of several NADPH-generating enzymes [159]. Interestingly, *Drosophila* lacks homologs to mammalian mitochondrial NADPH-generating isocitrate dehydrogenase (IDH2) and NADPH-generating mitochondrial nicotinamide nucleotide transhydrogenase (NNT), while homologs of both are present in *C. elegans*. However, a proteomics experiment identified the mostly cytoplasmic Idh protein as being present in *Drosophila* mitochondria [160]. Therefore, *Drosophila* likely depends heavily on malic enzyme (Men-b) and the mitochondrial localized fraction of Idh for mitochondrial NADPH production.

There are seven peroxiredoxin genes in *Drosophila*. Overexpression of three different *Drosophila* peroxiredoxin (thioredoxin peroxidase) genes has been shown to extend lifespan. When expressed in neurons dPrx1/Jafrac1, homologous to mammalian PRDX2, increased lifespan up to 29% [161]. *Drosophila* dPrx5 is endogenously localized to multiple subcellular compartments including the cytoplasm, nucleus, and mitochondria. Global overexpression increased lifespan by more than 30% [162]. Overexpression of dPrx5 specifically in mitochondria also extended lifespan [163]. dPrx3 is exclusively expressed in mitochondria. Although dPrx3 overexpression did not lead to lifespan extension, a dPrx3/dPrx5 double knockout showed premature aging phenotypes [164,165]. dPrx4 is endogenously localized to the ER, and moderate global overexpression or high level overexpression in neurons increased lifespan by greater than 30% [166]. Therefore, the NADPH-thioredoxin reductase-thioredoxin-peroxiredoxin network plays an important role in regulating aging in *Drosophila*.

9. Evidence for the Regulation of Longevity by the NADPH-Powered Redox Systems in Mammals

The study of NADPH synthesis in mammalian cells and tissues is complex as it synthesis is shared among at least 5 cytoplasmic enzymes including G6PD, 6PGD (6-phosphogluconate dehydrogenase), IDH1 (isocitrate dehydrogenase 1), ME1 (malic enzyme 1), and ALDH1L1 (10-formyltetrahydrofolate dehydrogenase) and 5 mitochondrial enzymes NNT, IDH2, ME3 (malic enzyme 3), ALDH1L2 (10-formyltetrahydrofolate dehydrogenase), and MTHFD1L (methylenetetrahydrofolate dehydrogenase 1 like) [167] (Figure 1). ALDH1L1, ALDH1L2, and MTHFD1L play a role in one-carbon and folate metabolism [167], and are an important source of NADPH in proliferating cells [168], where ribonucleotide reductase-mediated deoxynucleotide synthesis utilizes reducing equivalents from the NADPH-thioredoxin reductase-thioredoxin redox system. Overexpression of G6PD increased the mean lifespan of female mice [169].

Levels and activities of NADPH generating enzymes are altered by aging. For example, G6PD levels were shown to decline with aging in mouse brain [170], rat liver [171,172] and human erythrocytes [173], but not lymphocytes [174]. Activity of the PPP enzyme 6PGD was shown to decline by 26% with aging due to lysine oxidation, while malic enzyme activity declined 36% with aging due to histidine oxidation [175]. Activities of IDH1 and IDH2 decreased with aging in rat kidney, but increased with aging in rat testes [176]. Both of these changes were prevented by lifespan-extending calorie restriction (CR). The C57B/6J strain of mice was identified to contain a mutation in the NNT gene, but this strain has a longer lifespan than many other inbred strains. So it appears that the mice are able to compensate for the loss of NNT function and synthesize sufficient NADPH for proper mitochondrial function, at least under normal, non-stressed conditions [177].

Reducing the cytoplasmic $[NADP^+]/[NADPH]$ may not be beneficial for maintaining a reduced cellular redox environment in all cell types as NADPH oxidase enzymes use NADPH to produce superoxide, and sometimes also hydrogen peroxide [178]. For example, NADPH oxidase Nox2 complexes are present at high levels in macrophages and microglia and function to increase superoxide production. Most NADPH oxidase isoforms are not constitutively active, but require a signal such as increased Ca^{2+} levels for activation. However, the Nox4 isoform is widely expressed, constitutively active, and present in intracellular membranes such as those of mitochondria, ER, and the nucleus. Nox4 produces mostly hydrogen peroxide that is membrane permeable instead of superoxide that is not [179]. Nox4 has a K_m for NADPH of 55 μM [180], while human glutathione reductase has a K_m for NADPH of ~9 μM [181], and human cytoplasmic thioredoxin reductase (TXNRD1) has a K_m for NADPH of 18 μM. Cytoplasmic NADPH has been measured to be at a concentration of 3 μM in transformed cells, while mitochondrial NADPH was measured to be 37 μM in the same cells [61]. Therefore Nox4 activity is likely to be low under normal conditions, but would increase if Nox4 localized to the inner mitochondrial membrane with the active site facing the matrix space where increased levels of NADPH are present.

Stress increases Nox4 levels and increased Nox4 levels can lead to ETC complex I instability [182]. In addition dominant-negative Nox4 expression caused cytoplasmic reductive stress and increased mitochondrial ROS production, while Nox4 overexpression led to cytoplasmic oxidative stress. Although Nox4 appears to regulate mitochondrial ETC function and ROS production in heart and endothelial cells [183,184], Nox4 knockout mice have a normal lifespan [185]. This is likely due to the low levels of mitochondrial Nox4 in many tissues under normal, healthy conditions [186]. But increased Nox4 expression has been shown to contribute to hydrogen peroxide-induced senescence of endothelial cells [183].

10. Evidence for the Regulation of Longevity by the NADPH-Powered Redox Systems in Budding Yeast

When *S. cerevisiae* cells are cultured with glucose as the carbon source the majority of cytoplasmic NADPH was produced by the PPP enzyme Zwf1 (G6PD) and acetaldehyde dehydrogenase Ald6 [187], although the PPP 6PGD enzymes Gnd1 and Gnd2 also contributed to a certain extent [188]. When the yeast cells were cultured using a nonfermentable carbon source instead of glucose, levels of cytoplasmic isocitrate dehydrogenase Idp2 increased and it became an important source of cytoplasmic NADPH [189]. Deletion of Ald6 was shown to increase the chronological longevity of yeast [190].

Most mitochondrial NADPH in yeast is generated by the mitochondrial NADH kinase Pos5. Pos5 also contains an NAD^+ kinase activity and the Pos5 NAD^+ kinase activity followed by the activity of the NADPH-generating Ald4 acetaldehyde dehydrogenase, homologous to human ALDH2, was also shown to play a role in mitochondrial NADPH production. Deletion of Ald4 in yeast increased chronological lifespan [191]. Unlike multicellular eukaryotes, yeast mitochondrial malic enzyme Mae1 and mitochondrial $NADP^+$-dependent isocitrate dehydrogenase Idp1 only appeared to play minor roles in mitochondrial NADPH generation [187]. Like *Drosophila*, budding yeast lack a homolog to mammalian mitochondrial NNT. In yeast, mitochondrial transporters of NAD^+ (Ndt1 and Ndt2) provide the vast majority of NAD^+ for mitochondrial NADP(H) synthesis. Ndt1/Ndt2 double deletion mutants showed decreased mitochondrial and cellular NAD(H) levels and increased chronological lifespan, while Ndt1 overexpression resulted in increased mitochondrial and cellular NAD(H) levels and decreased chronological lifespan [192].

In chronologically aged *S. cerevisiae* cells, NADPH levels and levels of reduced cytoplasmic thioredoxin reductase drop before the majority of cysteine oxidation in proteins and before increased ROS production, while anti-aging dietary restriction (DR) delayed the oxidation of NADPH and thioredoxin reductase and extended lifespan [193]. Therefore, the drop in NADPH levels could be a key driving force in postmitotic cell aging that leads to redox stress. Consistent with this data, deletion of Zwf1 [194] or the cytoplasmic thioredoxin reductase Trr1 decreased chronological longevity when using a strain of the α haploid mating type (MATα), which may be a result of the inverse relationship between thioredoxin reductase activity and the activity of longevity controlling TORC1 kinase [195]. The chronologically short-lived MATα Zwf1 deletion strain had both increased $NADP^+/NADPH$ and increased $NAD^+/NADH$ demonstrating that the pro-aging effects of NADPH depletion were dominant over the pro-longevity effects of increased $NAD^+/NADH$ in this context [194]. However, deletion of the Zwf1 gene increased chronological lifespan when a strain of the a mating type (MATa) was used [196]. Since deletion of NADPH-generating enzymes in yeast generally led to increased longevity, a lifespan-extending signaling pathway appears to be activated by increased $NADP^+/NADPH$. Other studies in yeast have shown that the heat shock-induced increase in replicative longevity was due to a transient increase in superoxide levels that signaled for the redirection of metabolic flux from glycolysis to the PPP to increase NADPH synthesis and GSH levels [197].

There are three different NADPH-generating isocitrate dehydrogenase genes in *S. cerevisiae*. Idp1 is mitochondrial, Idp2 is cytoplasmic as mentioned above, and Idp3 is peroxisomal. Deletion of each of these 3 genes increased replicative lifespan in a MATα strain [198,199], while deletion of Idp2 or Idp3 decreased replicative lifespan in a MATa strain. Deletion of Idp1 increased chronological longevity in a MATa strain [196], while deletion of Idp2 decreased chronological longevity in a MATa strain [191]. As a comparison, deletions of Idh1 or Idh2 subunits of the mitochondrial NADH-generating isocitrate dehydrogenase complex led to increased replicative lifespans when using either MATa or MATα strains [198,199]. Since these replicative lifespan analyses were performed on glucose-containing media, where the NADPH-generating isocitrate dehydrogenases do not greatly control NADPH levels, the effects on lifespan are likely due to changes in citric acid cycle flux that may alter the $NAD^+/NADH$. Studies like these using a nonfermentable carbon source instead of glucose would be more informative regarding the influence of $[NADP^+]/[NADPH]$ on yeast replicative lifespan.

11. Evidence for the Regulation of Longevity by NADPH-Powered Redox Systems in *C. Elegans* Nematodes

The most commonly studied model of lifespan extension in *C. elegans* is the *daf-2* insulin receptor-deficient strain [200], which requires the DAF-16/FOXO transcriptional regulator and to a lesser extent the SKN-1/Nrf2 transcriptional regulator for the enhanced longevity [201]. The PPP enzyme GSPD-1/G6PD and the cytoplasmic $NADP^+$-dependent isocitrate dehydrogenase IDH-1 likely provide the vast majority of cytoplasmic NADPH in *C. elegans*, while the PPP enzyme T25B9.9/6PGD also likely contributes. Knockdown of *gspd-1* in an *idh-1* mutant strain led to severe growth, locomotion, and molting defects, although individual RNAi-mediated knockdown of *gspd-1* or individual knockout of *idh-1* had no effect on these phenotypes. The growth defect in *gspd-1* and *idh-1* double deficient animals was possibly mediated by alterations in amino acid metabolism as a result of NADPH depletion [202]. Decreased glutamate levels were found in these NADPH-deficient worms that may have been due to decreased glutamate dehydrogenase (GDH-1) activity, which relies upon NAD(P)H as a cofactor. However, GDH-1 is predicted to be localized to mitochondria [69], where GDH-1 would be less affected by GSPD-1 and IDH-1 deficiency than if it were localized to the cytoplasm. Folate metabolism could also contribute to a minor extent to cytoplasmic NADPH levels as *C. elegans* possesses two homologs to human MTHFD1 ($NADP^+$-dependent methylenetetrahydrofolate dehydrogenase 1), K07E3.4 and *dao-3*, the latter being transcriptionally regulated by DAF-16/FOXO [203].

Long-lived *daf-2* mutants showed increased IDH-1 activity [204], GSPD-1 levels [204,205], and levels of the mitochondrial citrate carrier (K11H3.3), a component of the mitochondrial NADPH shuttle [204]. The increase in IDH-1 activity may be especially important for longevity as we and others have shown that IDH-1 protein levels (as well as cytoplasmic aconitase (ACO-1) levels) decline greatly with aging [46,206]. Therefore, decreased cytoplasmic NADPH levels or decreased mitochondrial NADPH shuttle activity could contribute to aging phenotypes.

There are likely three major enzymes that contribute to mitochondrial NADPH generation in *C. elegans*, nicotinamide nucleotide transhydrogenase-1 (NNT-1), isocitrate dehydrogenase-2 (IDH-2), and malic enzyme (MEN-1) [69,157]. However, the localization of MEN-1 has yet to be confirmed experimentally. *Nnt-1* gene expression is induced mainly in the intestine and neurons by DAF-16 in the long-lived *daf-2* mutant worms [207,208]. Since knockdown of *nnt-1* by RNAi decreased lifespan by 18–20% in both N2 control and *daf-2* mutant worms [207], NNT-1 is likely a major regulator of mitochondrial NADPH levels. NADPH-generating malic enzyme (MEN-1) levels were not altered in long-lived *daf-2* mutants [206].

The increased longevity of *C. elegans daf-2* mutants required increased expression of *icl-1* (*gei-7*) [209], the bifunctional mitochondrial glyoxylate shunt enzyme possessing isocitrate lyase and malate synthase activity [210]. Increased ICL-1 activity decreases flux through mitochondrial IDH-2 and the heterotrimeric (IDHA-1, IDHB-1, and IDHG-1/IDHG-2) mitochondrial NADH-generating isocitrate dehydrogenase. ICL-1 expression levels also correlate with longevity in *eat-2* mutants that undergo dietary restriction and long-lived mitochondrial ETC mutants [211]. However, this correlation could be uncoupled for ETC deficiency, where knockout of the transcriptional regulator *nhr-49* prevented increased *icl-1* expression, but did not prevent increased lifespan [212]. With aging there is a strong decrease in the abundance of the IDHG-2 subunit of the NADH-generating isocitrate dehydrogenase complex [206] and a decrease in the NAD^+/NADH [46] that would likely increase flux through IDH-2 and counter aging-induced increases in the mitochondrial $NADP^+$/NADPH.

Knockdown of the *C. elegans* mitochondrial citric acid cycle genes aconitase (*aco-2*) [213], isocitrate dehydrogenase subunit *idha-1* [213], or alpha-ketoglutarate dehydrogenase subunits *ogdh-1* [214] or *dld-1* (dihydrolipoamide dehydrogenase) [215] extended lifespan. Knockdown of these enzymes could lead to accumulation of mitochondrial citrate, transport of citrate into the cytoplasm, its conversion into isocitrate (by ACO-1) and then into α-ketoglutarate by IDH-1 to reduce cytoplasmic $[NADP^+]/[NADPH]$ and increase lifespan.

C. elegans GSPD-1/G6PD may be a very important source of NADPH for removing old cuticle for molting during larval development [137]. Consistent with its important role in NADPH synthesis a *gspd-1* knockout is inviable [216]. Unexpectedly, knocking down each of four cytoplasmic PPP enzymes 6PGD (T25B9.9), transaldolase (*tald-1*), transketolase (*tkt-1*) [217], or *gspd-1* (G6PD) [205] or knocking down *idh-1* [213] extended lifespan. The lifespan extension may have been a result of upregulated expression of compensatory NADPH generating enzymes, through ROS-mediated activation of SKN-1/Nrf2 and/or through activation of the mitochondrial unfolded protein response (UPR^{mt}) [217,218]. UPR^{mt} is a stress response pathway that frequently, but not always, associates with lifespan extension [219] and is associated with activation of the transcriptional regulators ATFS-1 (ATF4, ATF5, and CHOP in mammals), DVE-1, and SKN-1/Nrf2 [220]. During larval development ATFS-1 was activated in ETC complex I *nuo-6* mutants that resulted in DAF-16/FOXO and HIF-1 activation and increased longevity [221].

In *Drosophila*, mutations that decreased Idh and malic enzyme (Men) activities were accompanied by a compensatory upregulation of G6PD activity [153,222], while in mice decreased G6PD activity leads to a compensatory increase in IDH1 levels [223]. G6PD is also allosterically activated by $NADP^+$ [224,225]. Perhaps due to these responses, knockdown of *C. elegans idh-1* [213], *gspd-1* (G6PD) [205] or T25B9.9 (6PGD) [217] led to lifespan extension. Knockdown of the PPP gene *tald-1*, beginning from the L1 larval stage extended lifespan, but not when knockdown was initiated during adulthood [217]. In contrast, knockdown of *gcs-1*, the rate limiting step of glutathione synthesis, had no effect on lifespan when initiated at the L1 larval stage, but extended lifespan when initiated at the L4 larval stage [226]. Low levels of the glutathione depleting compound diethyl maleate increased lifespan through a DAF-16 and SKN-1 dependent mechanism, but high diethyl maleate levels decreased lifespan [226]. These compensatory effects that modulate longevity partly driven by DAF-16 and SKN-1 make aging studies where the cytoplasmic redox state is oxidized in young individuals difficult to interpret unless detailed redox measurements are made in parallel.

A *C. elegans* RNAi screen identified 41 genes including *gspd-1*, other PPP genes, and glutathione reductase (*gsr-1*) as the strongest inducers of the SKN-1/Nrf2 target gene *gcs-1* [218]. SKN-1 is activated by oxidative stress and regulates expression of hundreds of genes. It decreases expression of insulin-like peptides to activate DAF-16/FOXO [227]. Together DAF-16 and SKN-1 induce several NADPH-generating enzymes and antioxidant enzymes. However, DAF-16 and SKN-1 activity greatly decline with aging [228], which may contribute to the increased $NADP^+$/NADPH with aging. Juglone, an oxidant that induces robust activation of the SKN-1 reporter *Pgst-4::gfp* in young worms was completely ineffective in activating the reporter by day 10 of the lifespan [228], while *daf-2* knockdown failed to extend lifespan when initiated at day 8 of adulthood or later [229]. Consistent with their important roles in longevity, *skn-1* or *daf-16* knockdown can slightly decrease normal lifespan [230].

Compensatory responses to NADPH depletion also likely occur in humans as G6PD deficiency is associated with long life [231]. As NADPH is a known activator of the class I histone deacetylases (HDACs) HDAC1 and HDAC2 [232], part of this compensatory response may involve decreased activity of class I HDACs, which extends lifespan in model organisms [233].

Some data do not support a role for NADPH levels to be limiting for lifespan. For example, deletion of the mitochondrial *nnt-1* in *C. elegans* increased the GSSG/GSH ratio, but did not decrease lifespan [234]. However, unexpectedly as referred to above, RNAi knockdown of *nnt-1* in *C. elegans* decreased lifespan by 18% [207]. The reasons for the different effects between knockout and knockdown of *nnt-1* on lifespan are not known. Completely knocking out *nnt-1* may lead to greater ROS production and activation of SKN-1 and DAF-16-mediated protective pathways than incompletely knocking it down. Not only does ROS-mediated SKN-1/Nrf2 activation induce expression of NADPH-generating enzymes to partially compensate for decreased NADPH levels [235], it also increases expression of other antioxidants including superoxide dismutase [236], catalase [237], and enzymes of glutathione metabolism [238]. Activation of SKN-1 by knocking out its endogenous inhibitor WDR-23 extended lifespan, but unexpectedly increased the GSSG/GSH ratio [239], yet another example of how the cellular GSSG/GSH ratio is not always predictive of lifespan. Determining the effects of SKN-1 activation or DAF-16 activation on cytoplasmic and mitochondrial [$NADP^+$]/[NADPH] may help to decipher the mechanisms through which each extends lifespan.

12. Calorie Restriction May Extend Lifespan In Part through the NADPH-Driven Redox Systems

Calorie restriction (CR) extends lifespan in the vast majority of eukaryotic organisms from yeasts to humans [240] and studies using mice have shown that the methionine restriction (MR) induced by the CR diet provides much of this longevity effect through decreasing mitochondrial ROS production [241] and increasing hydrogen sulfide production through the transulfuration pathway [242]. Flux from methionine degradation through the transulfuration pathway results in cysteine production. The majority of cysteine from the diet is oxidized to cystine and requires NADPH oxidation to reduce it to cysteine once it is taken up by cells [243]. Reduction of the extracellular cystine/cysteine has been shown to increase the intracellular levels of NADPH and GSH [244]. Therefore, use of cystine for cysteine synthesis decreases cellular NADPH levels and use of the transulfuration pathway for cysteine production conserves NADPH. Somewhat paradoxically, CR or MR increases expression of transulfuration pathway enzymes [245]. Long-lived Ames dwarf mice also show increased transulfuration pathway activity [246]. The increased cysteine production through this pathway likely leads to decreased cellular cystine uptake, decreased oxidation of NADPH to reduce cystine, and stabilization of the [$NADP^+$]/[NADPH] with aging leading to lifespan extension.

Methionine synthesis in yeast requires 3 NADPH molecules. Studies have shown that a Zwf1 (G6PD) mutant yeast strain becomes a methionine auxotroph as it is not able to produce the NADPH needed for methionine synthesis [247]. Genes of methionine metabolism appear to be co-regulated with PPP enzymes [248]. Methionine auxotrophs show extended replicative [249] and chronological longevity, while methionine supplementation decreases chronological longevity [250,251]. MR may provide an optimal level of cellular NADPH for longevity by minimizing methionine oxidation to methionine sulfoxide, which requires NADPH oxidation to repair, while maintaining high enough levels of methionine where methionine synthesis does not deplete NADPH levels. Arginine and lysine synthesis in yeast also require NADPH and synthesis becomes impaired when NADPH levels are low [252,253]. But, lysine auxotrophy does not increase chronological longevity [250].

Some of the largest consumers of NADPH include the enzymes for the biosynthesis of fatty acids, cholesterol, steroids, and deoxyribonucleotides [48]. During CR, AMP kinase (AMPK) becomes activated [254], prominently in the hypothalamus [255]. AMPK phosphorylates acetyl-CoA carboxylase to inhibit fatty acid synthesis [255]. This inhibition of fatty acid synthesis leads to the activation of fatty acid beta-oxidation (except in neurons that lack these enzymes) to provide cellular energy and prevent a futile cycle of fatty acid synthesis and breakdown. The inhibition of fatty acid synthesis preserves NADPH levels and contributes to the increased levels of redox defenses associated with the longevity benefits of CR. Stimulating AMPK using the AMP analog AICAR (5-Aminoimidazole-4-carboxamide ribonucleotide) increased the cellular NAD^+/NADH to activate the NAD^+-dependent sirtuin deacetylase SIRT1 [256], which deacetylates and activates the master regulator of mitochondrial gene expression PGC-1α to stimulate mitochondrial biogenesis and increase expression of SOD2 and catalase. Blocking mitochondrial fatty acid uptake with etomoxovir blocked the change in NAD^+/NADH [256]. The reduced [NADP+]/[NADPH] induced by AMPK activation functions together with the increased expression of SOD2 and catalase to maintain redox status in the presence of increased mitochondrial ETC function.

The effect of the anti-aging CR diet in rodents on antioxidant systems has been reviewed [257]. Overall, the majority of studies showed no overall change in mitochondrial ROS production or antioxidant enzyme levels by CR. However, GSH was increased, and the GSSG/GSH and oxidative damage were decreased in the vast majority of studies supporting the redox stress theory of aging. The Nrf2 transcriptional regulator was not required for lifespan extension by CR [258]. Two major mechanisms likely drive the reduced GSSG/GSH and decreased oxidative damage in CR mice. These include the CR-mediated increase in mitochondrial SIRT3 levels and the increased activity of FOXO transcriptional regulators due to decreased insulin signaling during CR. SIRT3 has been shown to deacetylate and activate mitochondrial IDH2 to increase mitochondrial NADPH production [259], while the FOXO3 transcriptional regulator increases PPP flux to increase cytoplasmic NADPH [260].

Neural progenitor cells from FOXO3 knockout mice showed increased $NADP^+$/NADPH and GSSG/GSH ratios due to decreased glucose uptake and PPP pathway activity. Furthermore SIRT1 overexpression, which mimics the increased expression of SIRT1 during CR in muscle and white adipose tissue [261], stimulated the formation of a FOXO3/PGC-1α complex that was shown to induce expression of the mitochondrial redox factors TXNRD2, TXN2, peroxiredoxin 3 (PRDX3), and peroxiredoxin 5 (PRDX5) [262].

CR was also shown to blunt the aging-related loss of cytoplasmic TXNRD1 and TXN protein levels in rat kidney [263]. In contrast, in rat cardiac and skeletal muscle aging and CR had no effect on TXNRD1 levels, while CR decreased the aging-related loss of TXN [264]. In muscle, mitochondria-localized TXNRD2 decreased with aging, while CR blunted this effect. Muscle mitochondrial TXN2 levels increased with aging with no effect of CR [264]. CR was also shown to decrease the skeletal muscle levels of TXNIP, an inhibitor of TXN, to enhance TXN function [265]. Extension of lifespan by DR in yeast also required the peroxiredoxin Tsa1 and increased expression of a sulfiredoxin gene to decrease the oxidation of Tsa1 with aging [266]. In *C. elegans*, lifespan extension by DR required the thioredoxin *trx-1* [267]. Global protein cysteine levels were shown not to be oxidized during aging in *Drosophila*, although 24 hours of fasting caused a major oxidation of protein cysteines [268], most likely by decreasing PPP flux and NADPH generation. However, the use of tissue-specific redox probes for H_2O_2 and GSSG/GSH were able to measure an aging-induced oxidation of the cytoplasm of midgut enterocytes [74]. Surprisingly long-lived *chico* (insulin receptor substrate) heterozygotes showed increased, not decreased midgut oxidation.

Some portion of the disease delaying effects of CR may be mediated by the increased levels of ketone bodies that occur as a result of the CR diet [55], as a ketogenic diet increased the mean lifespan of mice [269,270]. Excitingly, exogenous ketone body supplementation partially mimicked the protective redox changes induced by CR in the brain (i.e. reduced GSSG/GSH [257]) as exogenous ketone bodies were able to reduce the cytoplasmic [$NADP^+$]/[NADPH] in the cerebral cortex of 3XTgAD Alzheimer's mice, but not in their hippocampus [271]. However, oxidative damage as measured by protein carbonyl levels (2,4-dintrophenylhydrazine reactivity) and lipid peroxidation (4-hydroxynonenal levels) was decreased by ketone body treatment in the hippocampus, but not the cortex of these animals. The data suggest that hippocampal NADPH was oxidized to prevent oxidative damage in this region of the brain and this oxidation of NADPH was the likely mechanism through which no ketone body-induced change in the [$NADP^+$]/[NADPH] was found. However, the cerebral cortex of these mice may have lacked high enough NADPH-coupled redox enzyme levels to utilize the reduced [$NADP^+$]/[NADPH] for the prevention of oxidative damage. The exogenous ketone treatment also resulted in increased cytoplasmic [NAD^+]/[NADH] in both brain regions similar to CR and increased mitochondrial [NAD^+]/[NADH] only in the hippocampus [271].

13. Regulation of Aging by NADPH and the Circadian Clock

It has been clearly demonstrated in several model organisms that robust circadian rhythms are associated with longevity and that disrupting circadian oscillations in humans and other models is associated with aging and aging-related disorders [272,273]. It was found that 43% of mouse protein coding genes oscillated in expression in a circadian manner in at least one of twelve tissues studied [274], while the levels of roughly half of the mRNAs for these proteins oscillated [275] suggesting post-transcriptional events that regulate the circadian changes in the other half of these proteins. The NAD^+/NADH and the $NADP^+$/NADPH ratios oscillate over a 24 hour cycle [276,277] due in part to circadian regulation of NAMPT [278,279], NADK [280], and the PPP [281,282]. Therefore, loss of circadian rhythms could play an important role in the decreased NAD^+ [3] and NADPH [1,2] levels observed in aged tissues. Disruption of the PPP through the administration of 6-aminonicotinic acid was described to lengthen the circadian period in one study [282], while disruption of the PPP with the inhibitors diphenyleneiodonium (DPI) or dehydroepiandrosterone (DHEA) was described to alter the phase and amplitude of the circadian changes without affecting the period in another [281]. To limit the potential side effects of small molecule inhibitors, future studies could express the highly specific NADPH-oxidizing enzyme triphosphopyridine nucleotide oxidase (TPNOX) [283], an engineered mutant of *Lactobacillus brevis* NADH oxidase, in cells and target it to the mitochondria or to the cytoplasm to determine the compartment-specific role of changes in the [NADP$^+$]/[NADPH] on the circadian clock.

CR may extend longevity in part by restoring the loss of circadian rhythms. This may occur through the increased NAD$^+$/NADH and reduced NADP$^+$/NADPH conferred by CR, as dimerization of the circadian clock proteins CLOCK and BMAL1 is regulated by redox state [284]. Also, NADPH binds the circadian transcriptional regulator NPAS2 and modulates its dimerization with BMAL1 and DNA binding of the heterodimer [285,286]. In addition, circadian oscillations, especially in genes involved with metabolism, occur in *C. elegans* [287], *Drosophila* S2 cells [288], and budding yeast [289], organisms that lack essential components of the well-characterized circadian clock, suggesting an evolutionarily ancient uncharacterized circadian system regulating metabolism. It will be important to determine the influence of changes in the [NAD$^+$]/[NADH] and [NADP$^+$]/[NADPH] on this ancient circadian system.

14. NAD$^+$ Kinases as Possible Regulators of NADPH Levels and Longevity

The human cytoplasmic NAD$^+$ kinase (NADK) was identified in 2001 [290] and has been fairly well-characterized since then, including its regulation by Ca2+/calmodulin-dependent protein kinases [291] and the control of expression by the circadian clock [280]. Mice lacking NADK are not viable [292]. The *Drosophila melanogaster* genome contains two homologous genes, while the *C. elegans* genome contains no homologs of human NADK. So up until the year 2012, it was unknown how *C. elegans* obtained NADP(H). In 2012 a pivotal discovery of the human mitochondrial NAD$^+$ kinase (NADK2) was made [293,294]. The *C. elegans* genome contains two homologous uncharacterized genes, while the fruit fly genome contains one. Recently, studies using genetically encoded iNap fluorescent NADPH sensors have verified the exchange of NADPH equivalents between the cytoplasmic and mitochondrial compartments in mammalian cells [61]. Overexpression of cytoplasmic NADK resulted in a 4-fold increase in cytoplasmic [NADPH] and a 57% increase in mitochondrial [NADPH].

Like other eukaryotes, yeast rely on cytoplasmic and mitochondrial NAD(H) kinases to provide NADP(H). The two yeast cytoplasmic NAD(H) kinases, Yef1 and Utr1 appear to prefer NAD$^+$ as a substrate unlike mitochondrial Pos5, which prefers NADH [187]. In the filamentous fungus *Podospora anserine,* loss of a mitochondrial NADH kinase gene extended lifespan by apparently inducing expression of an ETC alternative oxidase that decreased ROS production [295].

15. Pharmacological Modulation of Cellular Redox Status to Prevent Cellular Senescence and Delay Aging

Methylene blue is a redox active compound that has been demonstrated to delay cellular senescence [296] and showed promise in a phase II clinical trial for Alzheimer's disease [297]. It has been shown to accept electrons from NADH or reduced flavins and pass them to ETC complex III [298] bypassing superoxide generation from ETC complexes I or II [299]. Presumably these redox properties are responsible at least in part for the many other protective cellular responses including inhibition of the NLRP3 inflammasome [300], activation of the proteasome [301], and stabilization of HSF1 [302]. Methylene blue treatment was shown to extend the lifespan of *C. elegans* [303] and female mice [304], but not *Drosophila* [305].

A screen of 2684 compounds identified the redox-active compounds violuric acid (VA) and 1-naphthoquinone-2-monoxime (N2N1) as the top hits that delayed cellular senescence [306]. These compounds were then shown to increase the lifespan of *C. elegans* and mice. VA greatly reduced the level of cellular protein disulfides by facilitating electron transfer from NADH (and NADPH to a lesser extent) to GSSG to increase GSH and the cellular NAD$^+$/NADH. VA also facilitated the transfer of electrons from NADH to H_2O_2 to form water, but did not transfer electrons from NADH to cytochrome

c. N2N1 was shown to pass electrons from NADH (and NADPH to a lesser extent) to CoQ_{10} and to cytochrome c with the NQO1 (NAD(P)H: quinone oxidoreductase 1) redox system as a major target. Consistent with these results, overexpression of NQO1 together with another NADH-oxidizing redox protein, cytochrome b_5 reductase 3 (CYB5R3), extended lifespan in mice and mimicked some phenotypes of CR [307]. However, invertebrates such as *C. elegans* lack the NQO1 system, so the longevity effects of N2N1 and methylene blue in nematodes may be due to stimulation of electron transfer from NADH to ETC complex III or to the *C. elegans* CYB5R3 homologs HPO-19 or T05H4.4. Increasing the NAD^+/NADH ratio is likely key to the longevity effects of these compounds, but VA may also stabilize the $NADP^+$/NADPH to provide longevity benefits. Compounds that facilitate the selective transfer of electrons from NADH to GSSG, H_2O_2, oxidized thioredoxin, and other electron acceptors could increase the NAD^+/NADH with aging and would therefore be compounds for the potential treatment of aging-related disorders. Compounds that facilitate the selective transfer of electrons from NADPH to these electron acceptors may also be beneficial at low levels, but at high levels they also have the potential to increase the [$NADP^+$]/[NADPH] leading to oxidative stress.

16. Summary and Future Perspectives

Evidence from model organisms strongly suggests that redox changes influence the rate of aging. However, both oxidizing and reducing changes can lead to increased longevity making redox measurements in both cytoplasmic and mitochondrial compartments especially important in when determining the mechanism for lifespan extension. In *S. cerevisiae* and *C. elegans*, deleting or knocking down NADPH-generating enzymes increased longevity more frequently than decreasing it, likely due to the active stress response pathways that have evolved in young cells to compensate for the loss of NADPH. Manipulations that lead to a reduction of the [$NADP^+$]/[NADPH] in the cytoplasm are especially linked with increased longevity. But reducing the redox potential of the cytoplasm frequently leads to reductive stress characterized by mitochondrial oxidation and ROS production. Mitochondrial ROS production and oxidation is linked with increased longevity when it occurs in young organisms capable of mounting robust longevity enhancing stress responses. The theory that mild reductive stress in the cytoplasm during development leads to increased mitochondrial superoxide production and lifespan extension should be tested in model organisms.

Another clear trend in the literature is the protective effects of the mitochondrial NADPH-linked redox systems. It would be helpful to explore potential molecular mechanisms behind the positive association between mitochondrial thioredoxin reductase activity and increased longevity. This could be accomplished in part through overexpression studies and measurements of mitochondrial superoxide or hydrogen peroxide production, GSSG/GSH, and [$NADP^+$]/[NADPH] measurements. However, overexpression of mitochondrial thioredoxin reductase on its own would be expected to have little effect on longevity, as was verified in studies using *Drosophila* [104], without a corresponding reduction of the mitochondrial [$NADP^+$]/[NADPH] that drives its enzymatic activity. Since little is known regarding the effects of a more reduced mitochondrial redox environment on longevity, future important experiments will be to overexpress a mitochondrial NADPH-generating enzyme, such as Men-b or mitochondrial targeted Idh in *Drosophila*, to determine the effects of reduced mitochondrial [$NADP^+$]/[NADPH] on lifespan.

Acknowledgments: I would like to thank the pioneers of research in the field of redox biology and aging including Dean Jones, Rajindar Sohal, and William Orr.

Abbreviations

ADP: adenosine diphosphate; AICAR, 5-aminoimidazole-4-carboxamide ribonucleotide; ALDH1L1, cytoplasmic 10-formyltetrahydrofolate dehydrogenase; ALDH1L2, mitochondrial 10-formyltetrahydrofolate dehydrogenase; AMP, adenosine monophosphate; AMPK, AMP kinase; ATP, adenosine triphosphate; CR, calorie restriction; CYB5R3, cytochrome b5 reductase 3; DAF-16, dauer formation-16; DAF-2, dauer formation-2; DHEA, dehydroepiandrosterone; DPI, diphenyleneiodonium; DR, dietary restriction; ER, endoplasmic reticulum; ETC, Electron transport chain; FOXO, forkhead box O; G6PD, glucose-6-phosphate dehydrogenase; GCL, glutamate-cysteine ligase; GDH-1, glutamate dehydrogenase-1; GPI-1, glucose-6-phosphate isomerase-1; GPX, glutathione peroxidase; GSH, glutathione; GSSG, glutathione disulfide; GSR, glutathione reductase; HDAC, histone deacetylase; HSF-1, heat shock factor-1; IDH1, isocitrate dehydrogenase 1 (cytoplasmic); IDH-1, *C. elegans* isocitrate dehydrogenase-1; IDH2, isocitrate dehydrogenase 2 (mitochondrial); IDH-2, *C. elegans* isocitrate dehydrogenase-2; Idh, *Drosophila* isocitrate dehydrogenase; ICL-1, isocitrate lyase-1; K_m, Michaelis constant; MATa, haploid mating type a; MATα, haploid mating type α; Men, *Drosophila* cytoplasmic malic enzyme; Men-b, *Drosophila* mitochondrial malic enzyme; MEN-1, *C. elegans* malic enzyme; ME1, malic enzyme 1; ME3, malic enzyme 3; MFRTA, Mitochondrial free radical theory of aging; MSRA, methionine sulfoxide reductase A; MSRB, methionine sulfoxide reductase B; MTAP, methylthioadenosine phosphorylase; MTHFD1L, methylenetetrahydrofolate dehydrogenase 1 like; mV, milliVolt; mM, milliMolar; N2N1, 1-naphthoquinone-2-monoxime; NAC, N-acetylcysteine; NAD^+, nicotinamide adenine dinucleotide (oxidized form); NADK, NAD^+ kinase; NADK2, mitochondrial NAD^+ kinase; NADH, nicotinamide adenine dinucleotide (reduced form); $NADP^+$, nicotinamide adenine dinucleotide phosphate (oxidized form); NADPH, nicotinamide adenine dinucleotide phosphate (reduced form); NAMPT, nicotinamide phosphoribosyl transferase; NQO1, NAD(P)H: quinone oxidoreductase 1; NNT, nicotinamide nucleotide transhydrogenase; Nox4, NADPH oxidase 4; Nrf2, Nuclear factor (erythroid-derived 2)-like 2; PARP, poly-ADP-ribose polymerase; 6PGD, 6-phosphogluconate dehydrogenase; PNP, purine nucleoside phosphorylase; PPP, pentose phosphate pathway; PRDX, peroxiredoxin; ROS, reactive oxygen species; SARM1, Sterile alpha and TIR motif containing 1; SKN-1, skinhead-1; SOD, superoxide dismutase; TFAM, mitochondrial transcription factor A; TPNOX, triphosphopyridine nucleotide oxidase; TRXR-1, *C. elegans* cytoplasmic thioredoxin reductase; TRXR-2, *C. elegans* mitochondrial thioredoxin reductase; TXN, cytoplasmic thioredoxin; TXN2, mitochondrial thioredoxin, TXNRD1, cytoplasmic thioredoxin reductase; TXNRD2, mitochondrial thioredoxin reductase; UPR^{mt}, mitochondrial unfolded protein response; VA, violuric acid; V_{max}, maximal velocity.

References

1. Aw, T.Y. Postnatal Changes in Pyridine Nucleotides in Rat Hepatocytes: Composition and O2 Dependence. *Pediatr. Res.* **1991**, *30*, 112–117. [CrossRef] [PubMed]
2. Ghosh, D.; Levault, K.R.; Brewer, G.J. Relative importance of redox buffers GSH and NAD(P)H in age-related neurodegeneration and Alzheimer disease-like mouse neurons. *Aging Cell* **2014**, *13*, 631–640. [CrossRef] [PubMed]
3. Zhu, X.H.; Lu, M.; Lee, B.Y.; Ugurbil, K.; Chen, W. In vivo NAD assay reveals the intracellular NAD contents and redox state in healthy human brain and their age dependences. *Proc. Natl. Acad. Sci. USA* **2015**, *112*, 2876–2881. [CrossRef] [PubMed]
4. Lenaz, G.; D'Aurelio, M.; Merlo Pich, M.; Genova, M.L.; Ventura, B.; Bovina, C.; Formiggini, G.; Parenti Castelli, G. Mitochondrial bioenergetics in aging. *Biochim. Biophys. Acta* **2000**, *1459*, 397–404. [CrossRef]
5. Baciou, L.; Masoud, R.; Souabni, H.; Serfaty, X.; Karimi, G.; Bizouarn, T.; Houee Levin, C. Phagocyte NADPH oxidase, oxidative stress and lipids: Anti- or pro ageing? *Mech. Ageing Dev.* **2018**, *172*, 30–34. [CrossRef] [PubMed]
6. Huang, Q.; Sun, M.; Li, M.; Zhang, D.; Han, F.; Wu, J.C.; Fukunaga, K.; Chen, Z.; Qin, Z.H. Combination of NAD(+) and NADPH Offers Greater Neuroprotection in Ischemic Stroke Models by Relieving Metabolic Stress. *Mol. Neurobiol.* **2018**, *55*, 6063–6075. [CrossRef] [PubMed]
7. Harman, D. The biologic clock: The mitochondria? *J. Am. Geriatr. Soc.* **1972**, *20*, 145–147. [CrossRef] [PubMed]
8. Barja, G. Updating the mitochondrial free radical theory of aging: An integrated view, key aspects, and confounding concepts. *Antioxid. Redox Signal.* **2013**, *19*, 1420–1445. [CrossRef] [PubMed]
9. Gems, D.; Doonan, R. Antioxidant defense and aging in *C. elegans*: Is the oxidative damage theory of aging wrong? *Cell Cycle* **2009**, *8*, 1681–1687. [CrossRef] [PubMed]
10. Jang, Y.C.; Perez, V.I.; Song, W.; Lustgarten, M.S.; Salmon, A.B.; Mele, J.; Qi, W.; Liu, Y.; Liang, H.; Chaudhuri, A.; et al. Overexpression of Mn superoxide dismutase does not increase life span in mice. *J. Gerontol. A Biol. Sci. Med. Sci.* **2009**, *64*, 1114–1125. [CrossRef] [PubMed]
11. Perez, V.I.; Van Remmen, H.; Bokov, A.; Epstein, C.J.; Vijg, J.; Richardson, A. The overexpression of major antioxidant enzymes does not extend the lifespan of mice. *Aging Cell* **2009**, *8*, 73–75. [CrossRef] [PubMed]
12. Selman, C.; McLaren, J.S.; Meyer, C.; Duncan, J.S.; Redman, P.; Collins, A.R.; Duthie, G.G.; Speakman, J.R. Life-long vitamin C supplementation in combination with cold exposure does not affect oxidative damage or lifespan in mice, but decreases expression of antioxidant protection genes. *Mech. Ageing Dev.* **2006**, *127*, 897–904. [CrossRef] [PubMed]

13. Ernst, I.M.; Pallauf, K.; Bendall, J.K.; Paulsen, L.; Nikolai, S.; Huebbe, P.; Roeder, T.; Rimbach, G. Vitamin E supplementation and lifespan in model organisms. *Ageing Res. Rev.* **2013**, *12*, 365–375. [CrossRef] [PubMed]
14. Desjardins, D.; Cacho-Valadez, B.; Liu, J.L.; Wang, Y.; Yee, C.; Bernard, K.; Khaki, A.; Breton, L.; Hekimi, S. Antioxidants reveal an inverted U-shaped dose-response relationship between reactive oxygen species levels and the rate of aging in Caenorhabditis elegans. *Aging Cell* **2017**, *16*, 104–112. [CrossRef] [PubMed]
15. Orr, W.C.; Sohal, R.S. Does overexpression of Cu,Zn-SOD extend life span in Drosophila melanogaster? *Exp. Gerontol.* **2003**, *38*, 227–230. [CrossRef]
16. Shibamura, A.; Ikeda, T.; Nishikawa, Y. A method for oral administration of hydrophilic substances to Caenorhabditis elegans: Effects of oral supplementation with antioxidants on the nematode lifespan. *Mech. Ageing Dev.* **2009**, *130*, 652–655. [CrossRef] [PubMed]
17. Schriner, S.E.; Linford, N.J.; Martin, G.M.; Treuting, P.; Ogburn, C.E.; Emond, M.; Coskun, P.E.; Ladiges, W.; Wolf, N.; Van Remmen, H.; et al. Extension of murine life span by overexpression of catalase targeted to mitochondria. *Science* **2005**, *308*, 1909–1911. [CrossRef] [PubMed]
18. Lebovitz, R.M.; Zhang, H.; Vogel, H.; Cartwright, J., Jr.; Dionne, L.; Lu, N.; Huang, S.; Matzuk, M.M. Neurodegeneration, myocardial injury, and perinatal death in mitochondrial superoxide dismutase-deficient mice. *Proc. Natl. Acad. Sci. USA* **1996**, *93*, 9782–9787. [CrossRef] [PubMed]
19. Kirkman, H.N.; Gaetani, G.F. Catalase: A tetrameric enzyme with four tightly bound molecules of NADPH. *Proc. Natl. Acad. Sci. USA* **1984**, *81*, 4343–4347. [CrossRef] [PubMed]
20. Sohal, R.S.; Orr, W.C. The redox stress hypothesis of aging. *Free Radic. Biol. Med.* **2012**, *52*, 539–555. [CrossRef] [PubMed]
21. Go, Y.M.; Jones, D.P. Redox theory of aging: Implications for health and disease. *Clin. Sci. (Lond. Engl. 1979)* **2017**, *131*, 1669–1688. [CrossRef]
22. Heidler, T.; Hartwig, K.; Daniel, H.; Wenzel, U. *Caenorhabditis elegans* lifespan extension caused by treatment with an orally active ROS-generator is dependent on DAF-16 and SIR-2.1. *Biogerontology* **2010**, *11*, 183–195. [CrossRef] [PubMed]
23. Schulz, T.J.; Zarse, K.; Voigt, A.; Urban, N.; Birringer, M.; Ristow, M. Glucose restriction extends *Caenorhabditis elegans* life span by inducing mitochondrial respiration and increasing oxidative stress. *Cell Metab.* **2007**, *6*, 280–293. [CrossRef] [PubMed]
24. Barja, G. Rate of generation of oxidative stress-related damage and animal longevity. *Free Radic. Biol. Med.* **2002**, *33*, 1167–1172. [CrossRef]
25. Schindeldecker, M.; Stark, M.; Behl, C.; Moosmann, B. Differential cysteine depletion in respiratory chain complexes enables the distinction of longevity from aerobicity. *Mech. Ageing Dev.* **2011**, *132*, 171–179. [CrossRef] [PubMed]
26. Pamplona, R.; Barja, G.; Portero-Otin, M. Membrane fatty acid unsaturation, protection against oxidative stress, and maximum life span: A homeoviscous-longevity adaptation? *Ann. N. Y. Acad. Sci.* **2002**, *959*, 475–490. [CrossRef] [PubMed]
27. Moosmann, B. Respiratory chain cysteine and methionine usage indicate a causal role for thiyl radicals in aging. *Exp. Gerontol.* **2011**, *46*, 164–169. [CrossRef] [PubMed]
28. Paradies, G.; Paradies, V.; Ruggiero, F.M.; Petrosillo, G. Cardiolipin and mitochondrial function in health and disease. *Antioxid. Redox Signal.* **2014**, *20*, 1925–1953. [CrossRef] [PubMed]
29. Ma, C.; Pi, C.; Yang, Y.; Lin, L.; Shi, Y.; Li, Y.; Li, Y.; He, X. Nampt Expression Decreases Age-Related Senescence in Rat Bone Marrow Mesenchymal Stem Cells by Targeting Sirt1. *PLoS ONE* **2017**, *12*, e0170930. [CrossRef] [PubMed]
30. Ahn, B.H.; Kim, H.S.; Song, S.; Lee, I.H.; Liu, J.; Vassilopoulos, A.; Deng, C.X.; Finkel, T. A role for the mitochondrial deacetylase Sirt3 in regulating energy homeostasis. *Proc. Natl. Acad. Sci. USA* **2008**, *105*, 14447–14452. [CrossRef] [PubMed]
31. Nemoto, S.; Fergusson, M.M.; Finkel, T. SIRT1 functionally interacts with the metabolic regulator and transcriptional coactivator PGC-1α. *J. Biol. Chem.* **2005**, *280*, 16456–16460. [CrossRef] [PubMed]
32. Braidy, N.; Guillemin, G.J.; Mansour, H.; Chan-Ling, T.; Poljak, A.; Grant, R. Age related changes in NAD+ metabolism oxidative stress and Sirt1 activity in wistar rats. *PLoS ONE* **2011**, *6*, e19194. [CrossRef] [PubMed]
33. Camacho-Pereira, J.; Tarrago, M.G.; Chini, C.C.S.; Nin, V.; Escande, C.; Warner, G.M.; Puranik, A.S.; Schoon, R.A.; Reid, J.M.; Galina, A.; et al. CD38 Dictates Age-Related NAD Decline and Mitochondrial Dysfunction through an SIRT3-Dependent Mechanism. *Cell Metab.* **2016**, *23*, 1127–1139. [CrossRef] [PubMed]

34. Boslett, J.; Helal, M.; Chini, E.; Zweier, J.L. Genetic deletion of CD38 confers post-ischemic myocardial protection through preserved pyridine nucleotides. *J. Mol. Cell. Cardiol.* **2018**, *118*, 81–94. [CrossRef] [PubMed]
35. Vu, C.Q.; Lu, P.J.; Chen, C.S.; Jacobson, M.K. 2′-Phospho-cyclic ADP-ribose, a calcium-mobilizing agent derived from NADP. *J. Biol. Chem.* **1996**, *271*, 4747–4754. [PubMed]
36. Andrabi, S.A.; Umanah, G.K.E.; Chang, C.; Stevens, D.A.; Karuppagounder, S.S.; Gagné, J.-P.; Poirier, G.G.; Dawson, V.L.; Dawson, T.M. Poly(ADP-ribose) polymerase-dependent energy depletion occurs through inhibition of glycolysis. *Proc. Natl. Acad. Sci. USA* **2014**, *111*, 10209–10214. [CrossRef] [PubMed]
37. Essuman, K.; Summers, D.W.; Sasaki, Y.; Mao, X.; DiAntonio, A.; Milbrandt, J. The SARM1 Toll/Interleukin-1 Receptor Domain Possesses Intrinsic NAD(+) Cleavage Activity that Promotes Pathological Axonal Degeneration. *Neuron* **2017**, *93*, 1334–1343.e5. [CrossRef]
38. Ferrero, E.; Malavasi, F. A Natural History of the Human CD38 Gene. In *Cyclic ADP-Ribose and NAADP: Structures, Metabolism and Functions*; Lee, H.C., Ed.; Springer: Boston, MA, USA, 2002; pp. 65–79.
39. Sur, M.; Dey, P.; Sarkar, A.; Bar, S.; Banerjee, D.; Bhat, S.; Mukherjee, P. Sarm1 induction and accompanying inflammatory response mediates age-dependent susceptibility to rotenone-induced neurotoxicity. *Cell Death Discov.* **2018**, *4*, 114. [CrossRef] [PubMed]
40. Navas, P.; Minnifield, N.; Sun, I.; Morre, D.J. NADP phosphatase as a marker in free-flow electrophoretic separations for cisternae of the Golgi apparatus midregion. *Biochim. Biophys. Acta* **1986**, *881*, 1–9. [CrossRef]
41. Richter, C. NADP+ phosphatase: A novel mitochondrial enzyme. *Biochem. Biophys. Res. Commun.* **1987**, *146*, 253–257. [CrossRef]
42. Balan, V.; Miller, G.S.; Kaplun, L.; Balan, K.; Chong, Z.Z.; Li, F.; Kaplun, A.; VanBerkum, M.F.; Arking, R.; Freeman, D.C.; et al. Life span extension and neuronal cell protection by Drosophila nicotinamidase. *J. Biol. Chem.* **2008**, *283*, 27810–27819. [CrossRef] [PubMed]
43. Vrablik, T.L.; Huang, L.; Lange, S.E.; Hanna-Rose, W. Nicotinamidase modulation of NAD+ biosynthesis and nicotinamide levels separately affect reproductive development and cell survival in *C. elegans*. *Development* **2009**, *136*, 3637–3646. [CrossRef] [PubMed]
44. McReynolds, M.R.; Wang, W.; Holleran, L.M.; Hanna-Rose, W. Uridine monophosphate synthetase enables eukaryotic de novo NAD+ biosynthesis from quinolinic acid. *J. Biol. Chem.* **2017**, *292*, 11147–11153. [CrossRef] [PubMed]
45. Breda, C.; Sathyasaikumar, K.V.; Sograte Idrissi, S.; Notarangelo, F.M.; Estranero, J.G.; Moore, G.G.; Green, E.W.; Kyriacou, C.P.; Schwarcz, R.; Giorgini, F. Tryptophan-2,3-dioxygenase (TDO) inhibition ameliorates neurodegeneration by modulation of kynurenine pathway metabolites. *Proc. Natl. Acad. Sci. USA* **2016**, *113*, 5435–5440. [CrossRef] [PubMed]
46. Copes, N.; Edwards, C.; Chaput, D.; Saifee, M.; Barjuca, I.; Nelson, D.; Paraggio, A.; Saad, P.; Lipps, D.; Stevens, S.M., Jr.; et al. Metabolome and proteome changes with aging in *Caenorhabditis elegans*. *Exp. Gerontol.* **2015**, *72*, 67–84. [CrossRef] [PubMed]
47. Sohal, R.S.; Arnold, L.; Orr, W.C. Effect of age on superoxide dismutase, catalase, glutathione reductase, inorganic peroxides, TBA-reactive material, GSH/GSSG, NADPH/NADP+ and NADH/NAD+ in Drosophila melanogaster. *Mech. Ageing Dev.* **1990**, *56*, 223–235. [CrossRef]
48. Pollak, N.; Dolle, C.; Ziegler, M. The power to reduce: Pyridine nucleotides—Small molecules with a multitude of functions. *Biochem. J.* **2007**, *402*, 205–218. [CrossRef] [PubMed]
49. Hashimoto, T.; Horikawa, M.; Nomura, T.; Sakamoto, K. Nicotinamide adenine dinucleotide extends the lifespan of *Caenorhabditis elegans* mediated by sir-2.1 and daf-16. *Biogerontology* **2010**, *11*, 31–43. [CrossRef]
50. Mouchiroud, L.; Houtkooper, R.H.; Moullan, N.; Katsyuba, E.; Ryu, D.; Canto, C.; Mottis, A.; Jo, Y.S.; Viswanathan, M.; Schoonjans, K.; et al. The NAD(+)/Sirtuin Pathway Modulates Longevity through Activation of Mitochondrial UPR and FOXO Signaling. *Cell* **2013**, *154*, 430–441. [CrossRef] [PubMed]
51. Belenky, P.; Christensen, K.C.; Gazzaniga, F.; Pletnev, A.A.; Brenner, C. Nicotinamide riboside and nicotinic acid riboside salvage in fungi and mammals. Quantitative basis for Urh1 and purine nucleoside phosphorylase function in NAD+ metabolism. *J. Boil. Chem.* **2009**, *284*, 158–164. [CrossRef]
52. Gomes, A.P.; Price, N.L.; Ling, A.J.; Moslehi, J.J.; Montgomery, M.K.; Rajman, L.; White, J.P.; Teodoro, J.S.; Wrann, C.D.; Hubbard, B.P.; et al. Declining NAD(+) induces a pseudohypoxic state disrupting nuclear-mitochondrial communication during aging. *Cell* **2013**, *155*, 1624–1638. [CrossRef] [PubMed]

53. Ren, X.; Zou, L.; Zhang, X.; Branco, V.; Wang, J.; Carvalho, C.; Holmgren, A.; Lu, J. Redox Signaling Mediated by Thioredoxin and Glutathione Systems in the Central Nervous System. *Antioxid. Redox Signal.* **2017**, *27*, 989–1010. [CrossRef] [PubMed]
54. Andziak, B.; Buffenstein, R. Disparate patterns of age-related changes in lipid peroxidation in long-lived naked mole-rats and shorter-lived mice. *Aging Cell* **2006**, *5*, 525–532. [CrossRef] [PubMed]
55. Veech, R.L.; Bradshaw, P.C.; Clarke, K.; Curtis, W.; Pawlosky, R.; King, M.T. Ketone bodies mimic the life span extending properties of caloric restriction. *IUBMB Life* **2017**, *69*, 305–314. [CrossRef] [PubMed]
56. Veech, R.L.; Eggleston, L.V.; Krebs, H.A. The redox state of free nicotinamide-adenine dinucleotide phosphate in the cytoplasm of rat liver. *Biochem. J.* **1969**, *115*, 609–619. [CrossRef] [PubMed]
57. Son, M.J.; Kwon, Y.; Son, T.; Cho, Y.S. Restoration of Mitochondrial NAD(+) Levels Delays Stem Cell Senescence and Facilitates Reprogramming of Aged Somatic Cells. *Stem Cells* **2016**, *34*, 2840–2851. [CrossRef] [PubMed]
58. Tischler, M.E.; Friedrichs, D.; Coll, K.; Williamson, J.R. Pyridine nucleotide distributions and enzyme mass action ratios in hepatocytes from fed and starved rats. *Arch. Biochem. Biophys.* **1977**, *184*, 222–236. [CrossRef]
59. Owen, J.B.; Butterfield, D.A. Measurement of oxidized/reduced glutathione ratio. *Methods Mol. Biol.* **2010**, *648*, 269–277. [CrossRef] [PubMed]
60. Chai, Y.C.; Ashraf, S.S.; Rokutan, K.; Johnston, R.B., Jr.; Thomas, J.A. S-thiolation of individual human neutrophil proteins including actin by stimulation of the respiratory burst: Evidence against a role for glutathione disulfide. *Arch. Biochem. Biophys.* **1994**, *310*, 273–281. [CrossRef] [PubMed]
61. Tao, R.; Zhao, Y.; Chu, H.; Wang, A.; Zhu, J.; Chen, X.; Zou, Y.; Shi, M.; Liu, R.; Su, N.; et al. Genetically encoded fluorescent sensors reveal dynamic regulation of NADPH metabolism. *Nat. Methods* **2017**, *14*, 720–728. [CrossRef] [PubMed]
62. Yap, L.P.; Garcia, J.V.; Han, D.; Cadenas, E. The energy-redox axis in aging and age-related neurodegeneration. *Adv. Drug Deliv. Rev.* **2009**, *61*, 1283–1298. [CrossRef] [PubMed]
63. Canepa, L.; Ferraris, A.M.; Miglino, M.; Gaetani, G.F. Bound and unbound pyridine dinucleotides in normal and glucose-6-phosphate dehydrogenase-deficient erythrocytes. *Biochim. Biophys. Acta* **1991**, *1074*, 101–104. [CrossRef]
64. Booty, L.M.; Gawel, J.M.; Cvetko, F.; Caldwell, S.T.; Hall, A.R.; Mulvey, J.F.; James, A.M.; Hinchy, E.C.; Prime, T.A.; Arndt, S.; et al. Selective Disruption of Mitochondrial Thiol Redox State in Cells and In Vivo. *Cell Chem. Boil.* **2019**. [CrossRef] [PubMed]
65. Jones, D.P.; Mody, V.C., Jr.; Carlson, J.L.; Lynn, M.J.; Sternberg, P., Jr. Redox analysis of human plasma allows separation of pro-oxidant events of aging from decline in antioxidant defenses. *Free Radic. Biol. Med.* **2002**, *33*, 1290–1300. [CrossRef]
66. Clement, J.; Wong, M.; Poljak, A.; Sachdev, P.; Braidy, N. The Plasma NAD(+) Metabolome Is Dysregulated in "Normal" Aging. *Rejuvenation Res.* **2018**. [CrossRef] [PubMed]
67. Dellinger, R.W.; Santos, S.R.; Morris, M.; Evans, M.; Alminana, D.; Guarente, L.; Marcotulli, E. Repeat dose NRPT (nicotinamide riboside and pterostilbene) increases NAD(+) levels in humans safely and sustainably: A randomized, double-blind, placebo-controlled study. *Npj Aging Mech. Dis.* **2017**, *3*, 17. [CrossRef] [PubMed]
68. Zhou, Y.; Wu, J.; Sheng, R.; Li, M.; Wang, Y.; Han, R.; Han, F.; Chen, Z.; Qin, Z.H. Reduced Nicotinamide Adenine Dinucleotide Phosphate Inhibits MPTP-Induced Neuroinflammation and Neurotoxicity. *Neuroscience* **2018**, *391*, 140–153. [CrossRef] [PubMed]
69. Horton, P.; Park, K.J.; Obayashi, T.; Fujita, N.; Harada, H.; Adams-Collier, C.J.; Nakai, K. WoLF PSORT: Protein localization predictor. *Nucleic Acids Res.* **2007**, *35*, W585–W587. [CrossRef] [PubMed]
70. Gutteridge, J.M.C.; Halliwell, B. Mini-Review: Oxidative stress, redox stress or redox success? *Biochem. Biophys. Res. Commun.* **2018**, *502*, 183–186. [CrossRef] [PubMed]
71. Zou, Y.; Wang, A.; Shi, M.; Chen, X.; Liu, R.; Li, T.; Zhang, C.; Zhang, Z.; Zhu, L.; Ju, Z.; et al. Analysis of redox landscapes and dynamics in living cells and in vivo using genetically encoded fluorescent sensors. *Nat. Protoc.* **2018**, *13*, 2362–2386. [CrossRef] [PubMed]
72. Hanson, G.T.; Aggeler, R.; Oglesbee, D.; Cannon, M.; Capaldi, R.A.; Tsien, R.Y.; Remington, S.J. Investigating mitochondrial redox potential with redox-sensitive green fluorescent protein indicators. *J. Biol. Chem.* **2004**, *279*, 13044–13053. [CrossRef] [PubMed]

73. Gutscher, M.; Pauleau, A.L.; Marty, L.; Brach, T.; Wabnitz, G.H.; Samstag, Y.; Meyer, A.J.; Dick, T.P. Real-time imaging of the intracellular glutathione redox potential. *Nat. Methods* **2008**, *5*, 553–559. [CrossRef] [PubMed]
74. Albrecht, S.C.; Barata, A.G.; Grosshans, J.; Teleman, A.A.; Dick, T.P. In vivo mapping of hydrogen peroxide and oxidized glutathione reveals chemical and regional specificity of redox homeostasis. *Cell Metab.* **2011**, *14*, 819–829. [CrossRef] [PubMed]
75. Zhang, H.; Limphong, P.; Pieper, J.; Liu, Q.; Rodesch, C.K.; Christians, E.; Benjamin, I.J. Glutathione-dependent reductive stress triggers mitochondrial oxidation and cytotoxicity. *FASEB J.* **2012**, *26*, 1442–1451. [CrossRef] [PubMed]
76. Booty, L.M.; King, M.S.; Thangaratnarajah, C.; Majd, H.; James, A.M.; Kunji, E.R.; Murphy, M.P. The mitochondrial dicarboxylate and 2-oxoglutarate carriers do not transport glutathione. *FEBS Lett.* **2015**, *589*, 621–628. [CrossRef] [PubMed]
77. Wadey, A.L.; Muyderman, H.; Kwek, P.T.; Sims, N.R. Mitochondrial glutathione uptake: Characterization in isolated brain mitochondria and astrocytes in culture. *J. Neurochem.* **2009**, *109* (Suppl. 1), 101–108. [CrossRef] [PubMed]
78. Blacker, T.S.; Duchen, M.R. Investigating mitochondrial redox state using NADH and NADPH autofluorescence. *Free Radic. Biol. Med.* **2016**, *100*, 53–65. [CrossRef] [PubMed]
79. Korge, P.; Calmettes, G.; Weiss, J.N. Increased reactive oxygen species production during reductive stress: The roles of mitochondrial glutathione and thioredoxin reductases. *Biochim. Biophys. Acta* **2015**, *1847*, 514–525. [CrossRef] [PubMed]
80. Ralser, M.; Benjamin, I.J. Reductive stress on life span extension in *C. elegans*. *BMC Res. Notes* **2008**, *1*, 19. [CrossRef] [PubMed]
81. Ralser, M.; Wamelink, M.M.; Kowald, A.; Gerisch, B.; Heeren, G.; Struys, E.A.; Klipp, E.; Jakobs, C.; Breitenbach, M.; Lehrach, H.; et al. Dynamic rerouting of the carbohydrate flux is key to counteracting oxidative stress. *J. Boil.* **2007**, *6*, 10. [CrossRef] [PubMed]
82. Breitenbach, M.; Laun, P.; Dickinson, J.R.; Klocker, A.; Rinnerthaler, M.; Dawes, I.W.; Aung-Htut, M.T.; Breitenbach-Koller, L.; Caballero, A.; Nystrom, T.; et al. The role of mitochondria in the aging processes of yeast. *Sub-Cell. Biochem.* **2012**, *57*, 55–78. [CrossRef]
83. Rajasekaran, N.S.; Connell, P.; Christians, E.S.; Yan, L.J.; Taylor, R.P.; Orosz, A.; Zhang, X.Q.; Stevenson, T.J.; Peshock, R.M.; Leopold, J.A.; et al. Human alpha B-crystallin mutation causes oxido-reductive stress and protein aggregation cardiomyopathy in mice. *Cell* **2007**, *130*, 427–439. [CrossRef] [PubMed]
84. Brand, M.D.; Goncalves, R.L.; Orr, A.L.; Vargas, L.; Gerencser, A.A.; Borch Jensen, M.; Wang, Y.T.; Melov, S.; Turk, C.N.; Matzen, J.T.; et al. Suppressors of Superoxide-H_2O_2 Production at Site IQ of Mitochondrial Complex I Protect against Stem Cell Hyperplasia and Ischemia-Reperfusion Injury. *Cell Metab.* **2016**, *24*, 582–592. [CrossRef] [PubMed]
85. Orr, A.L.; Vargas, L.; Turk, C.N.; Baaten, J.E.; Matzen, J.T.; Dardov, V.J.; Attle, S.J.; Li, J.; Quackenbush, D.C.; Goncalves, R.L.; et al. Suppressors of superoxide production from mitochondrial complex III. *Nat. Chem. Boil.* **2015**, *11*, 834–836. [CrossRef] [PubMed]
86. Lewis, K.N.; Andziak, B.; Yang, T.; Buffenstein, R. The naked mole-rat response to oxidative stress: Just deal with it. *Antioxid. Redox Signal.* **2013**, *19*, 1388–1399. [CrossRef] [PubMed]
87. Broniowska, K.A.; Diers, A.R.; Hogg, N. S-nitrosoglutathione. *Biochim. Biophys. Acta* **2013**, *1830*, 3173–3181. [CrossRef] [PubMed]
88. Ran, Q.; Liang, H.; Ikeno, Y.; Qi, W.; Prolla, T.A.; Roberts, L.J., 2nd; Wolf, N.; Van Remmen, H.; Richardson, A. Reduction in glutathione peroxidase 4 increases life span through increased sensitivity to apoptosis. *J. Gerontol. A Biol. Sci. Med. Sci.* **2007**, *62*, 932–942. [CrossRef] [PubMed]
89. Mockett, R.J.; Orr, W.C.; Rahmandar, J.J.; Sohal, B.H.; Sohal, R.S. Antioxidant status and stress resistance in long- and short-lived lines of Drosophila melanogaster. *Exp. Gerontol.* **2001**, *36*, 441–463. [CrossRef]
90. Lopez-Torres, M.; Perez-Campo, R.; Rojas, C.; Cadenas, S.; Barja, G. Maximum life span in vertebrates: Relationship with liver antioxidant enzymes, glutathione system, ascorbate, urate, sensitivity to peroxidation, true malondialdehyde, in vivo H_2O_2, and basal and maximum aerobic capacity. *Mech. Ageing Dev.* **1993**, *70*, 177–199. [CrossRef]
91. Heinze, I.; Bens, M.; Calzia, E.; Holtze, S.; Dakhovnik, O.; Sahm, A.; Kirkpatrick, J.M.; Szafranski, K.; Romanov, N.; Sama, S.N.; et al. Species comparison of liver proteomes reveals links to naked mole-rat longevity and human aging. *BMC Biol.* **2018**, *16*, 82. [CrossRef] [PubMed]

92. Hawkes, H.J.; Karlenius, T.C.; Tonissen, K.F. Regulation of the human thioredoxin gene promoter and its key substrates: A study of functional and putative regulatory elements. *Biochim. Biophys. Acta* **2014**, *1840*, 303–314. [CrossRef] [PubMed]
93. Munro, D.; Baldy, C.; Pamenter, M.E.; Treberg, J.R. The exceptional longevity of the naked mole-rat may be explained by mitochondrial antioxidant defenses. *Aging Cell* **2019**, e12916. [CrossRef] [PubMed]
94. Perez, L.M.; Pareja-Galeano, H.; Sanchis-Gomar, F.; Emanuele, E.; Lucia, A.; Galvez, B.G. 'Adipaging': Ageing and obesity share biological hallmarks related to a dysfunctional adipose tissue. *J. Physiol.* **2016**, *594*, 3187–3207. [CrossRef] [PubMed]
95. Tang, Y.; Purkayastha, S.; Cai, D. Hypothalamic microinflammation: A common basis of metabolic syndrome and aging. *Trends Neurosci.* **2015**, *38*, 36–44. [CrossRef] [PubMed]
96. Ribas, V.; García-Ruiz, C.; Fernández-Checa, J.C. Glutathione and mitochondria. *Front. Pharmacol.* **2014**, *5*, 151. [CrossRef] [PubMed]
97. Abdrakhmanova, A.; Zwicker, K.; Kerscher, S.; Zickermann, V.; Brandt, U. Tight binding of NADPH to the 39-kDa subunit of complex I is not required for catalytic activity but stabilizes the multiprotein complex. *Biochim. Biophys. Acta* **2006**, *1757*, 1676–1682. [CrossRef] [PubMed]
98. Fiedorczuk, K.; Letts, J.A.; Degliesposti, G.; Kaszuba, K.; Skehel, M.; Sazanov, L.A. Atomic structure of the entire mammalian mitochondrial complex I. *Nature* **2016**, *538*, 406–410. [CrossRef] [PubMed]
99. Lesnefsky, E.J.; Hoppel, C.L. Oxidative phosphorylation and aging. *Ageing Res. Rev.* **2006**, *5*, 402–433. [CrossRef] [PubMed]
100. Stefanatos, R.; Sanz, A. Mitochondrial complex I: A central regulator of the aging process. *Cell Cycle* **2011**, *10*, 1528–1532. [CrossRef] [PubMed]
101. Cunningham, G.M.; Flores, L.C.; Roman, M.G.; Cheng, C.; Dube, S.; Allen, C.; Valentine, J.M.; Hubbard, G.B.; Bai, Y.; Saunders, T.L.; et al. Thioredoxin overexpression in both the cytosol and mitochondria accelerates age-related disease and shortens lifespan in male C57BL/6 mice. *GeroScience* **2018**, *40*, 453–468. [CrossRef] [PubMed]
102. Cunningham, G.M.; Roman, M.G.; Flores, L.C.; Hubbard, G.B.; Salmon, A.B.; Zhang, Y.; Gelfond, J.; Ikeno, Y. The paradoxical role of thioredoxin on oxidative stress and aging. *Arch. Biochem. Biophys.* **2015**, *576*, 32–38. [CrossRef] [PubMed]
103. Flores, L.C.; Roman, M.G.; Cunningham, G.M.; Cheng, C.; Dube, S.; Allen, C.; Van Remmen, H.; Hubbard, G.B.; Saunders, T.L.; Ikeno, Y. Continuous overexpression of thioredoxin 1 enhances cancer development and does not extend maximum lifespan in male C57BL/6 mice. *Pathobiol. Aging Age Relat. Dis.* **2018**, *8*, 1533754. [CrossRef] [PubMed]
104. Pickering, A.M.; Lehr, M.; Gendron, C.M.; Pletcher, S.D.; Miller, R.A. Mitochondrial thioredoxin reductase 2 is elevated in long-lived primate as well as rodent species and extends fly mean lifespan. *Aging Cell* **2017**, *16*, 683–692. [CrossRef] [PubMed]
105. Orr, W.C.; Mockett, R.J.; Benes, J.J.; Sohal, R.S. Effects of overexpression of copper-zinc and manganese superoxide dismutases, catalase, and thioredoxin reductase genes on longevity in Drosophila melanogaster. *J. Biol. Chem.* **2003**, *278*, 26418–26422. [CrossRef] [PubMed]
106. Mockett, R.J.; Sohal, R.S.; Orr, W.C. Overexpression of glutathione reductase extends survival in transgenic Drosophila melanogaster under hyperoxia but not normoxia. *FASEB J.* **1999**, *13*, 1733–1742. [CrossRef] [PubMed]
107. Rojanathammanee, L.; Rakoczy, S.; Brown-Borg, H.M. Growth hormone alters the glutathione S-transferase and mitochondrial thioredoxin systems in long-living Ames dwarf mice. *J. Gerontol. A Biol. Sci. Med. Sci.* **2014**, *69*, 1199–1211. [CrossRef] [PubMed]
108. Drechsel, D.A.; Patel, M. Respiration-dependent H_2O_2 Removal in Brain Mitochondria via the Thioredoxin/Peroxiredoxin System. *J. Boil. Chem.* **2010**, *285*, 27850–27858. [CrossRef] [PubMed]
109. Calabrese, G.; Morgan, B.; Riemer, J. Mitochondrial Glutathione: Regulation and Functions. *Antioxid. Redox Signal.* **2017**, *27*, 1162–1177. [CrossRef] [PubMed]
110. May, J.M.; Mendiratta, S.; Hill, K.E.; Burk, R.F. Reduction of dehydroascorbate to ascorbate by the selenoenzyme thioredoxin reductase. *J. Biol. Chem.* **1997**, *272*, 22607–22610. [CrossRef] [PubMed]
111. Xia, L.; Nordman, T.; Olsson, J.M.; Damdimopoulos, A.; Bjorkhem-Bergman, L.; Nalvarte, I.; Eriksson, L.C.; Arner, E.S.; Spyrou, G.; Bjornstedt, M. The mammalian cytosolic selenoenzyme thioredoxin reductase reduces ubiquinone. A novel mechanism for defense against oxidative stress. *J. Biol. Chem.* **2003**, *278*, 2141–2146. [CrossRef] [PubMed]

112. Nalvarte, I.; Damdimopoulos, A.E.; Spyrou, G. Human mitochondrial thioredoxin reductase reduces cytochrome c and confers resistance to complex III inhibition. *Free Radic. Biol. Med.* **2004**, *36*, 1270–1278. [CrossRef] [PubMed]
113. Arner, E.S.; Nordberg, J.; Holmgren, A. Efficient reduction of lipoamide and lipoic acid by mammalian thioredoxin reductase. *Biochem. Biophys. Res. Commun.* **1996**, *225*, 268–274. [CrossRef] [PubMed]
114. Bjornstedt, M.; Hamberg, M.; Kumar, S.; Xue, J.; Holmgren, A. Human thioredoxin reductase directly reduces lipid hydroperoxides by NADPH and selenocystine strongly stimulates the reaction via catalytically generated selenols. *J. Biol. Chem.* **1995**, *270*, 11761–11764. [CrossRef] [PubMed]
115. Jee, C.; Vanoaica, L.; Lee, J.; Park, B.J.; Ahnn, J. Thioredoxin is related to life span regulation and oxidative stress response in Caenorhabditis elegans. *Genes Cells* **2005**, *10*, 1203–1210. [CrossRef] [PubMed]
116. Miranda-Vizuete, A.; Fierro Gonzalez, J.C.; Gahmon, G.; Burghoorn, J.; Navas, P.; Swoboda, P. Lifespan decrease in a *Caenorhabditis elegans* mutant lacking TRX-1, a thioredoxin expressed in ASJ sensory neurons. *FEBS Lett.* **2006**, *580*, 484–490. [CrossRef] [PubMed]
117. Li, W.; Bandyopadhyay, J.; Hwaang, H.S.; Park, B.J.; Cho, J.H.; Lee, J.I.; Ahnn, J.; Lee, S.K. Two thioredoxin reductases, trxr-1 and trxr-2, have differential physiological roles in Caenorhabditis elegans. *Mol. Cells* **2012**, *34*, 209–218. [CrossRef] [PubMed]
118. Cacho-Valadez, B.; Munoz-Lobato, F.; Pedrajas, J.R.; Cabello, J.; Fierro-Gonzalez, J.C.; Navas, P.; Swoboda, P.; Link, C.D.; Miranda-Vizuete, A. The characterization of the *Caenorhabditis elegans* mitochondrial thioredoxin system uncovers an unexpected protective role of thioredoxin reductase 2 in beta-amyloid peptide toxicity. *Antioxid. Redox Signal.* **2012**, *16*, 1384–1400. [CrossRef] [PubMed]
119. Arodin, L.; Miranda-Vizuete, A.; Swoboda, P.; Fernandes, A.P. Protective effects of the thioredoxin and glutaredoxin systems in dopamine-induced cell death. *Free Radic. Biol. Med.* **2014**, *73*, 328–336. [CrossRef] [PubMed]
120. Oláhová, M.; Veal, E.A. A peroxiredoxin, PRDX-2, is required for insulin secretion and insulin/IIS-dependent regulation of stress resistance and longevity. *Aging Cell* **2015**, *14*, 558–568. [CrossRef] [PubMed]
121. De Haes, W.; Frooninckx, L.; Van Assche, R.; Smolders, A.; Depuydt, G.; Billen, J.; Braeckman, B.P.; Schoofs, L.; Temmerman, L. Metformin promotes lifespan through mitohormesis via the peroxiredoxin PRDX-2. *Proc. Natl. Acad. Sci. USA* **2014**, *111*, E2501–E2509. [CrossRef] [PubMed]
122. Henderson, D.; Huebner, C.; Markowitz, M.; Taube, N.; Harvanek, Z.M.; Jakob, U.; Knoefler, D. Do developmental temperatures affect redox level and lifespan in *C. elegans* through upregulation of peroxiredoxin? *Redox Boil.* **2017**, *14*, 386–390. [CrossRef] [PubMed]
123. Thamsen, M.; Kumsta, C.; Li, F.; Jakob, U. Is overoxidation of peroxiredoxin physiologically significant? *Antioxid. Redox Signal.* **2011**, *14*, 725–730. [CrossRef] [PubMed]
124. Jiang, B.; Moskovitz, J. The Functions of the Mammalian Methionine Sulfoxide Reductase System and Related Diseases. *Antioxidants* **2018**, *7*, 122. [CrossRef] [PubMed]
125. Lee, B.C.; Lee, H.M.; Kim, S.; Avanesov, A.S.; Lee, A.; Chun, B.-H.; Vorbruggen, G.; Gladyshev, V.N. Expression of the methionine sulfoxide reductase lost during evolution extends Drosophila lifespan in a methionine-dependent manner. *Sci. Rep.* **2018**, *8*, 1010. [CrossRef] [PubMed]
126. Kim, H.Y.; Gladyshev, V.N. Methionine sulfoxide reductases: Selenoprotein forms and roles in antioxidant protein repair in mammals. *Biochem. J.* **2007**, *407*, 321–329. [CrossRef] [PubMed]
127. Minniti, A.N.; Cataldo, R.; Trigo, C.; Vasquez, L.; Mujica, P.; Leighton, F.; Inestrosa, N.C.; Aldunate, R. Methionine sulfoxide reductase A expression is regulated by the DAF-16/FOXO pathway in Caenorhabditis elegans. *Aging Cell* **2009**, *8*, 690–705. [CrossRef] [PubMed]
128. Bruce, L.; Singkornrat, D.; Wilson, K.; Hausman, W.; Robbins, K.; Huang, L.; Foss, K.; Binninger, D. In Vivo Effects of Methionine Sulfoxide Reductase Deficiency in Drosophila melanogaster. *Antioxidants* **2018**, *7*, 155. [CrossRef] [PubMed]
129. Ruan, H.; Tang, X.D.; Chen, M.L.; Joiner, M.L.; Sun, G.; Brot, N.; Weissbach, H.; Heinemann, S.H.; Iverson, L.; Wu, C.F.; et al. High-quality life extension by the enzyme peptide methionine sulfoxide reductase. *Proc. Natl. Acad. Sci. USA* **2002**, *99*, 2748–2753. [CrossRef] [PubMed]
130. Chung, H.; Kim, A.K.; Jung, S.A.; Kim, S.W.; Yu, K.; Lee, J.H. The Drosophila homolog of methionine sulfoxide reductase A extends lifespan and increases nuclear localization of FOXO. *FEBS Lett.* **2010**, *584*, 3609–3614. [CrossRef] [PubMed]

131. Salmon, A.B.; Kim, G.; Liu, C.; Wren, J.D.; Georgescu, C.; Richardson, A.; Levine, R.L. Effects of transgenic methionine sulfoxide reductase A (MsrA) expression on lifespan and age-dependent changes in metabolic function in mice. *Redox Boil.* **2016**, *10*, 251–256. [CrossRef] [PubMed]
132. Tarafdar, S.; Kim, G.; Levine, R.L. Drosophila methionine sulfoxide reductase A (MSRA) lacks methionine oxidase activity. *Free Radic. Biol. Med.* **2018**, *131*, 154–161. [CrossRef] [PubMed]
133. Barja, G.; Cadenas, S.; Rojas, C.; Lopez-Torres, M.; Perez-Campo, R. A decrease of free radical production near critical targets as a cause of maximum longevity in animals. *Comp. Biochem. Physiol. Part B* **1994**, *108*, 501–512. [CrossRef]
134. Kanzok, S.M.; Fechner, A.; Bauer, H.; Ulschmid, J.K.; Muller, H.M.; Botella-Munoz, J.; Schneuwly, S.; Schirmer, R.; Becker, K. Substitution of the thioredoxin system for glutathione reductase in Drosophila melanogaster. *Science* **2001**, *291*, 643–646. [CrossRef] [PubMed]
135. Mora-Lorca, J.A.; Saenz-Narciso, B.; Gaffney, C.J.; Naranjo-Galindo, F.J.; Pedrajas, J.R.; Guerrero-Gomez, D.; Dobrzynska, A.; Askjaer, P.; Szewczyk, N.J.; Cabello, J.; et al. Glutathione reductase gsr-1 is an essential gene required for *Caenorhabditis elegans* early embryonic development. *Free Radic. Biol. Med.* **2016**, *96*, 446–461. [CrossRef] [PubMed]
136. Luersen, K.; Stegehake, D.; Daniel, J.; Drescher, M.; Ajonina, I.; Ajonina, C.; Hertel, P.; Woltersdorf, C.; Liebau, E. The glutathione reductase GSR-1 determines stress tolerance and longevity in Caenorhabditis elegans. *PLoS ONE* **2013**, *8*, e60731. [CrossRef] [PubMed]
137. Stenvall, J.; Fierro-Gonzalez, J.C.; Swoboda, P.; Saamarthy, K.; Cheng, Q.; Cacho-Valadez, B.; Arner, E.S.; Persson, O.P.; Miranda-Vizuete, A.; Tuck, S. Selenoprotein TRXR-1 and GSR-1 are essential for removal of old cuticle during molting in Caenorhabditis elegans. *Proc. Natl. Acad. Sci. USA* **2011**, *108*, 1064–1069. [CrossRef] [PubMed]
138. Guerrero-Gomez, D.; Mora-Lorca, J.A.; Saenz-Narciso, B.; Naranjo-Galindo, F.J.; Munoz-Lobato, F.; Parrado-Fernandez, C.; Goikolea, J.; Cedazo-Minguez, A.; Link, C.D.; Neri, C.; et al. Loss of glutathione redox homeostasis impairs proteostasis by inhibiting autophagy-dependent protein degradation. *Cell Death Differ.* **2019**. [CrossRef] [PubMed]
139. Luchak, J.M.; Prabhudesai, L.; Sohal, R.S.; Radyuk, S.N.; Orr, W.C. Modulating longevity in Drosophila by over- and underexpression of glutamate-cysteine ligase. *Ann. N. Y. Acad. Sci.* **2007**, *1119*, 260–273. [CrossRef] [PubMed]
140. Orr, W.C.; Radyuk, S.N.; Prabhudesai, L.; Toroser, D.; Benes, J.J.; Luchak, J.M.; Mockett, R.J.; Rebrin, I.; Hubbard, J.G.; Sohal, R.S. Overexpression of glutamate-cysteine ligase extends life span in Drosophila melanogaster. *J. Biol. Chem.* **2005**, *280*, 37331–37338. [CrossRef] [PubMed]
141. Li, F.; Ma, X.; Cui, X.; Li, J.; Wang, Z. Recombinant buckwheat glutaredoxin intake increases lifespan and stress resistance via hsf-1 upregulation in Caenorhabditis elegans. *Exp. Gerontol.* **2018**, *104*, 86–97. [CrossRef] [PubMed]
142. Andziak, B.; O'Connor, T.P.; Qi, W.; DeWaal, E.M.; Pierce, A.; Chaudhuri, A.R.; Van Remmen, H.; Buffenstein, R. High oxidative damage levels in the longest-living rodent, the naked mole-rat. *Aging Cell* **2006**, *5*, 463–471. [CrossRef] [PubMed]
143. Go, Y.M.; Jones, D.P. Redox compartmentalization in eukaryotic cells. *Biochim. Biophys. Acta* **2008**, *1780*, 1273–1290. [CrossRef] [PubMed]
144. Cai, J.; Jones, D.P. Superoxide in apoptosis. Mitochondrial generation triggered by cytochrome c loss. *J. Biol. Chem.* **1998**, *273*, 11401–11404. [CrossRef] [PubMed]
145. Kemp, M.; Go, Y.M.; Jones, D.P. Nonequilibrium thermodynamics of thiol/disulfide redox systems: A perspective on redox systems biology. *Free Radic. Biol. Med.* **2008**, *44*, 921–937. [CrossRef] [PubMed]
146. Rebrin, I.; Sohal, R.S. Comparison of thiol redox state of mitochondria and homogenates of various tissues between two strains of mice with different longevities. *Exp. Gerontol.* **2004**, *39*, 1513–1519. [CrossRef] [PubMed]
147. Legan, S.K.; Rebrin, I.; Mockett, R.J.; Radyuk, S.N.; Klichko, V.I.; Sohal, R.S.; Orr, W.C. Overexpression of glucose-6-phosphate dehydrogenase extends the life span of Drosophila melanogaster. *J. Biol. Chem.* **2008**, *283*, 32492–32499. [CrossRef] [PubMed]
148. Luckinbill, L.S.; Riha, V.; Rhine, S.; Grudzien, T.A. The role of glucose-6-phosphate dehydrogenase in the evolution of longevity in Drosophila melanogaster. *Heredity* **1990**, *65 Pt 1*, 29–38. [CrossRef]

149. Wang, C.-T.; Chen, Y.-C.; Wang, Y.-Y.; Huang, M.-H.; Yen, T.-L.; Li, H.; Liang, C.-J.; Sang, T.-K.; Ciou, S.-C.; Yuh, C.-H.; et al. Reduced neuronal expression of ribose-5-phosphate isomerase enhances tolerance to oxidative stress, extends lifespan, and attenuates polyglutamine toxicity in Drosophila. *Aging Cell* **2012**, *11*, 93–103. [CrossRef] [PubMed]
150. Farkas, R.; Danis, P.; Medved'ova, L.; Mechler, B.M.; Knopp, J. Regulation of cytosolic malate dehydrogenase by juvenile hormone in Drosophila melanogaster. *Cell Biochem. Biophys.* **2002**, *37*, 37–52. [CrossRef]
151. Kim, G.H.; Lee, Y.E.; Lee, G.H.; Cho, Y.H.; Lee, Y.N.; Jang, Y.; Paik, D.; Park, J.J. Overexpression of malic enzyme in the larval stage extends Drosophila lifespan. *Biochem. Biophys. Res. Commun.* **2015**, *456*, 676–682. [CrossRef] [PubMed]
152. Paik, D.; Jang, Y.G.; Lee, Y.E.; Lee, Y.N.; Yamamoto, R.; Gee, H.Y.; Yoo, S.; Bae, E.; Min, K.J.; Tatar, M.; et al. Misexpression screen delineates novel genes controlling Drosophila lifespan. *Mech. Ageing Dev.* **2012**, *133*, 234–245. [CrossRef] [PubMed]
153. Merritt, T.J.S.; Kuczynski, C.; Sezgin, E.; Zhu, C.-T.; Kumagai, S.; Eanes, W.F. Quantifying interactions within the NADP(H) enzyme network in Drosophila melanogaster. *Genetics* **2009**, *182*, 565–574. [CrossRef] [PubMed]
154. Rong, Y.S.; Golic, K.G. A targeted gene knockout in Drosophila. *Genetics* **2001**, *157*, 1307–1312. [PubMed]
155. Tremblay, G.B.; Sohi, S.S.; Retnakaran, A.; MacKenzie, R.E. NAD-dependent methylenetetrahydrofolate dehydrogenase-methenyltetrahydrofolate cyclohydrolase is targeted to the cytoplasm in insect cell lines. *FEBS Lett.* **1995**, *368*, 177–182. [CrossRef]
156. Yu, S.; Jang, Y.; Paik, D.; Lee, E.; Park, J.J. Nmdmc overexpression extends Drosophila lifespan and reduces levels of mitochondrial reactive oxygen species. *Biochem. Biophys. Res. Commun.* **2015**, *465*, 845–850. [CrossRef] [PubMed]
157. Gaudet, P.; Livstone, M.S.; Lewis, S.E.; Thomas, P.D. Phylogenetic-based propagation of functional annotations within the Gene Ontology consortium. *Brief. Bioinform.* **2011**, *12*, 449–462. [CrossRef] [PubMed]
158. Da Cunha, G.L.; de Oliveira, A.K. Citric acid cycle: A mainstream metabolic pathway influencing life span in Drosophila melanogaster? *Exp. Gerontol.* **1996**, *31*, 705–715. [CrossRef]
159. Arking, R.; Burde, V.; Graves, K.; Hari, R.; Feldman, E.; Zeevi, A.; Soliman, S.; Saraiya, A.; Buck, S.; Vettraino, J.; et al. Forward and reverse selection for longevity in Drosophila is characterized by alteration of antioxidant gene expression and oxidative damage patterns. *Exp. Gerontol.* **2000**, *35*, 167–185. [CrossRef]
160. Alonso, J.; Rodriguez, J.M.; Baena-Lopez, L.A.; Santaren, J.F. Characterization of the Drosophila melanogaster mitochondrial proteome. *J. Proteome Res.* **2005**, *4*, 1636–1645. [CrossRef] [PubMed]
161. Lee, K.S.; Iijima-Ando, K.; Iijima, K.; Lee, W.J.; Lee, J.H.; Yu, K.; Lee, D.S. JNK/FOXO-mediated neuronal expression of fly homologue of peroxiredoxin II reduces oxidative stress and extends life span. *J. Biol. Chem.* **2009**, *284*, 29454–29461. [CrossRef] [PubMed]
162. Radyuk, S.N.; Michalak, K.; Klichko, V.I.; Benes, J.; Rebrin, I.; Sohal, R.S.; Orr, W.C. Peroxiredoxin 5 confers protection against oxidative stress and apoptosis and also promotes longevity in Drosophila. *Biochem. J.* **2009**, *419*, 437–445. [CrossRef] [PubMed]
163. Odnokoz, O.; Nakatsuka, K.; Klichko, V.I.; Nguyen, J.; Solis, L.C.; Ostling, K.; Badinloo, M.; Orr, W.C.; Radyuk, S.N. Mitochondrial peroxiredoxins are essential in regulating the relationship between Drosophila immunity and aging. *Biochim. Biophys. Acta Mol. Basis Dis.* **2017**, *1863*, 68–80. [CrossRef] [PubMed]
164. Orr, W.C.; Radyuk, S.N.; Sohal, R.S. Involvement of redox state in the aging of Drosophila melanogaster. *Antioxid. Redox Signal.* **2013**, *19*, 788–803. [CrossRef] [PubMed]
165. Radyuk, S.N.; Rebrin, I.; Klichko, V.I.; Sohal, B.H.; Michalak, K.; Benes, J.; Sohal, R.S.; Orr, W.C. Mitochondrial peroxiredoxins are critical for the maintenance of redox state and the survival of adult Drosophila. *Free Radic. Biol. Med.* **2010**, *49*, 1892–1902. [CrossRef] [PubMed]
166. Klichko, V.I.; Orr, W.C.; Radyuk, S.N. The role of peroxiredoxin 4 in inflammatory response and aging. *Biochim. Biophys. Acta* **2016**, *1862*, 265–273. [CrossRef] [PubMed]
167. Fernandez-Marcos, P.J.; Nóbrega-Pereira, S. NADPH: New oxygen for the ROS theory of aging. *Oncotarget* **2016**, *7*, 50814–50815. [CrossRef] [PubMed]
168. Fan, J.; Ye, J.; Kamphorst, J.J.; Shlomi, T.; Thompson, C.B.; Rabinowitz, J.D. Quantitative flux analysis reveals folate-dependent NADPH production. *Nature* **2014**, *510*, 298–302. [CrossRef] [PubMed]

169. Nobrega-Pereira, S.; Fernandez-Marcos, P.J.; Brioche, T.; Gomez-Cabrera, M.C.; Salvador-Pascual, A.; Flores, J.M.; Vina, J.; Serrano, M. G6PD protects from oxidative damage and improves healthspan in mice. *Nat. Commun.* **2016**, *7*, 10894. [CrossRef] [PubMed]
170. Dietzmann, K. Histochemical demonstration of enzyme activity changes in the regio postcentralis of the mouse brain under the effect of the aging process. *J. Hirnforsch.* **1981**, *22*, 405–408. [PubMed]
171. Kaliman, P.A.; Konovalova, E.O. Age-dependent characteristics of the regulation of cytoplasmic NADP+-dehydrogenases in the liver of rats on different diets. *Ukrainskii Biokhimicheskii Zhurnal (1978)* **1985**, *57*, 38–42.
172. Lemeshko, V.V.; Nikitchenko Iu, V.; Kaliman, P.A. Enzymes of the antioxidant system of rat liver during aging. *Ukrainskii Biokhimicheskii Zhurnal (1978)* **1983**, *55*, 523–528.
173. Maurya, P.K.; Kumar, P.; Chandra, P. Age-dependent detection of erythrocytes glucose-6-phosphate dehydrogenase and its correlation with oxidative stress. *Arch. Physiol. Biochem.* **2016**, *122*, 61–66. [CrossRef] [PubMed]
174. Gartler, S.M.; Hornung, S.K.; Motulsky, A.G. Effect of chronologic age on induction of cystathionine synthase, uroporphyrinogen I synthase, and glucose-6-phosphate dehydrogenase activities in lymphocytes. *Proc. Natl. Acad. Sci. USA* **1981**, *78*, 1916–1919. [CrossRef] [PubMed]
175. Machado, A.; Ayala, A.; Gordillo, E.; Revilla, E.; Santa Maria, C. Relationship between enzymatic activity loss and post-translational protein modification in aging. *Arch. Gerontol. Geriatr.* **1991**, *12*, 187–197. [CrossRef]
176. Kil, I.S.; Lee, Y.S.; Bae, Y.S.; Huh, T.L.; Park, J.W. Modulation of NADP(+)-dependent isocitrate dehydrogenase in aging. *Redox Rep.* **2004**, *9*, 271–277. [CrossRef] [PubMed]
177. Wong, N.; Blair, A.R.; Morahan, G.; Andrikopoulos, S. The deletion variant of nicotinamide nucleotide transhydrogenase (Nnt) does not affect insulin secretion or glucose tolerance. *Endocrinology* **2010**, *151*, 96–102. [CrossRef] [PubMed]
178. Serrander, L.; Cartier, L.; Bedard, K.; Banfi, B.; Lardy, B.; Plastre, O.; Sienkiewicz, A.; Fórró, L.; Schlegel, W.; Krause, K.-H. NOX4 activity is determined by mRNA levels and reveals a unique pattern of ROS generation. *Biochem. J.* **2007**, *406*, 105–114. [CrossRef] [PubMed]
179. Nisimoto, Y.; Diebold, B.A.; Cosentino-Gomes, D.; Lambeth, J.D. Nox4: A hydrogen peroxide-generating oxygen sensor. *Biochemistry* **2014**, *53*, 5111–5120. [CrossRef] [PubMed]
180. Nisimoto, Y.; Jackson, H.M.; Ogawa, H.; Kawahara, T.; Lambeth, J.D. Constitutive NADPH-dependent electron transferase activity of the Nox4 dehydrogenase domain. *Biochemistry* **2010**, *49*, 2433–2442. [CrossRef] [PubMed]
181. Worthington, D.J.; Rosemeyer, M.A. Glutathione reductase from human erythrocytes. Catalytic properties and aggregation. *Eur. J. Biochem.* **1976**, *67*, 231–238. [CrossRef] [PubMed]
182. Koziel, R.; Pircher, H.; Kratochwil, M.; Lener, B.; Hermann, M.; Dencher, N.A.; Jansen-Durr, P. Mitochondrial respiratory chain complex I is inactivated by NADPH oxidase Nox4. *Biochem. J.* **2013**, *452*, 231–239. [CrossRef] [PubMed]
183. Goy, C.; Czypiorski, P.; Altschmied, J.; Jakob, S.; Rabanter, L.L.; Brewer, A.C.; Ale-Agha, N.; Dyballa-Rukes, N.; Shah, A.M.; Haendeler, J. The imbalanced redox status in senescent endothelial cells is due to dysregulated Thioredoxin-1 and NADPH oxidase 4. *Exp. Gerontol.* **2014**, *56*, 45–52. [CrossRef] [PubMed]
184. Handy, D.E.; Loscalzo, J. Responses to reductive stress in the cardiovascular system. *Free Radic. Boil. Med.* **2017**, *109*, 114–124. [CrossRef] [PubMed]
185. Rezende, F.; Schürmann, C.; Schütz, S.; Harenkamp, S.; Herrmann, E.; Seimetz, M.; Weißmann, N.; Schröder, K. Knock out of the NADPH oxidase Nox4 has no impact on life span in mice. *Redox Boil.* **2016**, *11*, 312–314. [CrossRef] [PubMed]
186. Hirschhauser, C.; Bornbaum, J.; Reis, A.; Bohme, S.; Kaludercic, N.; Menabo, R.; Di Lisa, F.; Boengler, K.; Shah, A.M.; Schulz, R.; et al. NOX4 in Mitochondria: Yeast Two-Hybrid-Based Interaction with Complex I Without Relevance for Basal Reactive Oxygen Species? *Antioxid. Redox Signal.* **2015**, *23*, 1106–1112. [CrossRef] [PubMed]
187. Miyagi, H.; Kawai, S.; Murata, K. Two sources of mitochondrial NADPH in the yeast Saccharomyces cerevisiae. *J. Biol. Chem.* **2009**, *284*, 7553–7560. [CrossRef] [PubMed]
188. He, W.; Wang, Y.; Liu, W.; Zhou, C.Z. Crystal structure of Saccharomyces cerevisiae 6-phosphogluconate dehydrogenase Gnd1. *BMC Struct. Boil.* **2007**, *7*, 38. [CrossRef] [PubMed]

189. Minard, K.I.; McAlister-Henn, L. Sources of NADPH in yeast vary with carbon source. *J. Biol. Chem.* **2005**, *280*, 39890–39896. [CrossRef] [PubMed]
190. Garay, E.; Campos, S.E.; Gonzalez de la Cruz, J.; Gaspar, A.P.; Jinich, A.; Deluna, A. High-resolution profiling of stationary-phase survival reveals yeast longevity factors and their genetic interactions. *PLoS Genet.* **2014**, *10*, e1004168. [CrossRef] [PubMed]
191. Laschober, G.T.; Ruli, D.; Hofer, E.; Muck, C.; Carmona-Gutierrez, D.; Ring, J.; Hutter, E.; Ruckenstuhl, C.; Micutkova, L.; Brunauer, R.; et al. Identification of evolutionarily conserved genetic regulators of cellular aging. *Aging Cell* **2010**, *9*, 1084–1097. [CrossRef] [PubMed]
192. Orlandi, I.; Stamerra, G.; Vai, M. Altered Expression of Mitochondrial NAD(+) Carriers Influences Yeast Chronological Lifespan by Modulating Cytosolic and Mitochondrial Metabolism. *Front. Genet.* **2018**, *9*, 676. [CrossRef] [PubMed]
193. Brandes, N.; Tienson, H.; Lindemann, A.; Vitvitsky, V.; Reichmann, D.; Banerjee, R.; Jakob, U. Time line of redox events in aging postmitotic cells. *eLife* **2013**, *2*, e00306. [CrossRef] [PubMed]
194. Kwolek-Mirek, M.; Maslanka, R.; Molon, M. Disorders in NADPH generation via pentose phosphate pathway influence the reproductive potential of the Saccharomyces cerevisiae yeast due to changes in redox status. *J. Cell. Biochem.* **2018**. [CrossRef] [PubMed]
195. Picazo, C.; Matallana, E.; Aranda, A. Yeast thioredoxin reductase Trr1p controls TORC1-regulated processes. *Sci. Rep.* **2018**, *8*, 16500. [CrossRef] [PubMed]
196. Matecic, M.; Smith, D.L.; Pan, X.; Maqani, N.; Bekiranov, S.; Boeke, J.D.; Smith, J.S. A microarray-based genetic screen for yeast chronological aging factors. *PLoS Genet.* **2010**, *6*, e1000921. [CrossRef] [PubMed]
197. Musa, M.; Peric, M.; Bou Dib, P.; Sobocanec, S.; Saric, A.; Lovric, A.; Rudan, M.; Nikolic, A.; Milosevic, I.; Vlahovicek, K.; et al. Heat-induced longevity in budding yeast requires respiratory metabolism and glutathione recycling. *Aging* **2018**, *10*, 2407–2427. [CrossRef] [PubMed]
198. Managbanag, J.R.; Witten, T.M.; Bonchev, D.; Fox, L.A.; Tsuchiya, M.; Kennedy, B.K.; Kaeberlein, M. Shortest-path network analysis is a useful approach toward identifying genetic determinants of longevity. *PLoS ONE* **2008**, *3*, e3802. [CrossRef] [PubMed]
199. Smith, E.D.; Tsuchiya, M.; Fox, L.A.; Dang, N.; Hu, D.; Kerr, E.O.; Johnston, E.D.; Tchao, B.N.; Pak, D.N.; Welton, K.L.; et al. Quantitative evidence for conserved longevity pathways between divergent eukaryotic species. *Genome Res.* **2008**, *18*, 564–570. [CrossRef] [PubMed]
200. Kenyon, C.; Chang, J.; Gensch, E.; Rudner, A.; Tabtiang, R. A *C. elegans* mutant that lives twice as long as wild type. *Nature* **1993**, *366*, 461–464. [CrossRef] [PubMed]
201. Tullet, J.M.; Hertweck, M.; An, J.H.; Baker, J.; Hwang, J.Y.; Liu, S.; Oliveira, R.P.; Baumeister, R.; Blackwell, T.K. Direct inhibition of the longevity-promoting factor SKN-1 by insulin-like signaling in *C. elegans*. *Cell* **2008**, *132*, 1025–1038. [CrossRef] [PubMed]
202. Yang, H.C.; Yu, H.; Liu, Y.C.; Chen, T.L.; Stern, A.; Lo, S.J.; Chiu, D.T. IDH-1 deficiency induces growth defects and metabolic alterations in GSPD-1-deficient *Caenorhabditis elegans*. *J. Mol. Med.* **2019**, *366*, 461–464. [CrossRef] [PubMed]
203. Yu, H.; Larsen, P.L. DAF-16-dependent and independent expression targets of DAF-2 insulin receptor-like pathway in *Caenorhabditis elegans* include FKBPs. *J. Mol. Biol.* **2001**, *314*, 1017–1028. [CrossRef] [PubMed]
204. Depuydt, G.; Xie, F.; Petyuk, V.A.; Smolders, A.; Brewer, H.M.; Camp, D.G., 2nd; Smith, R.D.; Braeckman, B.P. LC-MS Proteomics Analysis of the Insulin/IGF-1-Deficient *Caenorhabditis elegans* daf-2(e1370) Mutant Reveals Extensive Restructuring of Intermediary Metabolism. *J. Proteome Res.* **2014**, *13*, 1938–1956. [CrossRef] [PubMed]
205. Martell, J.; Seo, Y.; Bak, D.W.; Kingsley, S.F.; Tissenbaum, H.A.; Weerapana, E. Global Cysteine-Reactivity Profiling during Impaired Insulin/IGF-1 Signaling in *C. elegans* Identifies Uncharacterized Mediators of Longevity. *Cell Chem. Boil.* **2016**, *23*, 955–966. [CrossRef] [PubMed]
206. Walther, D.M.; Kasturi, P.; Zheng, M.; Pinkert, S.; Vecchi, G.; Ciryam, P.; Morimoto, R.I.; Dobson, C.M.; Vendruscolo, M.; Mann, M.; et al. Widespread Proteome Remodeling and Aggregation in Aging *C. elegans*. *Cell* **2015**, *161*, 919–932. [CrossRef] [PubMed]
207. Pinkston-Gosse, J.; Kenyon, C. DAF-16/FOXO targets genes that regulate tumor growth in *Caenorhabditis elegans*. *Nat. Genet.* **2007**, *39*, 1403–1409. [CrossRef] [PubMed]
208. Zhang, P.; Judy, M.; Lee, S.J.; Kenyon, C. Direct and indirect gene regulation by a life-extending FOXO protein in *C. elegans*: Roles for GATA factors and lipid gene regulators. *Cell Metab.* **2013**, *17*, 85–100. [CrossRef]

209. Murphy, C.T.; McCarroll, S.A.; Bargmann, C.I.; Fraser, A.; Kamath, R.S.; Ahringer, J.; Li, H.; Kenyon, C. Genes that act downstream of DAF-16 to influence the lifespan of *Caenorhabditis elegans*. *Nature* **2003**, *424*, 277–283. [CrossRef] [PubMed]
210. Erkut, C.; Gade, V.R.; Laxman, S.; Kurzchalia, T.V. The glyoxylate shunt is essential for desiccation tolerance in *C. elegans* and budding yeast. *eLife* **2016**, *5*, e13614. [CrossRef] [PubMed]
211. Gallo, M.; Park, D.; Riddle, D.L. Increased longevity of some *C. elegans* mitochondrial mutants explained by activation of an alternative energy-producing pathway. *Mech. Ageing Dev.* **2011**, *132*, 515–518. [CrossRef]
212. Zuryn, S.; Kuang, J.; Tuck, A.; Ebert, P.R. Mitochondrial dysfunction in *Caenorhabditis elegans* causes metabolic restructuring, but this is not linked to longevity. *Mech. Ageing Dev.* **2010**, *131*, 554–561. [CrossRef] [PubMed]
213. Hamilton, B.; Dong, Y.; Shindo, M.; Liu, W.; Odell, I.; Ruvkun, G.; Lee, S.S. A systematic RNAi screen for longevity genes in *C. elegans*. *Genes Dev.* **2005**, *19*, 1544–1555. [CrossRef] [PubMed]
214. Chin, R.M.; Fu, X.; Pai, M.Y.; Vergnes, L.; Hwang, H.; Deng, G.; Diep, S.; Lomenick, B.; Meli, V.S.; Monsalve, G.C.; et al. The metabolite alpha-ketoglutarate extends lifespan by inhibiting ATP synthase and TOR. *Nature* **2014**, *510*, 397–401. [CrossRef] [PubMed]
215. Kim, Y.; Sun, H. Functional genomic approach to identify novel genes involved in the regulation of oxidative stress resistance and animal lifespan. *Aging Cell* **2007**, *6*, 489–503. [CrossRef] [PubMed]
216. Chen, T.L.; Yang, H.C.; Hung, C.Y.; Ou, M.H.; Pan, Y.Y.; Cheng, M.L.; Stern, A.; Lo, S.J.; Chiu, D.T. Impaired embryonic development in glucose-6-phosphate dehydrogenase-deficient *Caenorhabditis elegans* due to abnormal redox homeostasis induced activation of calcium-independent phospholipase and alteration of glycerophospholipid metabolism. *Cell Death Dis.* **2017**, *8*, e2545. [CrossRef] [PubMed]
217. Bennett, C.F.; Kwon, J.J.; Chen, C.; Russell, J.; Acosta, K.; Burnaevskiy, N.; Crane, M.M.; Bitto, A.; Vander Wende, H.; Simko, M.; et al. Transaldolase inhibition impairs mitochondrial respiration and induces a starvation-like longevity response in Caenorhabditis elegans. *PLoS Genet.* **2017**, *13*, e1006695. [CrossRef] [PubMed]
218. Wang, J.; Robida-Stubbs, S.; Tullet, J.M.; Rual, J.F.; Vidal, M.; Blackwell, T.K. RNAi screening implicates a SKN-1-dependent transcriptional response in stress resistance and longevity deriving from translation inhibition. *PLoS Genet.* **2010**, *6*, e1001048. [CrossRef] [PubMed]
219. Bennett, C.F.; Kaeberlein, M. The mitochondrial unfolded protein response and increased longevity: Cause, consequence, or correlation? *Exp. Gerontol.* **2014**, *56*, 142–146. [CrossRef] [PubMed]
220. Melber, A.; Haynes, C.M. UPR(mt) regulation and output: A stress response mediated by mitochondrial-nuclear communication. *Cell Res.* **2018**, *28*, 281–295. [CrossRef] [PubMed]
221. Wu, Z.; Senchuk, M.M.; Dues, D.J.; Johnson, B.K.; Cooper, J.F.; Lew, L.; Machiela, E.; Schaar, C.E.; DeJonge, H.; Blackwell, T.K.; et al. Mitochondrial unfolded protein response transcription factor ATFS-1 promotes longevity in a long-lived mitochondrial mutant through activation of stress response pathways. *BMC Biol.* **2018**, *16*, 147. [CrossRef] [PubMed]
222. Rzezniczak, T.Z.; Merritt, T.J. Interactions of NADP-reducing enzymes across varying environmental conditions: A model of biological complexity. *G3 Genes Genomes Genet.* **2012**, *2*, 1613–1623. [CrossRef] [PubMed]
223. White, K.; Kim, M.J.; Ding, D.; Han, C.; Park, H.J.; Meneses, Z.; Tanokura, M.; Linser, P.; Salvi, R.; Someya, S. G6pd Deficiency Does Not Affect the Cytosolic Glutathione or Thioredoxin Antioxidant Defense in Mouse Cochlea. *J. Neurosci.* **2017**, *37*, 5770–5781. [CrossRef] [PubMed]
224. Au, S.W.; Gover, S.; Lam, V.M.; Adams, M.J. Human glucose-6-phosphate dehydrogenase: The crystal structure reveals a structural NADP(+) molecule and provides insights into enzyme deficiency. *Structure (Lond. Engl. 1993)* **2000**, *8*, 293–303.
225. Pandolfi, P.P.; Sonati, F.; Rivi, R.; Mason, P.; Grosveld, F.; Luzzatto, L. Targeted disruption of the housekeeping gene encoding glucose 6-phosphate dehydrogenase (G6PD): G6PD is dispensable for pentose synthesis but essential for defense against oxidative stress. *EMBO J.* **1995**, *14*, 5209–5215. [CrossRef] [PubMed]
226. Urban, N.; Tsitsipatis, D.; Hausig, F.; Kreuzer, K.; Erler, K.; Stein, V.; Ristow, M.; Steinbrenner, H.; Klotz, L.O. Non-linear impact of glutathione depletion on *C. elegans* life span and stress resistance. *Redox Boil.* **2017**, *11*, 502–515. [CrossRef] [PubMed]
227. Okuyama, T.; Inoue, H.; Ookuma, S.; Satoh, T.; Kano, K.; Honjoh, S.; Hisamoto, N.; Matsumoto, K.; Nishida, E. The ERK-MAPK pathway regulates longevity through SKN-1 and insulin-like signaling in *Caenorhabditis elegans*. *J. Biol. Chem.* **2010**, *285*, 30274–30281. [CrossRef] [PubMed]

228. Przybysz, A.J.; Choe, K.P.; Roberts, L.J.; Strange, K. Increased age reduces DAF-16 and SKN-1 signaling and the hormetic response of *Caenorhabditis elegans* to the xenobiotic juglone. *Mech. Ageing Dev.* **2009**, *130*, 357–369. [CrossRef] [PubMed]
229. Dillin, A.; Crawford, D.K.; Kenyon, C. Timing requirements for insulin/IGF-1 signaling in *C. elegans*. *Science* **2002**, *298*, 830–834. [CrossRef] [PubMed]
230. Edwards, C.; Canfield, J.; Copes, N.; Rehan, M.; Lipps, D.; Bradshaw, P.C. D-β-hydroxybutyrate extends lifespan in *C. elegans*. *Aging (Albany Ny)* **2014**, *6*, 621–644.
231. Schwartz, A.G.; Pashko, L.L. Dehydroepiandrosterone, glucose-6-phosphate dehydrogenase, and longevity. *Ageing Res. Rev.* **2004**, *3*, 171–187. [CrossRef] [PubMed]
232. Vogelauer, M.; Krall, A.S.; McBrian, M.A.; Li, J.Y.; Kurdistani, S.K. Stimulation of histone deacetylase activity by metabolites of intermediary metabolism. *J. Biol. Chem.* **2012**, *287*, 32006–32016. [CrossRef] [PubMed]
233. Pasyukova, E.G.; Vaiserman, A.M. HDAC inhibitors: A new promising drug class in anti-aging research. *Mech. Ageing Dev.* **2017**, *166*, 6–15. [CrossRef] [PubMed]
234. Arkblad, E.L.; Tuck, S.; Pestov, N.B.; Dmitriev, R.I.; Kostina, M.B.; Stenvall, J.; Tranberg, M.; Rydstrom, J. A *Caenorhabditis elegans* mutant lacking functional nicotinamide nucleotide transhydrogenase displays increased sensitivity to oxidative stress. *Free Radic. Biol. Med.* **2005**, *38*, 1518–1525. [CrossRef] [PubMed]
235. Wu, K.C.; Cui, J.Y.; Klaassen, C.D. Beneficial role of Nrf2 in regulating NADPH generation and consumption. *Toxicol. Sci.* **2011**, *123*, 590–600. [CrossRef] [PubMed]
236. Yang, W.; Hekimi, S. Two modes of mitochondrial dysfunction lead independently to lifespan extension in *Caenorhabditis elegans*. *Aging Cell* **2010**, *9*, 433–447. [CrossRef] [PubMed]
237. Dues, D.J.; Schaar, C.E.; Johnson, B.K.; Bowman, M.J.; Winn, M.E.; Senchuk, M.M.; Van Raamsdonk, J.M. Uncoupling of oxidative stress resistance and lifespan in long-lived isp-1 mitochondrial mutants in *Caenorhabditis elegans*. *Free Radic. Biol. Med.* **2017**, *108*, 362–373. [CrossRef] [PubMed]
238. An, J.H.; Blackwell, T.K. SKN-1 links *C. elegans* mesendodermal specification to a conserved oxidative stress response. *Genes Dev.* **2003**, *17*, 1882–1893. [CrossRef] [PubMed]
239. Tang, L.; Choe, K.P. Characterization of skn-1/wdr-23 phenotypes in *Caenorhabditis elegans*; pleiotrophy, aging, glutathione, and interactions with other longevity pathways. *Mech. Ageing Dev.* **2015**, *149*, 88–98. [CrossRef] [PubMed]
240. Sohal, R.S.; Weindruch, R. Oxidative stress, caloric restriction, and aging. *Science* **1996**, *273*, 59–63. [CrossRef] [PubMed]
241. Sanchez-Roman, I.; Barja, G. Regulation of longevity and oxidative stress by nutritional interventions: Role of methionine restriction. *Exp. Gerontol.* **2013**, *48*, 1030–1042. [CrossRef] [PubMed]
242. Hine, C.; Mitchell, J.R. Calorie restriction and methionine restriction in control of endogenous hydrogen sulfide production by the transsulfuration pathway. *Exp. Gerontol.* **2015**, *68*, 26–32. [CrossRef] [PubMed]
243. Eriksson, S.; Prigge, J.R.; Talago, E.A.; Arner, E.S.; Schmidt, E.E. Dietary methionine can sustain cytosolic redox homeostasis in the mouse liver. *Nat. Commun.* **2015**, *6*, 6479. [CrossRef] [PubMed]
244. Ghosh, D.; Brewer, G.J. External cys/cySS redox state modification controls the intracellular redox state and neurodegeneration via Akt in aging and Alzheimer's disease mouse model neurons. *J. Alzheimers Dis.* **2014**, *42*, 313–324. [CrossRef] [PubMed]
245. McIsaac, R.S.; Lewis, K.N.; Gibney, P.A.; Buffenstein, R. From yeast to human: Exploring the comparative biology of methionine restriction in extending eukaryotic life span. *Ann. N. Y. Acad. Sci.* **2016**, *1363*, 155–170. [CrossRef] [PubMed]
246. Uthus, E.O.; Brown-Borg, H.M. Methionine flux to transsulfuration is enhanced in the long living Ames dwarf mouse. *Mech. Ageing Dev.* **2006**, *127*, 444–450. [CrossRef] [PubMed]
247. Slekar, K.H.; Kosman, D.J.; Culotta, V.C. The Yeast Copper/Zinc Superoxide Dismutase and the Pentose Phosphate Pathway Play Overlapping Roles in Oxidative Stress Protection. *J. Boil. Chem.* **1996**, *271*, 28831–28836. [CrossRef]
248. Campbell, K.; Vowinckel, J.; Keller, M.A.; Ralser, M. Methionine Metabolism Alters Oxidative Stress Resistance via the Pentose Phosphate Pathway. *Antioxid. Redox Signal.* **2016**, *24*, 543–547. [CrossRef] [PubMed]
249. Lee, B.C.; Kaya, A.; Ma, S.; Kim, G.; Gerashchenko, M.V.; Yim, S.H.; Hu, Z.; Harshman, L.G.; Gladyshev, V.N. Methionine restriction extends lifespan of Drosophila melanogaster under conditions of low amino-acid status. *Nat. Commun.* **2014**, *5*, 3592. [CrossRef] [PubMed]

250. Johnson, J.E.; Johnson, F.B. Methionine restriction activates the retrograde response and confers both stress tolerance and lifespan extension to yeast, mouse and human cells. *PLoS ONE* **2014**, *9*, e97729. [CrossRef] [PubMed]
251. Ruckenstuhl, C.; Netzberger, C.; Entfellner, I.; Carmona-Gutierrez, D.; Kickenweiz, T.; Stekovic, S.; Gleixner, C.; Schmid, C.; Klug, L.; Sorgo, A.G.; et al. Lifespan extension by methionine restriction requires autophagy-dependent vacuolar acidification. *PLoS Genet.* **2014**, *10*, e1004347. [CrossRef] [PubMed]
252. Wipf, B.; Leisinger, T. Compartmentation of arginine biosynthesis in Saccharomyces cerevisiae. *Fems Microbiol. Lett.* **1977**, *2*, 239–242. [CrossRef]
253. Zabriskie, T.M.; Jackson, M.D. Lysine biosynthesis and metabolism in fungi. *Nat. Prod. Rep.* **2000**, *17*, 85–97. [CrossRef] [PubMed]
254. Canto, C.; Auwerx, J. Calorie restriction: Is AMPK a key sensor and effector? *Physiol.* **2011**, *26*, 214–224. [CrossRef] [PubMed]
255. Iio, W.; Tokutake, Y.; Koike, H.; Matsukawa, N.; Tsukahara, T.; Chohnan, S.; Toyoda, A. Effects of chronic mild food restriction on behavior and the hypothalamic malonyl-CoA signaling pathway. *Anim. Sci. J.* **2015**, *86*, 181–188. [CrossRef] [PubMed]
256. Canto, C.; Gerhart-Hines, Z.; Feige, J.N.; Lagouge, M.; Noriega, L.; Milne, J.C.; Elliott, P.J.; Puigserver, P.; Auwerx, J. AMPK regulates energy expenditure by modulating NAD+ metabolism and SIRT1 activity. *Nature* **2009**, *458*, 1056–1060. [CrossRef] [PubMed]
257. Walsh, M.E.; Shi, Y.; Van Remmen, H. The effects of dietary restriction on oxidative stress in rodents. *Free Radic. Boil. Med.* **2014**, *66*, 88–99. [CrossRef] [PubMed]
258. Pearson, K.J.; Lewis, K.N.; Price, N.L.; Chang, J.W.; Perez, E.; Cascajo, M.V.; Tamashiro, K.L.; Poosala, S.; Csiszar, A.; Ungvari, Z.; et al. Nrf2 mediates cancer protection but not prolongevity induced by caloric restriction. *Proc. Natl. Acad. Sci. USA* **2008**, *105*, 2325–2330. [CrossRef] [PubMed]
259. Someya, S.; Yu, W.; Hallows, W.C.; Xu, J.; Vann, J.M.; Leeuwenburgh, C.; Tanokura, M.; Denu, J.M.; Prolla, T.A. Sirt3 mediates reduction of oxidative damage and prevention of age-related hearing loss under caloric restriction. *Cell* **2010**, *143*, 802–812. [CrossRef] [PubMed]
260. Yeo, H.; Lyssiotis, C.A.; Zhang, Y.; Ying, H.; Asara, J.M.; Cantley, L.C.; Paik, J.H. Fo_xO_3 coordinates metabolic pathways to maintain redox balance in neural stem cells. *EMBO J.* **2013**, *32*, 2589–2602. [CrossRef] [PubMed]
261. Chen, D.; Bruno, J.; Easlon, E.; Lin, S.J.; Cheng, H.L.; Alt, F.W.; Guarente, L. Tissue-specific regulation of SIRT1 by calorie restriction. *Genes Dev.* **2008**, *22*, 1753–1757. [CrossRef] [PubMed]
262. Olmos, Y.; Sanchez-Gomez, F.J.; Wild, B.; Garcia-Quintans, N.; Cabezudo, S.; Lamas, S.; Monsalve, M. SirT1 regulation of antioxidant genes is dependent on the formation of a FoxO3a/PGC-1alpha complex. *Antioxid. Redox Signal.* **2013**, *19*, 1507–1521. [CrossRef] [PubMed]
263. Cho, C.G.; Kim, H.J.; Chung, S.W.; Jung, K.J.; Shim, K.H.; Yu, B.P.; Yodoi, J.; Chung, H.Y. Modulation of glutathione and thioredoxin systems by calorie restriction during the aging process. *Exp. Gerontol.* **2003**, *38*, 539–548. [CrossRef]
264. Rohrbach, S.; Gruenler, S.; Teschner, M.; Holtz, J. The thioredoxin system in aging muscle: Key role of mitochondrial thioredoxin reductase in the protective effects of caloric restriction? *Am. J. Physiol. Regul. Integr. Comp. Physiol.* **2006**, *291*, R927–R935. [CrossRef] [PubMed]
265. Johnson, M.L.; Distelmaier, K.; Lanza, I.R.; Irving, B.A.; Robinson, M.M.; Konopka, A.R.; Shulman, G.I.; Nair, K.S. Mechanism by Which Caloric Restriction Improves Insulin Sensitivity in Sedentary Obese Adults. *Diabetes* **2016**, *65*, 74–84. [CrossRef] [PubMed]
266. Molin, M.; Yang, J.; Hanzen, S.; Toledano, M.B.; Labarre, J.; Nystrom, T. Life span extension and H(2)O(2) resistance elicited by caloric restriction require the peroxiredoxin Tsa1 in Saccharomyces cerevisiae. *Mol. Cell* **2011**, *43*, 823–833. [CrossRef] [PubMed]
267. Fierro-Gonzalez, J.C.; Gonzalez-Barrios, M.; Miranda-Vizuete, A.; Swoboda, P. The thioredoxin TRX-1 regulates adult lifespan extension induced by dietary restriction in Caenorhabditis elegans. *Biochem. Biophys. Res. Commun.* **2011**, *406*, 478–482. [CrossRef] [PubMed]
268. Menger, K.E.; James, A.M.; Cocheme, H.M.; Harbour, M.E.; Chouchani, E.T.; Ding, S.; Fearnley, I.M.; Partridge, L.; Murphy, M.P. Fasting, but Not Aging, Dramatically Alters the Redox Status of Cysteine Residues on Proteins in Drosophila melanogaster. *Cell Rep.* **2015**, *11*, 1856–1865. [CrossRef] [PubMed]

269. Newman, J.C.; Covarrubias, A.J.; Zhao, M.; Yu, X.; Gut, P.; Ng, C.P.; Huang, Y.; Haldar, S.; Verdin, E. Ketogenic Diet Reduces Midlife Mortality and Improves Memory in Aging Mice. *Cell Metab.* **2017**, *26*, 547–557.e8. [CrossRef]
270. Roberts, M.N.; Wallace, M.A.; Tomilov, A.A.; Zhou, Z.; Marcotte, G.R.; Tran, D.; Perez, G.; Gutierrez-Casado, E.; Koike, S.; Knotts, T.A.; et al. A Ketogenic Diet Extends Longevity and Healthspan in Adult Mice. *Cell Metab.* **2017**, *26*, 539–546.e5. [CrossRef]
271. Pawlosky, R.J.; Kemper, M.F.; Kashiwaya, Y.; King, M.T.; Mattson, M.P.; Veech, R.L. Effects of a dietary ketone ester on hippocampal glycolytic and tricarboxylic acid cycle intermediates and amino acids in a 3xTgAD mouse model of Alzheimer's disease. *J. Neurochem.* **2017**, *141*, 195–207. [CrossRef] [PubMed]
272. De Nobrega, A.K.; Lyons, L.C. Aging and the clock: Perspective from flies to humans. *Eur. J. Neurosci.* **2018**. [CrossRef] [PubMed]
273. Froy, O. Circadian rhythms, aging, and life span in mammals. *Physiology* **2011**, *26*, 225–235. [CrossRef] [PubMed]
274. Zhang, R.; Lahens, N.F.; Ballance, H.I.; Hughes, M.E.; Hogenesch, J.B. A circadian gene expression atlas in mammals: Implications for biology and medicine. *Proc. Natl. Acad. Sci. USA* **2014**, *111*, 16219–16224. [CrossRef] [PubMed]
275. Mauvoisin, D.; Wang, J.; Jouffe, C.; Martin, E.; Atger, F.; Waridel, P.; Quadroni, M.; Gachon, F.; Naef, F. Circadian clock-dependent and -independent rhythmic proteomes implement distinct diurnal functions in mouse liver. *Proc. Natl. Acad. Sci. USA* **2014**, *111*, 167–172. [CrossRef] [PubMed]
276. Mendez, I.; Vazquez-Martinez, O.; Hernandez-Munoz, R.; Valente-Godinez, H.; Diaz-Munoz, M. Redox regulation and pro-oxidant reactions in the physiology of circadian systems. *Biochimie* **2016**, *124*, 178–186. [CrossRef] [PubMed]
277. Peek, C.B.; Affinati, A.H.; Ramsey, K.M.; Kuo, H.Y.; Yu, W.; Sena, L.A.; Ilkayeva, O.; Marcheva, B.; Kobayashi, Y.; Omura, C.; et al. Circadian clock NAD+ cycle drives mitochondrial oxidative metabolism in mice. *Science* **2013**, *342*, 1243417. [CrossRef] [PubMed]
278. Nakahata, Y.; Sahar, S.; Astarita, G.; Kaluzova, M.; Sassone-Corsi, P. Circadian control of the NAD+ salvage pathway by CLOCK-SIRT1. *Science* **2009**, *324*, 654–657. [CrossRef] [PubMed]
279. Ramsey, K.M.; Yoshino, J.; Brace, C.S.; Abrassart, D.; Kobayashi, Y.; Marcheva, B.; Hong, H.K.; Chong, J.L.; Buhr, E.D.; Lee, C.; et al. Circadian clock feedback cycle through NAMPT-mediated NAD+ biosynthesis. *Science* **2009**, *324*, 651–654. [CrossRef] [PubMed]
280. Goodman, R.P.; Calvo, S.E.; Mootha, V.K. Spatiotemporal compartmentalization of hepatic NADH and NADPH metabolism. *J. Boil. Chem.* **2018**, *293*, 7508–7516. [CrossRef] [PubMed]
281. Putker, M.; Crosby, P.; Feeney, K.A.; Hoyle, N.P.; Costa, A.S.H.; Gaude, E.; Frezza, C.; O'Neill, J.S. Mammalian Circadian Period, But Not Phase and Amplitude, Is Robust Against Redox and Metabolic Perturbations. *Antioxid. Redox Signal.* **2018**, *28*, 507–520. [CrossRef] [PubMed]
282. Rey, G.; Valekunja, U.K.; Feeney, K.A.; Wulund, L.; Milev, N.B.; Stangherlin, A.; Ansel-Bollepalli, L.; Velagapudi, V.; O'Neill, J.S.; Reddy, A.B. The Pentose Phosphate Pathway Regulates the Circadian Clock. *Cell Metab.* **2016**, *24*, 462–473. [CrossRef] [PubMed]
283. Cracan, V.; Titov, D.V.; Shen, H.; Grabarek, Z.; Mootha, V.K. A genetically encoded tool for manipulation of NADP(+)/NADPH in living cells. *Nat. Chem. Boil.* **2017**, *13*, 1088–1095. [CrossRef] [PubMed]
284. Sandbichler, A.M.; Jansen, B.; Peer, B.A.; Paulitsch, M.; Pelster, B.; Egg, M. Metabolic Plasticity Enables Circadian Adaptation to Acute Hypoxia in Zebrafish Cells. *Cell. Physiol. Biochem.* **2018**, *46*, 1159–1174. [CrossRef] [PubMed]
285. Rutter, J.; Reick, M.; Wu, L.C.; McKnight, S.L. Regulation of clock and NPAS2 DNA binding by the redox state of NAD cofactors. *Science* **2001**, *293*, 510–514. [CrossRef] [PubMed]
286. Yoshii, K.; Tajima, F.; Ishijima, S.; Sagami, I. Changes in pH and NADPH regulate the DNA binding activity of neuronal PAS domain protein 2, a mammalian circadian transcription factor. *Biochemistry* **2015**, *54*, 250–259. [CrossRef] [PubMed]
287. Goya, M.E.; Romanowski, A.; Caldart, C.S.; Benard, C.Y.; Golombek, D.A. Circadian rhythms identified in *Caenorhabditis elegans* by in vivo long-term monitoring of a bioluminescent reporter. *Proc. Natl. Acad. Sci. USA* **2016**, *113*, E7837–E7845. [CrossRef] [PubMed]

288. Rey, G.; Milev, N.B.; Valekunja, U.K.; Ch, R.; Ray, S.; Silva Dos Santos, M.; Nagy, A.D.; Antrobus, R.; MacRae, J.I.; Reddy, A.B. Metabolic oscillations on the circadian time scale in Drosophila cells lacking clock genes. *Mol. Syst. Biol.* **2018**, *14*, e8376. [CrossRef] [PubMed]
289. Causton, H.C.; Feeney, K.A.; Ziegler, C.A.; O'Neill, J.S. Metabolic Cycles in Yeast Share Features Conserved among Circadian Rhythms. *Curr. Biol.* **2015**, *25*, 1056–1062. [CrossRef] [PubMed]
290. Lerner, F.; Niere, M.; Ludwig, A.; Ziegler, M. Structural and functional characterization of human NAD kinase. *Biochem. Biophys. Res. Commun.* **2001**, *288*, 69–74. [CrossRef] [PubMed]
291. Love, N.R.; Pollak, N.; Dolle, C.; Niere, M.; Chen, Y.; Oliveri, P.; Amaya, E.; Patel, S.; Ziegler, M. NAD kinase controls animal NADP biosynthesis and is modulated via evolutionarily divergent calmodulin-dependent mechanisms. *Proc. Natl. Acad. Sci. USA* **2015**, *112*, 1386–1391. [CrossRef] [PubMed]
292. Shianna, K.V.; Marchuk, D.A.; Strand, M.K. Genomic characterization of POS5, the Saccharomyces cerevisiae mitochondrial NADH kinase. *Mitochondrion* **2006**, *6*, 94–101. [CrossRef] [PubMed]
293. Ohashi, K.; Kawai, S.; Murata, K. Identification and characterization of a human mitochondrial NAD kinase. *Nat. Commun.* **2012**, *3*, 1248. [CrossRef] [PubMed]
294. Zhang, R. MNADK, a novel liver-enriched mitochondrion-localized NAD kinase. *Boil. Open* **2013**, *2*, 432–438. [CrossRef] [PubMed]
295. El-Khoury, R.; Sainsard-Chanet, A. Deletion of the mitochondrial NADH kinase increases mitochondrial DNA stability and life span in the filamentous fungus *Podospora anserina*. *Exp. Gerontol.* **2010**, *45*, 543–549. [CrossRef] [PubMed]
296. Xiong, Z.M.; O'Donovan, M.; Sun, L.; Choi, J.Y.; Ren, M.; Cao, K. Anti-Aging Potentials of Methylene Blue for Human Skin Longevity. *Sci. Rep.* **2017**, *7*, 2475. [CrossRef] [PubMed]
297. Gura, T. Hope in Alzheimer's fight emerges from unexpected places. *Nat. Med.* **2008**, *14*, 894. [CrossRef] [PubMed]
298. Gureev, A.P.; Shaforostova, E.A.; Popov, V.N.; Starkov, A.A. Methylene blue does not bypass Complex III antimycin block in mouse brain mitochondria. *FEBS Lett.* **2019**. [CrossRef] [PubMed]
299. Wen, Y.; Li, W.; Poteet, E.C.; Xie, L.; Tan, C.; Yan, L.J.; Ju, X.; Liu, R.; Qian, H.; Marvin, M.A.; et al. Alternative mitochondrial electron transfer as a novel strategy for neuroprotection. *J. Biol. Chem.* **2011**, *286*, 16504–16515. [CrossRef] [PubMed]
300. Ahn, H.; Kang, S.G.; Yoon, S.I.; Ko, H.J.; Kim, P.H.; Hong, E.J.; An, B.S.; Lee, E.; Lee, G.S. Methylene blue inhibits NLRP3, NLRC4, AIM2, and non-canonical inflammasome activation. *Sci. Rep.* **2017**, *7*, 12409. [CrossRef] [PubMed]
301. Medina, D.X.; Caccamo, A.; Oddo, S. Methylene blue reduces abeta levels and rescues early cognitive deficit by increasing proteasome activity. *Brain Pathol.* **2011**, *21*, 140–149. [CrossRef] [PubMed]
302. Huang, C.; Wu, J.; Xu, L.; Wang, J.; Chen, Z.; Yang, R. Regulation of HSF1 protein stabilization: An updated review. *Eur. J. Pharm.* **2018**, *822*, 69–77. [CrossRef] [PubMed]
303. Copes, N. *High-Throughput Screening of Age-Related Changes in Caenorhabditis elegans*; University of South Florida: Tampa, FL, USA, 2015.
304. Harrison, D.E.; Strong, R.; Allison, D.B.; Ames, B.N.; Astle, C.M.; Atamna, H.; Fernandez, E.; Flurkey, K.; Javors, M.A.; Nadon, N.L.; et al. Acarbose, 17-α-estradiol, and nordihydroguaiaretic acid extend mouse lifespan preferentially in males. *Aging Cell* **2014**, *13*, 273–282. [CrossRef] [PubMed]
305. Massie, H.R.; Aiello, V.R.; Williams, T.R. Influence of photosensitizers and light on the life span of Drosophila. *Mech. Ageing Dev.* **1993**, *68*, 175–182. [CrossRef]
306. Vatolin, S.; Radivoyevitch, T.; Maciejewski, J.P. New drugs for pharmacological extension of replicative life span in normal and progeroid cells. *Npj Aging Mech. Dis.* **2019**, *5*, 2. [CrossRef] [PubMed]
307. Diaz-Ruiz, A.; Lanasa, M.; Garcia, J.; Mora, H.; Fan, F.; Martin-Montalvo, A.; Di Francesco, A.; Calvo-Rubio, M.; Salvador-Pascual, A.; Aon, M.A.; et al. Overexpression of CYB5R3 and NQO1, two NAD(+) -producing enzymes, mimics aspects of caloric restriction. *Aging Cell* **2018**, *17*, e12767. [CrossRef] [PubMed]

17

Using an Overlapping Time Interval Strategy to Study Diagnostic Instability in Mild Cognitive Impairment Subtypes

David Facal [1,*], Joan Guàrdia-Olmos [2], Arturo X. Pereiro [1], Cristina Lojo-Seoane [1], Maribel Peró [2] and Onésimo Juncos-Rabadán [1]

1 Department of Developmental Psychology, University de Santiago de Compostela, 15782 Santiago de Compostela, Galicia, Spain; arturoxose.pereiro@usc.es (A.X.P.); cristina.lojo@usc.es (C.L.-S.); onesimo.juncos@usc.es (O.J.-R.)

2 Department of Methodology of Behavioural Sciences, University of Barcelona, 08035 Barcelona, Catalunya, Spain; jguardia@ub.edu (J.G.-O.); mpero@ub.edu (M.P.)

* Correspondence: david.facal@usc.es

Abstract: (1) Background: Mild cognitive impairment (MCI) is a diagnostic label in which stability is typically low. The aim of this study was to examine temporal changes in the diagnosis of MCI subtypes by using an overlapping-time strategy; (2) Methods: The study included 435 participants aged over 50 years with subjective cognitive complaints and who completed at least one follow-up evaluation. The probability of transition was estimated using Bayesian odds ratios; (3) Results: Within the different time intervals, the controls with subjective cognitive complaints represented the largest proportion of participants, followed by sda-MCI at baseline and in the first five intervals of the follow-up, but not in the last eight intervals. The odds ratios indicated higher odds of conversion to dementia in sda-MCI and mda-MCI groups relative to na-MCI (e.g., interval 9–15 months—sda-MCI OR = 9 and mda-MCI OR = 3.36; interval 27–33—sda-MCI OR = 16 and mda-MCI = 5.06; interval 42–48—sda-MCI OR = 8.16 and mda-MCI = 3.45; interval 45–51—sda-MCI OR = 3.31 and mda-MCI = 1); (4) Conclusions: Notable patterns of instability consistent with the current literature were observed. The limitations of a prospective approach in the study of MCI transitions are discussed.

Keywords: cognitive aging; mild cognitive impairment; subjective cognitive complaints; conversion to dementia; Bayesian odds ratios; time overlapping intervals; screening and diagnosis

1. Introduction

Mild cognitive impairment (MCI) is the diagnostic entity used to describe a condition in middle-aged and old adults who experience cognitive decline but without impaired daily functioning [1]. MCI has been indicated as a focal concept for understanding pre-dementia stages in relation to cognitive ageing [2]. Despite some controversy, the following are generally accepted as the core MCI criteria: (i) Evidence of subjective cognitive complaints from patients or their close contacts; (ii) evidence of cognitive impairment in one or more cognitive domains that is greater than expected for the patient's age and educational background; (iii) preservation or minimal impairment of instrumental activities of daily living; and (iv) non-fulfillment of diagnostic criteria for dementia [3–7]. This consensus also extends to the different subtypes of MCI (amnestic and non-amnestic, single and multi-domain) proposed by Petersen and colleagues [3,6]. Apart from its importance in research on cognitive impairment, MCI is also a multifaceted clinical label, characterized by complex cognitive changes and diagnostic instability in MCI subtypes, conversion to dementia and recovery to normal cognitive aging [8–10].

Although major advances in research have led to corresponding changes in the diagnostic criteria for MCI, it remains unclear how cognitive deficits increase over time and how these deficits affect progression to dementia in different MCI subtypes [1,11]. According to Gersteneker and Mast [1], the relationship between MCI subtypes and transition and conversion patterns is not as linear as initially proposed. Amnestic MCI is considered to be the MCI subtype most likely to progress to AD. The diagnostic guidelines produced by the National Institute on Aging- Alzheimer's disease working groups [5] indicate that the 'MCI, due to AD', refers to the symptomatic pre-dementia phase of AD and is characterized by impairment in one or more cognitive domains, typically including episodic memory. Different studies have already shown that multi-domain amnestic MCI (mda-MCI) is the most reliable MCI subtype, with a lower chance of reversion and a higher risk of conversion to dementia over time [12,13].

Although MCI is understood to be an unstable stage and the passage of the time is relevant in its cognitive and clinical manifestations, scant attention has been given in the literature to the time between assessments -but see [9,14]. Establishing this interval may have a considerable impact on the findings of MCI research. For example, longitudinal studies have developed non-linear, plateau models of decline that are dependent on the time of measurement [15]. In the current literature on MCI, the date of initial diagnosis and subsequent measurement points are determined as a function of the study start date; this is problematic as the moment at which participants report subjective cognitive complaints (SCCs) is intrinsically variable [6]. To address this problem, Cloutier et al. [11] suggested aligning the moment retrospectively according to the year in which participants received their diagnosis of AD. Facal et al. [9] proposed an alternative, complementary approach involving an overlapping interval strategy that considers different mid-point stages depending on the time between the baseline and follow-up assessment.

The aim of the present study was to test the capacity of an overlapping time interval strategy to address changes in MCI, by including supplementary follow-up evaluations and broader time intervals. The overlapping interval strategy was applied in the current sample of each time interval to explore whether changes (decline, stability, recovery) are temporally stable or vary according to different time intervals, and also to examine the trajectories of cognitive function in different MCI subtypes within different intervals.

2. Materials and Methods

2.1. Participants

The current research included 435 participants over 50 years old (range 50–88) included in the on-going Compostela aging study and who completed baseline and at least one follow-up evaluation [16]. All participants were referred to us by general practitioners after attending primary care health centers with subjective cognitive complaints, but with no prior diagnosis of dementia, psychiatric or neurological disorders.

At baseline, the sample comprised 40 participants in the mda-MCI group (multi-domain amnestic MCI), 34 participants in the na-MCI group (no amnestic MCI), 68 participants in the sda-MCI, and 293 participants in the control group with subjective cognitive complaints (SCCs). Age, years of education and results of the cognitive assessment at baseline are shown in Table 1. Group differences were calculated using non-parametric tests (Kruskal-Wallis and Mann-Whitney test) given the differences in sample size between the groups. Diagnoses were made following the Petersen criteria [3,4] updated by Albert et al. [5] and were reached by consensus at research team diagnostic meetings.

Table 1. Mean values and standard deviations (in parentheses) of the demographic and cognitive measures in each group at baseline.

	mda-MCI	na-MCI	sda-MCI	SCCs	Group Differences χ^2 (gl)	Group Comparisons
Age	72.42 (8.33)	67.12 (8.82)	69.29 (9.36)	65.49 (9.05)	24.83 **	mda-MCI > naMCI, SCCs; sda-MCI>SCCs
Years of education	9.68 (8.82)	8.29 (3.75)	9.40 (4.17)	9.92 (4.70)	1.81	
Memory complaints—participant	19.43 (4.69)	20.35 (3.45)	19.03 (4.69)	18.81 (4.51)	8.53 *	naMCI > SCCs
Memory complaints—proxy	17.97 (4.54)	18.03 (4.76)	16.84 (4.46)	15.49 (4.23)	17.03 **	mda-MCI, naMCI > sdaMCI, SCCs; sda-MCI > SCCs
CVLT Short Delay Free Recall	3.10 (2.03)	9.18 (2.21)	3.88 (2.05)	10.34 (2.70)	228.58 **	SCCs, na-MCI > mda-MCI, sda-MCI; sda-MCI > mda-MCI
CVLT Long Delay Free Recall	3.82 (3.19)	9.76 (2.69)	5.12 (3.06)	11.14 (2.83)	184.80 **	SCCs, sda-MCI, na-MCI > mdaMCI; SCCs> na-MCI, sda-MCI; na-MCI>sda-MCI
CAMCOG-R memory	15.50 (3.80)	18.56 (2.87)	18.53 (3.88)	21.26 (2.78)	99.18 **	SCCs, sda-MCI, na-MCI > mdaMCI; SCCs > na-MCI, sda-MCI
CAMCOG-R orientation	7.98 (1.46)	9.29 (0.80)	9.31 (0.83)	9.64 (0.63)	79.19 **	SCCs, sda-MCI, na-MCI > mdaMCI; SCCs > na-MCI, sda-MCI
CAMCOG-R language	22.77 (2.36)	23.53 (2.00)	24.90 (2.43)	25.60 (2.40)	54.55 **	SCCs, sda-MCI > mdaMCI, na-MCI
CAMCOG-R attention - calculation	5.03 (2.21)	4.29 (1.73)	7.25 (1.70)	7.05 (1.97)	100.90 **	SCCs, sda-MCI > mdaMCI, na-MCI
CAMCOG-R praxis	9.10 (2.53)	10.03 (1.71)	10.71 (1.47)	11.14 (1.19)	48.01 **	SCCs, sda-MCI > mdaMCI, na-MCI
CAMCOG-R perception	5.97 (1.64)	6.50 (1.28)	6.53 (1.48)	7.06 (1.44)	21.68 **	SCCs, sda-MCI > mdaMCI; SCCs > na-MCI, sda-MCI
CAMCOG-R executive function	13.22 (3.94)	15.35 (4.20)	15.93 (4.28)	18.42 (4.20)	58.84 **	SCCs, sda-MCI > mdaMCI; SCCs > na-MCI, sda-MCI

** $p < 0.01$ * $p < 0.05$. Note: CVLT = california verbal learning test; CAMCOG-R = cambridge cognitive assessment-revised; mda-MCI = multi-domain amnestic Mild Cognitive Impairment; na MCI = non amnestic mild cognitive impairment; sda-MCI = single-domain amnestic mild cognitive impairment; SCCs = subjective cognitive complaints.

In the final sample that completed at least one follow up evaluation, 415 participants completed the first follow-up around $1_{1/2}$ year after baseline (mean = 17.92 months, S.D. = 3.87, range 10–31 months), and 330 participants completed the second follow up assessment around 3 years after baseline (mean = 37.13 months, S.D. = 5.43, range 27–51 months; this includes 20 participants who did not complete the first follow-up assessment, but who did participate in the second follow-up). Reasons for deviation from the reference times include holidays, health issues and work issues.

2.2. Procedure

The baseline evaluations were made between 2 January 2008 and 11 November 2012. Participants undertook wide-ranging cognitive and neuropsychological evaluations, including the Spanish versions of the California Verbal Learning Test (CVLT) [17], the Mini-Mental State Examination (MMSE) [18] and the Cambridge Cognitive Examination—Revised (CAMCOG-R), which include subscales in several cognitive domains (memory, orientation, language, attention and calculation, praxis, perception and executive functioning) [19]. Within the follow-up assessments, all participants again underwent the assessment and were re-diagnosed by the same research team, again by consensus at specific meetings.

At all three evaluation times, the cut-off was 1.5 standard deviations (SDs) below age and education norms on the corresponding tests. All participants who displayed normal cognitive performance (scores higher than cut-off scores on cognitive status and cognitive functioning, including memory) were included in the SCCs group, as they all reported subjective memory complaints. For all MCI participants, the general criteria outlined by Albert et al. [5] were applied: (a) Presence of complaints corroborated by an informant; (b) impairment in one or more cognitive functions; (c) independence in daily living with minimum support or help; and (d) absence of dementia according to the NINCDS-ADRDA and DSM-IV standards. For the specific diagnosis of MCI subtypes, the criteria proposed by Petersen and colleagues [3,6] were applied, including (b1) a score of 1.5 SDs below age standards for short-term and long-term recall measures of the Spanish version of the CVLT for amnestic MCI (aMCI). Two different types of aMCI were diagnosed: Sda-MCI in those participants (b2) who performed 1.5 SDs below age norms in the Spanish version of the CVLT, but performed normally in the MMSE and the CAMCOG-R subscales; and mda-MCI in those participants (b3) who performed 1.5 SDs below norms in the MMSE and at least two sub-scores of the CAMCOG-R representing at least two cognitive functions. Finally, na-MCI was diagnosed in those participants (b4) who performed within the normal range in the Spanish version of the CVLT, but 1.5 SDs below average in at least one of the other subscales of the CAMCOG-R. Single- and multi-domain na-MCI were not differentiated, because of the small sample size in the single-domain na-MCI group. Probable AD or other types of dementia were diagnosed according to the NINCDS-ADRDA and DMS-IV criteria. Progression to dementia was confirmed by consultation of the medical history, and the date of neurological diagnosis was recorded.

The study received approval from the Ethics in Clinical Research Committee of the Galician Government and was conducted in accordance with the provisions of the Declaration of Helsinki as revised in Brazil 2013. Written informed consent was obtained from all participants.

2.3. *Overlapping Intervals Procedure*

According to the variability in the time between the baseline and follow-up evaluations, and the potential effect of time in the study of MCI according to its variability, a time-overlapping interval approach was taken [20] considering 13 mid-point time intervals with a range of 6 months across each interval. This approach enabled a wide range of time distributions to be covered between assessments and also consideration of all participants evaluated, irrespective of the time at which the follow-up was carried out and whether they participated in the first follow up assessment (about one year and a half after the baseline assessment) and/or the second follow up (about three years after the baseline). Seven intervals were included within the time-lapse established for the first follow up assessment (9–15, 12–18, 15–21, 18–24, 21–27, 24–30, 27–33), and seven intervals were also included within the time-lapse established for the second follow up assessment (27–33, 30–36, 33–39, 36–42, 39–45, 42–48, 45–51).

According to this overlapping-interval design, and in order to maximize sample sizes and temporal distributions across successive evaluations, the sample size was different for each interval (see Table 2). According to the reference times for the first (18 months) and the second (36 months) follow-up assessments, the sample sizes tended to be larger in the intervals closer to these times and smaller in the intervening intervals. This approach allows overlapping counts between time intervals, avoiding double-counting of participants by considering the participants only once in those intervals in which months between assessments are included. The range around each mid-point interval was six months, so that adjacent intervals differ in mean time between assessments, but overlap in the time range. Therefore, the mid-point of the 9–15 month group was 12, the mid-point for the 12–18 month group was 15, and so on. The results can, thus, be consulted with the maximum temporal continuum (13 time groups) or with the minimum overlap (seven and six time groups, 9–15, 15–21, 21–27, 27–33, 33–39, 39–45, 45–51 months and 12–18, 18–24, 24–30, 30–36, 36–42, 42–48, respectively). Overlapping intervals are used as independent sample estimates.

Table 2. Sample size in each overlapped time interval.

Interval	mda-MCI	na-MCI	sda-MCI	SCCs
9–15 months	6	3	10	35
12–18 months	14	15	30	125
15–21 months	16	16	31	155
18–24 months	13	11	22	105
21–27 months	5	8	13	49
24–30 months	4	4	7	25
27–33 months	6	3	11	47
30–36 months	9	7	21	98
33–39 months	10	15	21	98
36–42 months	8	12	14	56
39–45 months	8	8	9	51
42–48 months	6	3	9	27
45–51 months	4	4	9	18

2.4. Statistical Analysis

The probability of transition from one state to another was estimated using Bayesian estimates, calculated as follows:

$$P(A_i|B) = p(B|A_i)P(A_i)/\Sigma_{k=1}\ P(B|A_k)P(A_k),$$

where P(Ai) represents the a priori probability, P(B|Ai) represents the probability of transition from Ai to B and, finally, P(Ai|B) represents the a-posteriori probability. In the present study, event Ai assumes the state of the diagnosis at a given time (t), and B is the state of diagnosis at time (t +1). Evidently, transitions from states Ai to Ak and then to the next state B draw all combinations existing between the diagnostic categories at a given moment and the same categories at the next time. Models of these transitions were generated using P(Ai) and P(Ai|B) from estimates of the proportions observed in the original distributions.

In addition, as the demands of the Bayes' theorem require exhaustiveness, the odds ratio was obtained from the contrasts, as follows:

$$ORij = P(Ai|B)/P(Aj|B),$$

with the aim of evaluating the most probable transitions of the pair (i,j) as in the previous expression. Thus, apart from the estimated values of the Bayesian probabilities, more applied values of higher clinical value were obtained. Details of all of the calculations, including those made to obtain Odds Ratios in each interval, are available to readers in Supplementary File S1.

All the mathematical procedures were generated by Excel routines and specific programming in MatLab.

3. Results

The diagnostic probabilities for the different MCI subtypes are presented in Figures 1 and 2. Figure 3 shows those participants whose diagnosis did not change in the follow-up assessments and those participants in the different groups who progressed to dementia. The number of participants in the mda-MCI group who progressed to dementia was 4 at the first follow-up assessment and 7 at the second follow-up assessment; the corresponding numbers in the na-MCI group were 0 at the first follow-up and 1 at the second follow-up assessment; the numbers in the sda-MCI group were 3 at the first follow-up and 5 at the second follow-up; and finally, the corresponding numbers in the SCCs group were 0 at the first follow-up and 4 at the second follow-up. Cases recorded at the first follow-up were also counted at the second follow-up, so that the numbers are cumulative.

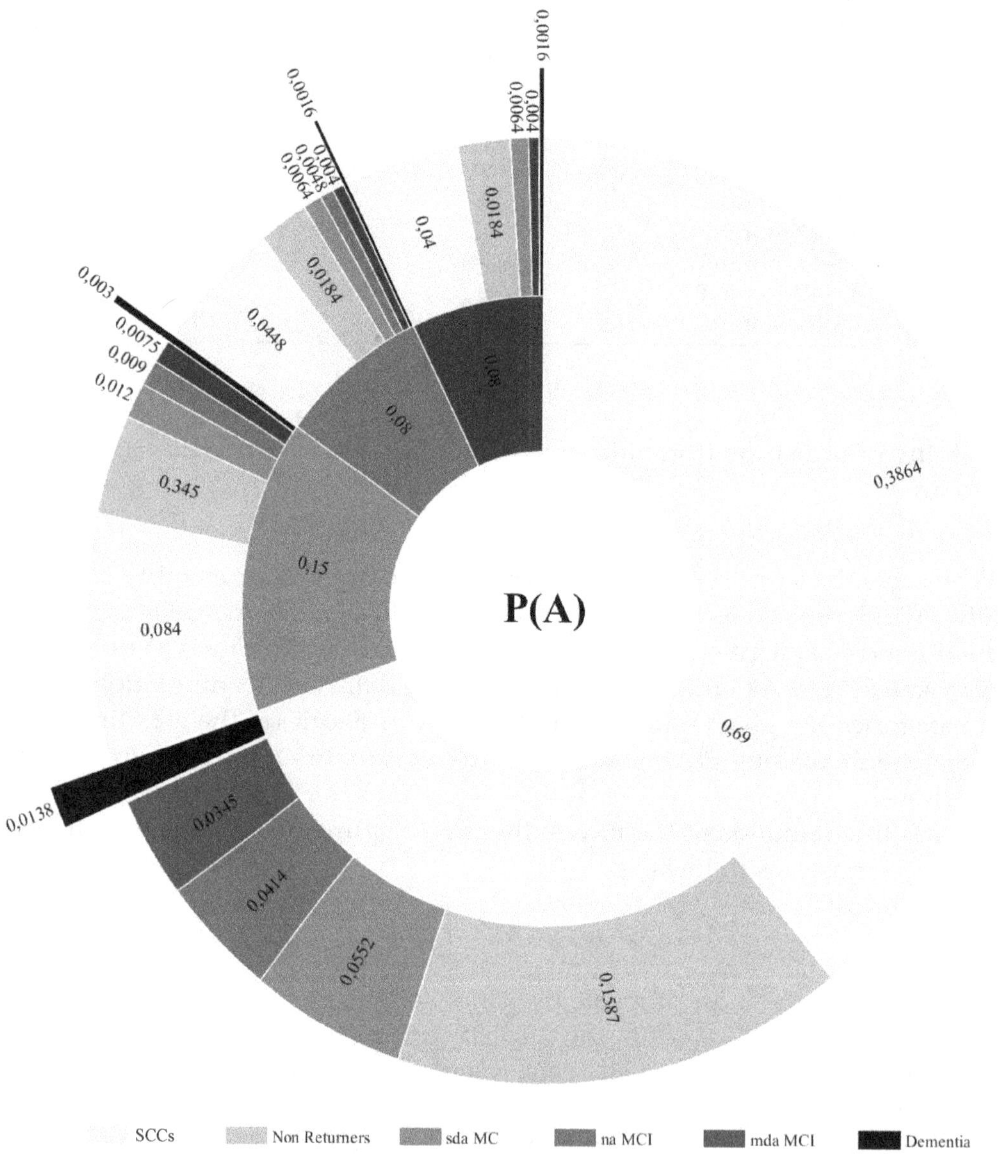

Figure 1. Diagnostic probabilities at baseline (inner circle) and at first follow-up (outer circle). Diagnostic probabilities are presented numerically, as proportions, with the total sum of proportions in the inner and outer circles equaling 1. The naMCI group is absent from the outer circle, but corresponds to the mdaMCI group in the inner circle as no transitions from mdaMCI to naMCI were recorded. SCCs = Subjective cognitive complaints; MCI = mild cognitive impairment; mda = multidomain amnestic; na = non-amnestic; sda = single domain amnestic.

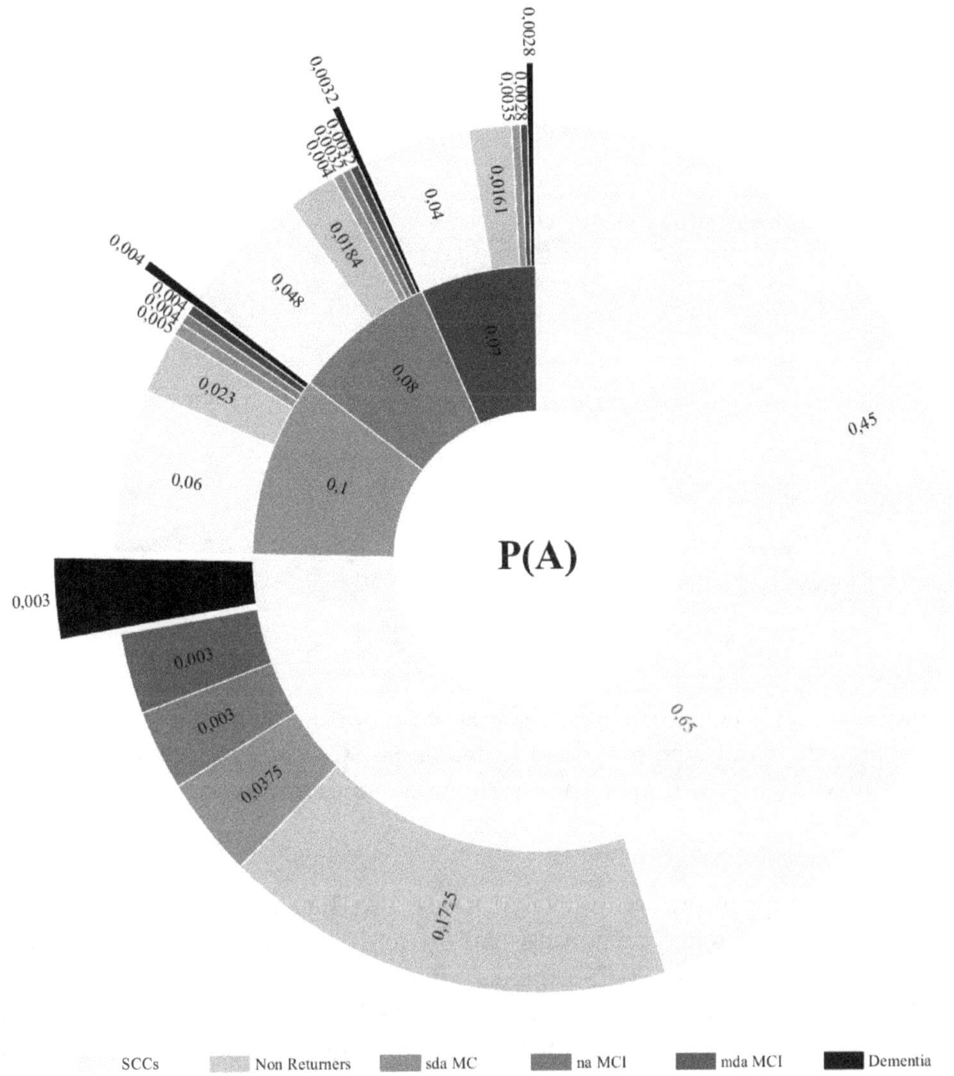

Figure 2. Diagnostic probabilities at first follow-up (inner circle) and at second follow-up (outer circle). Diagnostic probabilities are presented numerically, as proportions, with the total sum of proportions in the inner and outer circles equaling 1. The naMCI group is absent from the outer circle, but corresponds to the mdaMCI group in the inner circle as no transitions from mdaMCI no naMCI were recorded. SCCs = Subjective cognitive complaints; MCI = mild cognitive impairment; mda = multi-domain amnestic; na = non-amnestic; sda = single domain amnestic.

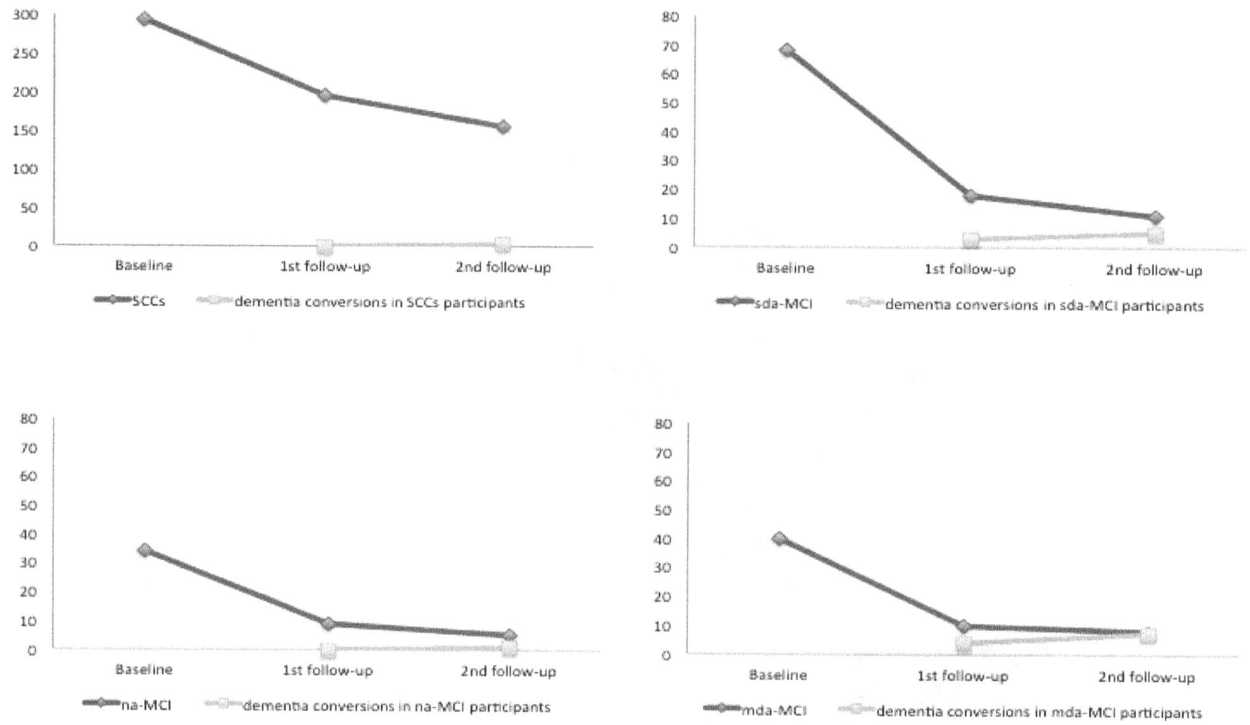

Figure 3. The number of participants whose diagnosis did not change at the follow-up assessments, and the number of participants who converted to dementia. SCCs = Subjective cognitive complaints; MCI = mild cognitive impairment; mda = multi-domain amnestic; na = non-amnestic; sda = single domain amnestic.

According to the overlapping time interval strategy, the diagnostic probabilities for the different MCI subtypes at different times are presented in Figure 4. Similar trends were observed for the different time intervals, as follows: (a) SCCs represented the largest proportion of participants, and the proportion tended to increase at follow-up assessments; (b) sda-MCI participants comprised the second largest group at baseline and in the first five intervals of the follow-up, but not in the last eight intervals of the follow-up continuum; (c) the probabilities of diagnosis of mda-MCI and na-MCI were similar at both baseline and follow-up, with slight variations across the time intervals; and (d) there was a small, but increasing, probability of conversion to dementia, represented in the right column of the follow-up section in Figure 3. In this figure, only the cases of conversion to dementia recorded during each time interval are counted.

According to the higher, but temporally variable, probability of sda-MCI at follow-up and to test the theoretical relevance of mda-MCI as the closest point to dementia within the MCI continuum, odds ratios were calculated for each time interval and for sda-MCI and mda-MCI relative to na-MCI. This enabled the probability of conversion to dementia to be determined by comparing the two different amnestic subtypes and considering the non-amnestic subtype as the reference subtype. The conversion odds (Table 3) revealed a higher probability of conversion to dementia in sda-MCI than in na-MCI, which would be expected according to the higher proportion of sda-MCI participants at baseline, and also a higher probability of conversion to dementia in mda-MCI than in na-MCI.

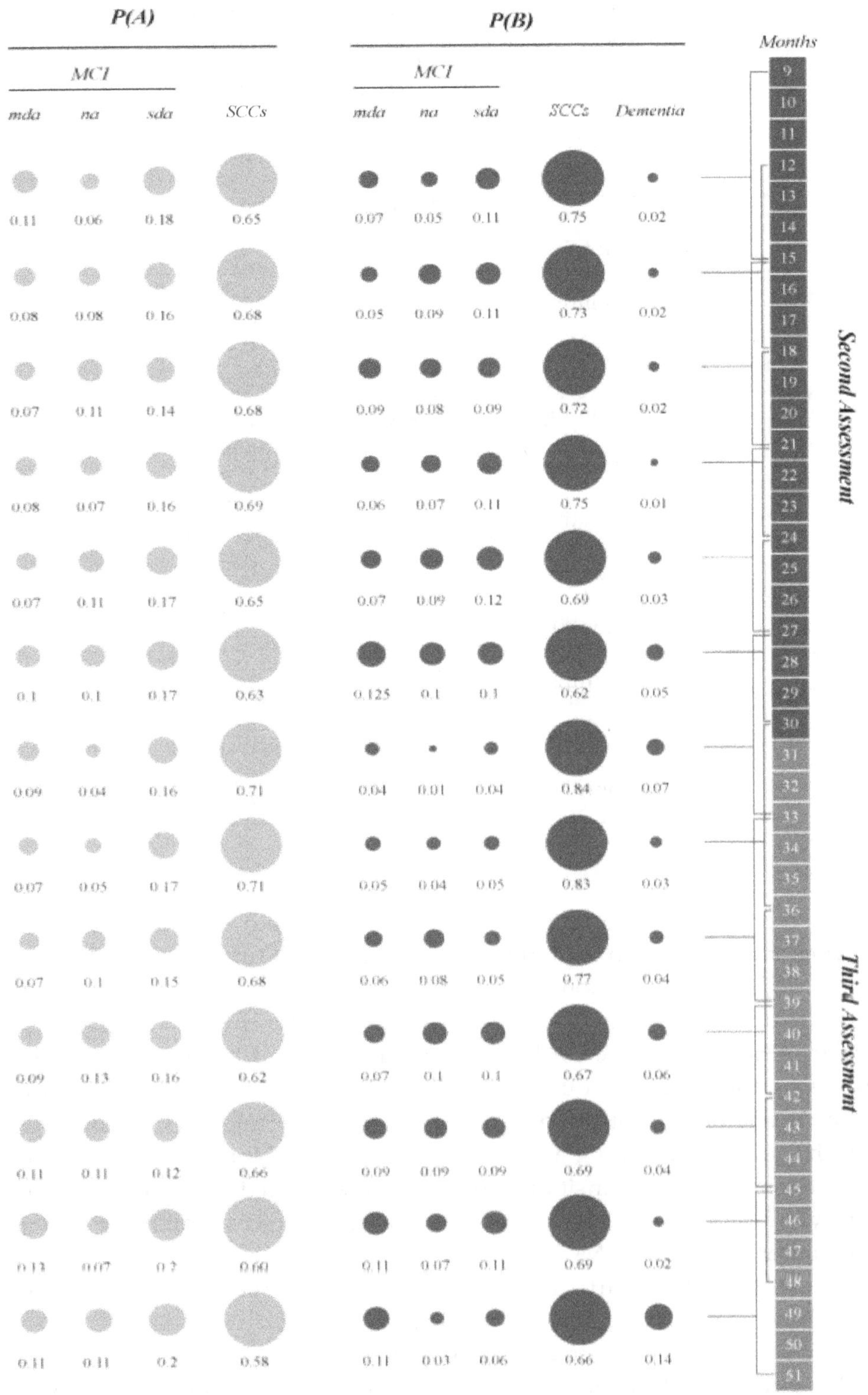

Figure 4. Diagnostic probabilities at baseline **P(A)** and at follow-up **P(B)**. Months between baseline and follow-up assessments are represented on the right-hand side of the diagram. Each line represents one time interval, with brackets in the column on the right showing the overlapping nature of the intervals (e.g., time interval 1 is indicated by the bracket encompassing months 9 to 15 and overlaps with interval 2, indicated by the bracket encompassing months 12 to 18). Diagnostic probabilities are represented at baseline in light grey and at follow-up in dark grey. SCCs = subjective cognitive complaints; MCI = mild cognitive impairment; mda = multidomain amnestic; na = non-amnestic; sda = single domain amnestic.

Table 3. Odds ratios for conversion to dementia in sda-MCI and mda-MCI groups relative to na-MCI.

Interval	sda-MCI OR (95% CI)	mda-MCI OR (95% CI)
9–15 months	9 (8.20–9.80)	3.36 (3.06–3.66)
12–18 months	4 (3.35–4.65)	1 (1.00–2.12)
15–21 months	1.62 (1.22–2.02)	0.41 (0–1.21)
18–24 months	5.22 (4.67–5.77)	1.31 (1.08–1.34)
21–27 months	2.39 (1.45–3.34)	0.41 (0–1.21)
24–30 months	2.89 (2.10–3.68)	1 (1.00–2.12)
27–33 months	16 (12.10–19.90)	5.06 (4.85–5.27)
30–36 months	11.56 (10.10–12.45)	1.96 (1.52–2.40)
33–39 months	2.25 (1,10–3.40)	0.49 (0–1.21)
36–42 months	1.51 (1.10–1.92)	0.48 (0–1.21)
39–45 months	1.19 (1.00–1.77)	1 (1.00–2.12)
42–48 months	8.16 (6.80–9.54)	3.45 (2.90–4.05)
45–51 months	3.31 (2.80–3.82)	1 (1.00–2.12)

4. Discussion

This study overcomes some limitations of previous research considering diagnostic transition within MCI subtypes and conversion to dementia within different time frames. For example, it includes longer follow-up periods than in previous studies e.g., [9,13] and it uses Bayesian estimates to illustrate the diagnostic transitions more clearly and accurately, representing the reality of daily practice by avoiding an artificial balance of the probability of diagnosis at baseline. In daily gerontological and geriatric practice, longitudinal follow-up and serial cognitive assessments are recommended as they provide a clearer picture of the patient's baseline and trajectory of cognitive function over time [21], although the optimal timing and cost-effectiveness of longitudinal cognitive assessments remain unclear. In this regard, the transition probabilities calculated using the Bayesian approach with overlapping-interval design are similar to current daily practice in which the time of assessment is variable (i.e., the higher odds in sda-MCI than in mda-MCI compared to na-MCI can be explained by the higher proportion of sda-MCI participants at baseline, in parallel to the higher number of patients with sda-MCI that professionals diagnose in daily practice).

The increase in number of participants classified as SCCs and the decrease in those diagnosed as sda-MCI in the second part of the follow-up assessments indicates the instability of this MCI subtype, as previously highlighted by Malek-Ahmadi in a meta-analysis [22], in which the rate of reversion to normal cognition was approximately 24%. The increase may indicate an excess number of false-positives in diagnosing this particular MCI subtype, which includes patients with impairments only in memory. Nonetheless, the higher odds ratios for conversion to dementia of sda-MCI relative to na-MCI also indicate an important risk of progression of cognitive impairment in the sda-MCI subtype [5,7]. The current clinical criteria, which include a cut-off of <1.5 SD below mean only in memory scores, indicate an unstable subtype, especially when the follow-up assessments are carried out after short intervals. This confirms that other functional, behavioral and biological markers should be included for more accurate diagnosis, as recommended by the American Academy of Neurology (AAN) guidelines on MCI [7]. Follow-up studies are needed because studies that test the actual cognitive status of middle-aged and older adults living in the community with subjective memory complaints appear to be susceptible to false-positive diagnostic errors, mainly regarding single domain MCI subtypes. In this respect, Han et al. [10] recommended considering the diagnostic stability over time and the multiplicity of impaired cognitive domains for managing MCI.

Regarding the rates of conversion to dementia, longitudinal studies have found that non-linear, plateau models of decline (initial decline in memory, followed by a temporary plateau occurring prior to a final rapid decline immediately prior to AD diagnosis) are more accurate than linear models, at least for memory performance [15]. The small, but increasing, probability of conversion to dementia between time intervals observed in our study does not support these findings, although the intervals are relatively short and a slight increase in the case of cognitive decline was detected in the final intervals. However, the rates of conversion to dementia in this study are relatively low [9,23]. Accordingly, adjusting the overlapping time interval strategy included here by including longer intervals and successive follow-up assessments may help to clarify these trends in conversion, e.g., [24].

As already mentioned, this study has some limitations, due to the temporal approach and the rate of variability in the diagnosis of MCI subtypes. Regarding the first limitation, this study used a prospective approach to the complex phenomena of MCI transition and conversion to dementia, adopting overlapping intervals to study the role of time in the MCI diagnostic process. Although the prospective approach has traditionally been used in this field, retrospective approaches involving analysis of data from the moment when patients are diagnosed with Alzheimer's disease or other types of dementia are increasingly common [6]. For the diagnosis of MCI subtypes, Klekociuk and Summers [13] indicate that it may be necessary to wait until single-domain variants transition to multiple-domain variants in order to identify genuine cases, particularly when recruiting prospective samples with subjective memory complaints—as in the present study. Regarding the variability in diagnosis of MCI subtypes, in this study, we measured verbal learning and memory with the Spanish version of the CVLT [9] and other cognitive functions with the CAMCOG-R. The use of other specific cognitive measures of memory and non-memory functions [25,26], as well as functional, behavioral and biological measures, could minimize the diagnostic instability [7]. It has been suggested that the number of false-positive can also be reduced by using empirical statistical approaches to identify MCI, such as cluster analysis based on the actual cognitive performance of the participants rather than previously established cut-off scores [27–29]. In this regard, Edmonds et al. [27] suggest that the inclusion of self-reported cognitive complaints as a core MCI diagnostic criterion may yield higher false-positive rates, as amnestic MCI participants tend to underestimate the level of cognitive impairment.

5. Conclusions

In summary, use of the time-overlapping intervals strategy enabled us to study the diagnostic instability in MCI subtypes, contributing further knowledge about temporal effects and the time between follow-up assessment on MCI trajectories, and revealing distinctive trajectories of diagnostic changes, especially in the sda-MCI subtype. Nevertheless, the classical prospective approach has some limitations in relation to studying diagnostic instability in MCI. These limitations must be addressed in future studies by using a more comprehensive neuropsychological and biological approaches, longer time intervals between successive follow-ups, and combining prospective and retrospective diagnostic approaches.

Author Contributions: Conceptualization, D.F., J.G.-O. and O.J.-R.; Methodology, D.F., J.G.-O., M.P.; Software, J.G.-O., M.P.; Data acquisition, D.F., C.L.-S., O.J.-R. and A.X.P.; Data Processing, C.L.-S. and O.J.-R.; Writing—Original Draft Preparation, D.F.; Writing—Review and Editing, all; Visualization, D.F., J.G.-O. and O.J.-R.; Project Administration, O.J.-R. and A.X.P.; Funding Acquisition, O.J.-R. and A.X.P.

References

1. Gerstenecker, A.; Mast, B. Mild cognitive impairment: A history and the state of current diagnostic criteria. *Int. Psychogeriatr.* **2015**, *27*, 199–211. [CrossRef]
2. Peters, K.R.; Katz, S. Voices from the field: Expert reflections on mild cognitive impairment. *Dementia* **2015**, *14*, 285–297. [CrossRef] [PubMed]
3. Petersen, R.C. Mild cognitive impairment as a diagnostic entity. *J. Intern. Med.* **2004**, *256*, 183–194. [CrossRef] [PubMed]
4. Winblad, B.; Palmer, K.; Kiyipelto, M. Mild cognitive impairment–beyond controversies, towards a consensus: Report of the International Working Group on Mild Cognitive Impairment. *J. Intern. Med.* **2004**, *256*, 240–246. [CrossRef] [PubMed]
5. Albert, M.S.; DeKosky, S.T.; Dickson, D.; Dubois, B.; Feldman, H.H.; Fox, N.C.; Gamst, A.; Holtzman, D.M.; Jagust, W.J.; Petersen, R.C.; et al. The diagnosis of mild cognitive impairment due to Alzheimer's disease: Recommendations from the National Institute on Aging and Alzheimer's Association workgroup. *Alzheimer's Dement.* **2011**, *7*, 270–279. [CrossRef]
6. Dubois, B.; Feldman, H.H.; Jacova, C.; DeKosky, S.T.; Barberger-Gateau, P.; Cummings, J.; Delacourte, A.; Galasko, D.; Gauthier, S.; Jicha, G.; et al. Research criteria for the diagnosis of Alzheimer's disease: Revising the NINCDS-ADRDA criteria. *Lancet Neurol.* **2007**, *6*, 734–746. [CrossRef]
7. Petersen, R.C.; Lopez, O.; Armstrong, M.J.; Getchius, T.S.; Ganguli, M.; Gloss, D.; Gronseth, G.S.; Marson, D.; Pringsheim, T.; Day, G.S.; et al. Practice guideline update summary: Mild cognitive impairment: Report of the Guideline Development, Dissemination, and Implementation Subcommittee of the American Academy of Neurology. *Neurology* **2018**, *90*, 126–135. [CrossRef]
8. Díaz-Mardomingo, M.D.C.; García-Herranz, S.; Rodríguez-Fernández, R.; Venero, C.; Peraita, H. Problems in classifying mild cognitive impairment (MCI): One or multiple syndromes. *Brain Sci.* **2017**, *7*, 111. [CrossRef]
9. Facal, D.; Guàrdia-Olmos, J.; Juncos-Rabadán, O. Diagnostic transitions in mild cognitive impairment by use of simple Markov models. *Int. J. Geriatr. Psychiatry* **2015**, *30*, 669–676. [CrossRef]
10. Han, J.W.; Kim, T.H.; Lee, S.B.; Park, J.H.; Lee, J.J.; Huh, Y.; Park, J.E.; Jhoo, J.H.; Lee, D.Y.; Kim, K.W. Predictive validity and diagnostic stability of mild cognitive impairment subtypes. *Alzheimer's Dement.* **2012**, *8*, 553–559. [CrossRef]
11. Cloutier, S.; Chertkow, H.; Kergoat, M.J.; Gauthier, S.; Belleville, S. Patterns of cognitive decline prior to dementia in persons with mild cognitive impairment. *J. Alzheimer's Dis.* **2015**, *47*, 901–913. [CrossRef] [PubMed]
12. Ding, D.; Zhao, Q.; Guo, Q. Progression and predictors of mild cognitive impairment in Chinese elderly: A prospective follow-up in the Shanghai Aging Study. *Alzheimer's Dement.* **2016**, *4*, 28–36. [CrossRef]
13. Klekociuk, S.Z.; Summers, M.J. Exploring the validity of mild cognitive impairment (MCI) subtypes: Multipledomain amnestic MCI is the only identifiable subtype at longitudinal follow-up. *J. Clin. Exp. Neuropsychol.* **2014**, *36*, 290–301. [CrossRef] [PubMed]
14. Cui, Y.; Liu, B.; Luo, S.; Zhen, X.; Fan, M.; Liu, T.; Zhu, W.; Park, M.; Jiang, T.; Jin, J.S.; et al. Identification of conversion from mild cognitive impairment to Alzheimer's disease using multivariate predictors. *PLoS ONE* **2011**, *6*, e21896. [CrossRef] [PubMed]
15. Smith, G.E.; Pankratz, V.S.; Negash, S.; Machulda, M.M.; Petersen, R.C.; Boeve, B.F.; Knopman, D.S.; Lucas, J.A.; Ferman, T.J.; Graff-Radford, N.; et al. A plateau in pre-Alzheimer memory decline: Evidence for compensatory mechanisms? *Neurology* **2007**, *69*, 133–139. [CrossRef] [PubMed]
16. Juncos-Rabadan, O.; Pereiro, A.X.; Facal, D.; Lojo, C.; Caamaño, J.A.; Sueiro, J.; Boveda, J.; Eiroa, P. Prevalence and correlates of mild cognitive impairment in adults aged over 50 years with subjective cognitive complaints in primary care centers. *Geriatr. Gerontol. Int.* **2014**, *14*, 667–673. [CrossRef] [PubMed]
17. Benedet, M.J.; Alejandre, M.A. *TAVEC: Test de Aprendizaje Verbal España-Complutense (TAVEC: Spanish-Complutense Verbal Learning Test)*; TEA Ediciones: Madrid, Spain, 1998.

18. Lobo, A.; Saz, P.; Marcos, G.; Día, J.L.; de la Cámara, C.; Ventura, T.; Morales Asín, F.; Pascual, L.F.; Montañés, J.A.; Aznar, S. Revalidación y normalización del mini-examen cognoscitivo (primera versión en Castellano del mini-mental status examination) en la población general geriatrica. (Revalidation and standardization of the cognition mini-exam (first Spanish version of the mini-mental status examination) in the general geriatric population). *Med. Clin.* **1999**, *112*, 767–774.
19. López-Pousa, S. *CAMDEX-R: Prueba de Exploración Cambridge Revisada Para la Valoración de los Trastornos Mentales en la Vejez. Adaptación Española (CAMDEX-R: Revised Cambridge Screening Test for the Assessment of Mental Disorders in Old Age. Spanish Adaptation)*; TEA Ediciones: Madrid, Spain, 2003.
20. Pauker, J.D. Constructing overlapping cell tables to maximize the clinical usefulness of normative test data: Rationale and an example from neuropsychology. *J. Clin. Psychol.* **1988**, *44*, 930–933. [CrossRef]
21. Langa, K.M.L.; Levine, D.A. The diagnosis and management of mild cognitive impairment: A clinical review. *JAMA* **2014**, *312*, 2551–2562. [CrossRef] [PubMed]
22. Malek-Ahmadi, M. Reversion from mild cognitive impairment to normal cognition. *Alzheimer Dis. Assoc. Dis.* **2016**, *30*, 324–330. [CrossRef] [PubMed]
23. Forlenza, O.V.; Diniz, B.S.; Nunes, P.V.; Memória, C.M.; Yassuda, M.S.; Gattaz, W.F. Diagnostic transitions in mild cognitive impairment subtypes. *Int. Psychoger.* **2009**, *21*, 1088–1095. [CrossRef] [PubMed]
24. Reisberg, B.; Shulman, M.B.; Torossian, C.; Leng, L.; Zhu, W. Outcome over seven years of healthy adults with and without subjective cognitive impairment. *Alzheimer's Dement.* **2010**, *6*, 11–24. [CrossRef] [PubMed]
25. Klekociuk, S.Z.; Summers, J.J.; Vickers, J.C.; Summers, M.J. Reducing false positive diagnoses in mild cognitive impairment: The importance of comprehensive neuropsychological assessment. *Eur. J. Neurol.* **2014**, *21*, 1330–1336. [CrossRef] [PubMed]
26. Edmonds, E.C.; Delano-Woods, L.; Jak, A.J.; Galasko, D.R.; Salmon, D.P.; Bondi, M.W. "Missed" mild cognitive impairment: High false-negative error rate based on conventional diagnostic criteria. *J. Alzheimer's Dis.* **2016**, *52*, 685–691. [CrossRef] [PubMed]
27. Edmonds, E.C.; Delano-Wood, L.; Galasko, D.R.; Salmon, D.P.; Bondi, M.W. Subjective cognitive complaints contribute to misdiagnosis of mild cognitive impairment. *J. Int. Neuropsychol. Soc.* **2014**, *20*, 836–847. [CrossRef] [PubMed]
28. Edmonds, E.C.; Delano-Woods, L.; Clark, L.R.; Jaka, A.J.; Nationd, D.A.; McDonald, C.R.; Libone, D.J.; Auf, R.; Galasko, D.; Salmonh, D.P.; et al. Susceptibility of the conventional criteria for mild cognitive impairment to false-positive diagnostic errors. *Alzheimer's Dement.* **2015**, *11*, 415–424. [CrossRef] [PubMed]
29. Campos-Magdaleno, M.; Facal, D.; Juncos-Rabadán, O.; Picón, E.; Pereiro, A.X. Comparison between an empirically derived and a standard classification of amnestic mild cognitive impairment from a sample of adults with subjective cognitive complaints. *J. Aging Health* **2016**, *28*, 1105–1115. [CrossRef]

Permissions

All chapters in this book were first published by MDPI; hereby published with permission under the Creative Commons Attribution License or equivalent. Every chapter published in this book has been scrutinized by our experts. Their significance has been extensively debated. The topics covered herein carry significant findings which will fuel the growth of the discipline. They may even be implemented as practical applications or may be referred to as a beginning point for another development.

The contributors of this book come from diverse backgrounds, making this book a truly international effort. This book will bring forth new frontiers with its revolutionizing research information and detailed analysis of the nascent developments around the world.

We would like to thank all the contributing authors for lending their expertise to make the book truly unique. They have played a crucial role in the development of this book. Without their invaluable contributions this book wouldn't have been possible. They have made vital efforts to compile up to date information on the varied aspects of this subject to make this book a valuable addition to the collection of many professionals and students.

This book was conceptualized with the vision of imparting up-to-date information and advanced data in this field. To ensure the same, a matchless editorial board was set up. Every individual on the board went through rigorous rounds of assessment to prove their worth. After which they invested a large part of their time researching and compiling the most relevant data for our readers.

The editorial board has been involved in producing this book since its inception. They have spent rigorous hours researching and exploring the diverse topics which have resulted in the successful publishing of this book. They have passed on their knowledge of decades through this book. To expedite this challenging task, the publisher supported the team at every step. A small team of assistant editors was also appointed to further simplify the editing procedure and attain best results for the readers.

Apart from the editorial board, the designing team has also invested a significant amount of their time in understanding the subject and creating the most relevant covers. They scrutinized every image to scout for the most suitable representation of the subject and create an appropriate cover for the book.

The publishing team has been an ardent support to the editorial, designing and production team. Their endless efforts to recruit the best for this project, has resulted in the accomplishment of this book. They are a veteran in the field of academics and their pool of knowledge is as vast as their experience in printing. Their expertise and guidance has proved useful at every step. Their uncompromising quality standards have made this book an exceptional effort. Their encouragement from time to time has been an inspiration for everyone.

The publisher and the editorial board hope that this book will prove to be a valuable piece of knowledge for researchers, students, practitioners and scholars across the globe.

List of Contributors

Lucy Youngmin Eun and Jae Young Choi
Division of Pediatric Cardiology, Department of Pediatrics, Yonsei University College of Medicine, Seoul 03722, Korea

Han Ki Park
Division of Cardiovascular Surgery, Department of Thoracic and Cardiovascular Surgery, Yonsei University College of Medicine, Seoul 03722, Korea

Hui-Chuan Hsu
School of Public Health, Research Center of Health Equity, College of Public Health, Taipei Medical University, Taipei 11031, Taiwan

Maria F. Masana
Parc Sanitari Sant Joan de Déu, Universitat de Barcelona, Fundació Sant Joan de Déu, 08007 Barcelona, Spain
Instituto de Salud Carlos III, Centro de Investigación Biomédica en Red de Salud Mental, CIBERSAM, Monforte de Lemos 3-5, Pabellón 11, 28029 Madrid, Spain
Facultat de Medicina, Universitat de Barcelona, Casanova, 143, 08036 Barcelona, Spain

Stefanos Tyrovolas
Parc Sanitari Sant Joan de Déu, Universitat de Barcelona, Fundació Sant Joan de Déu, 08007 Barcelona, Spain
Instituto de Salud Carlos III, Centro de Investigación Biomédica en Red de Salud Mental, CIBERSAM, Monforte de Lemos 3-5, Pabellón 11, 28029 Madrid, Spain
Department of Science of Dietetics and Nutrition, School of Health Science and Education, Harokopio University, 17671 Athens, Greece

Josep Maria Haro
Parc Sanitari Sant Joan de Déu, Universitat de Barcelona, Fundació Sant Joan de Déu, 08007 Barcelona, Spain
Instituto de Salud Carlos III, Centro de Investigación Biomédica en Red de Salud Mental, CIBERSAM, Monforte de Lemos 3-5, Pabellón 11, 28029 Madrid, Spain

Natasa Kollia and Demosthenes B. Panagiotakos
Department of Science of Dietetics and Nutrition, School of Health Science and Education, Harokopio University, 17671 Athens, Greece

Christina Chrysohoou, John Skoumas, Dimitrios Tousoulis and Christos Pitsavos
First Cardiology Clinic, School of Medicine, University of Athens, 15772 Athens, Greece

Charalambos Papageorgiou
First Psychiatry Clinic, School of Medicine, University of Athens, 15772 Athens, Greece

Chien-Ying Lee
Department of Pharmacology, Chung Shan Medical University, Taichung 40201, Taiwan
Department of Pharmacy, Chung Shan Medical University Hospital, Taichung 40201, Taiwan

Yih-Dih Cheng
School of pharmacy, China Medical University, Taichung 40402, Taiwan
Department of Pharmacy, China Medical University Hospital, Taichung 40402, Taiwan

Wei-Yuan Cheng
Taso-Tun Psychiatric Center, Ministry of Health and Welfare, Nantou 54249, Taiwan

Tung-Han Tsai and Kuang-Hua Huang
Department of Health Services Administration, China Medical University, Taichung 40402, Taiwan

Ai Koyanagi
Research and Development Unit, Parc Sanitari Sant Joan de Déu, Universitat de Barcelona, Fundació Sant Joan de Déu, 08830 Barcelona, Spain
Instituto de Salud Carlos III, Centro de Investigación Biomédica en Red de Salud Mental, CIBERSAM, 28029 Madrid, Spain
ICREA, Pg. Lluis Companys 23, 08010 Barcelona, Spain

Nicola Veronese
Aging Branch, Neuroscience Institute, National Research Council, 35128 Padova, Italy
National Institute of Gastroenterology "S. De Bellis" Research Hospital, Castellana Grotte, 70013 Bari, Italy

Brendon Stubbs
Physiotherapy Department, South London and Maudsley NHS Foundation Trust, Denmark Hill, London SE5 8AZ, UK
Department of Psychological Medicine, Institute of Psychiatry, Psychology and Neuroscience, King's College London, London WC2R 2LS, UK
Faculty of Health, Social Care and Education, Anglia Ruskin University, Chelmsford CM1 1SQ, UK

Davy Vancampfort
Department of Rehabilitation Sciences, KU Leuven, 3001 Leuven, Belgium
University Psychiatric Center KU Leuven, KU Leuven, 3000 Leuven, Belgium

Andrew Stickley
Department of Preventive Intervention for Psychiatric Disorders, National Institute of Mental Health, National Center of Neurology and Psychiatry, Kodaira, Tokyo 187-8553, Japan
The Stockholm Center for Health and Social Change (SCOHOST), Södertörn University, 141 89 Huddinge, Sweden

Hans Oh
School of Social Work, University of Southern California, CA 90015, USA

Jae Il Shin
Department of Pediatrics, Yonsei University College of Medicine, Yonsei-ro 50, Seodaemun-gu, Seoul 03722, Korea
Division of Pediatric Nephrology, Severance Children's Hospital, Seoul 03722, Korea
Institute of Kidney Disease Research, Yonsei University College of Medicine, Seoul 03722, Korea

Sarah Jackson
Department of Behavioural Science and Health, University College London, London WC1E 7HB, UK

Lee Smith
The Cambridge Centre for Sport and Exercise Sciences, Anglia Ruskin University, Cambridge CB1 1PT, UK

Elvira Lara
Instituto de Salud Carlos III, Centro de Investigación Biomédica en Red de Salud Mental, CIBERSAM, 28029 Madrid, Spain
Department of Psychiatry, Hospital Universitario de La Princesa, Instituto de Investigación Sanitaria Princesa (IIS-Princesa), 28006 Madrid, Spain

Jonathan Roberts and Zoe Adler
Division of Medicine, Brighton and Sussex University Hospitals NHS Trust, UK

Tom Levett
Division of Medicine, Brighton and Sussex University Hospitals NHS Trust, UK
Department of Clinical and Experimental Medicine, Brighton and Sussex Medical School, Falmer, Brighton BN1 9PX, UK

Katie Alford
Department of Global Health and Infection, Brighton and Sussex Medical School, Falmer, Brighton BN1 9PX, UK

Jaime H. Vera
Division of Medicine, Brighton and Sussex University Hospitals NHS Trust, UK
Department of Global Health and Infection, Brighton and Sussex Medical School, Falmer, Brighton BN1 9PX, UK

Juliet Wright
Division of Medicine, Brighton and Sussex University Hospitals NHS Trust, UK
Department of Medical Education, Brighton and Sussex Medical School, Falmer, Brighton BN1 9PX, UK

Melissa E. Meade, John G. Meade and Myra A. Fernandes
Department of Psychology, University of Waterloo, Waterloo, ON N2L 3G1, Canada

Hélène Sauzeon
Lab EA413-Handicap, Activité, Cognition & Santé, Université de Bordeaux, F-33000 Bordeaux, France
Flowers Team-INRIA Center, F-33405 Talence, France

Akiko Mizuno
Department of Psychiatry, University of Pittsburgh, Pittsburgh, PA 15213, USA

Maria Ly
Department of Psychiatry, University of Pittsburgh, Pittsburgh, PA 15213, USA
Department of Neuroscience, University of Pittsburgh, Pittsburgh, PA 15213, USA

Howard J. Aizenstein
Department of Psychiatry, University of Pittsburgh, Pittsburgh, PA 15213, USA
Department of Bioengineering, University of Pittsburgh, Pittsburgh, PA 15213, USA

Romy Conzade
Australian Institute for Musculoskeletal Science (AIMSS), The University of Melbourne and Western Health, St. Albans, Victoria 3021, Australia
Department of Medicine—Western Health, Melbourne Medical School, The University of Melbourne, St. Albans, Victoria 3021, Australia
Institute of Epidemiology, Helmholtz Zentrum München, German Research Center for Environmental Health (GmbH), 85764 Neuherberg, Germany

Walter Sepúlveda-Loyola
Australian Institute for Musculoskeletal Science (AIMSS), The University of Melbourne and Western Health, St. Albans, Victoria 3021, Australia
Department of Medicine—Western Health, Melbourne Medical School, The University of Melbourne, St. Albans, Victoria 3021, Australia
Department of Physiotherapy, Londrina State University (UEL) and University North of Paraná (UNOPAR), Londrina, Paraná 86041-120, Brazil

Steven Phu, Sara Vogrin, Ebrahim Bani Hassan and Gustavo Duque
Australian Institute for Musculoskeletal Science (AIMSS), The University of Melbourne and Western Health, St. Albans, Victoria 3021, Australia
Department of Medicine—Western Health, Melbourne Medical School, The University of Melbourne, St. Albans, Victoria 3021, Australia

Barbara Thorand
Institute of Epidemiology, Helmholtz Zentrum München, German Research Center for Environmental Health (GmbH), 85764 Neuherberg, Germany

Lucy Morse, Linda Xiong, Vanessa Ramirez-Zohfeld and Lee A. Lindquist
Division of General Internal Medicine & Geriatrics, Northwestern University Feinberg School of Medicine, Chicago, IL 60611, USA

Scott Dresden
Department of Emergency Medicine, Northwestern University Feinberg School of Medicine, Chicago, IL 60611, USA

Sara Estéfani S. Sousa
Postgraduate Program in Nutrition, Federal University of Rio Grande do Norte, Av. Senador Salgado Filho, 3000, Lagoa Nova, 59078970 Natal, RN, Brazil

Márcia Cristina Sales
School of Medicine, State University of Roraima, Rua Sete de Setembro, 231, Canarinho, 69306530 Boa Vista, RR, Brazil

José Rodolfo T. Araújo
Postgraduate Program of Health Sciences, Federal University of Rio Grande do Norte, Rua General Gustavo Cordeiro de Farias, Petrópolis, 59010180 Natal, RN, Brazil

Karine C.M. Sena-Evangelista
Postgraduate Program in Nutrition, Federal University of Rio Grande do Norte, Av. Senador Salgado Filho, 3000, Lagoa Nova, 59078970 Natal, RN, Brazil
Department of Nutrition, Federal University of Rio Grande do Norte, Av. Senador Salgado Filho, 3000, Lagoa Nova, 59078970 Natal, Brazil

Kenio C. Lima
Postgraduate Program of Health Sciences, Federal University of Rio Grande do Norte, Rua General Gustavo Cordeiro de Farias, Petrópolis, 59010180 Natal, RN, Brazil
Department of Dentistry, Federal University of Rio Grande do Norte, Av. Senador Salgado Filho, 1787, Lagoa Nova, 59056000 Natal, RN, Brazil

Lucia F.C. Pedrosa
Postgraduate Program in Nutrition, Federal University of Rio Grande do Norte, Av. Senador Salgado Filho, 3000, Lagoa Nova, 59078970 Natal, RN, Brazil
Postgraduate Program of Health Sciences, Federal University of Rio Grande do Norte, Rua General Gustavo Cordeiro de Farias, Petrópolis, 59010180 Natal, RN, Brazil
Department of Nutrition, Federal University of Rio Grande do Norte, Av. Senador Salgado Filho, 3000, Lagoa Nova, 59078970 Natal, Brazil

Dorina Cadar
Department of Behavioural Science and Health, University College London, London WC1E 7HB, UK

Marius Usher
Department of Psychology, Tel-Aviv University, Tel-Aviv 69978, Israel

Eddy J. Davelaar
Department of Psychological Sciences, Birkbeck, University of London, London WC1E 7HX, UK

Ho-Jin Shin and Sung-Hyeon Kim
Department of Health Science, Gachon University Graduate School, Incheon 21936, Korea

Suk-Chan Hahm
Graduate School of Integrative Medicine, CHA University, Seongnam 13488, Korea

Hwi-Young Cho
Department of Health Science, Gachon University Graduate School, Incheon 21936, Korea
Department of Physical Therapy, Gachon University, Incheon 21936, Korea

Christina Daskalopoulou, Martin Prince and A. Matthew Prina
Department of Health Service and Population Research, Institute of Psychiatry, Psychology and Neuroscience, King's College London, London SE5 8AF, UK

Artemis Koukounari
Department of Infectious Disease Epidemiology, London School of Hygiene & Tropical Medicine, Faculty of Epidemiology and Population Health, London WC1E 7HT, UK

José Luis Ayuso-Mateos
Department of Psychiatry, Universidad Autónoma de Madrid, 28029 Madrid, Spain
Instituto de Salud Carlos III, Centro de Investigación Biomedica en Red de Salud Mental (CIBERSAM), 28029 Madrid, Spain
Department of Psychiatry, Hospital Universitario de La Princesa, Instituto de Investigación Sanitaria Princesa (IIS-Princesa), 28006 Madrid, Spain

Tao Yang
Department of Psychology, Tsinghua University, Beijing 100084, China
Department of Psychology, Goldsmiths, University of London, London SE14 6NW, UK

Caroline Di Bernardi Luft
School of Biological and Chemical Sciences, Queen Mary University of London, London E1 4NS, UK

Pei Sun
Department of Psychology, Tsinghua University, Beijing 100084, China

Joydeep Bhattacharya and Michael J. Banissy
Department of Psychology, Goldsmiths, University of London, London SE14 6NW, UK

Patrick C. Bradshaw
Department of Biomedical Sciences, James H. Quillen College of Medicine, East Tennessee State University, Johnson City, TN 37614, USA

David Facal, Arturo X. Pereiro, Cristina Lojo-Seoane and Onésimo Juncos-Rabadán
Department of Developmental Psychology, University de Santiago de Compostela, 15782 Santiago de Compostela, Galicia, Spain

Joan Guàrdia-Olmos and Maribel Peró
Department of Methodology of Behavioural Sciences, University of Barcelona, 08035 Barcelona, Catalunya, Spain

Index

O

P

Q

R

S

T

V

W

www.ingramcontent.com/pod-product-compliance
Lightning Source LLC
LaVergne TN
LVHW060539210926
848485LV00005B/1226